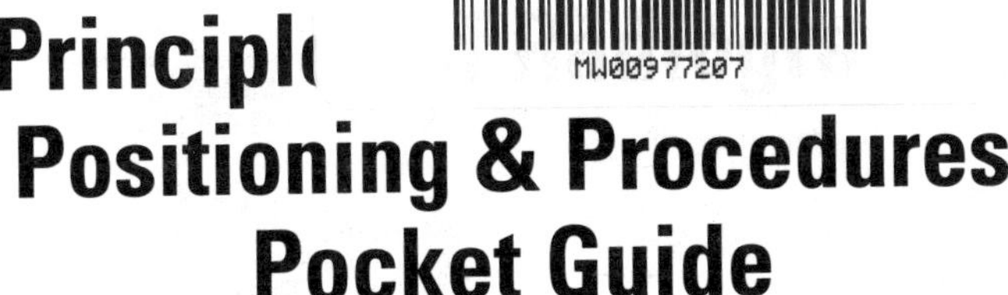

Principl
Positioning & Procedures Pocket Guide

Richard R. Carlton, M.S., R.T.(R)(CV), FAERS
Assistant Professor of Radiologic Sciences
Arkansas State University

Joanne S. Greathouse, EdS., R.T.(R), FASRT
Chief Executive Officer
Joint Review Committee on Education in Radiologic Technology

Arlene Adler, M.Ed., R.T.(R)
Director, Radiologic Technology
Indiana University Northwest
Gary, Indiana

Ray Winters, M.S., R.T.(R)(CT)
Program Director and Assistant Professor of Radiologic Sciences
Arkansas State University

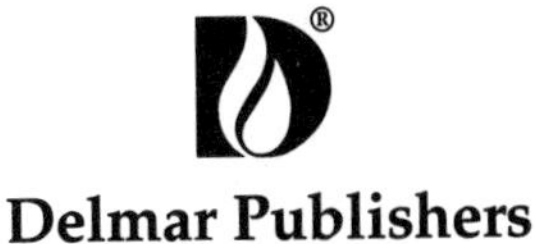

Delmar Publishers

an International Thomson Publishing company 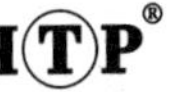

Albany • Bonn • Boston • Cincinnati • Detroit • London • Madrid
Melbourne • Mexico City • New York • Pacific Grove • Paris • San Francisco
Singapore • Tokyo • Toronto • Washington

NOTICE TO THE READER

Publisher does not warrant or guarantee any of the products described herein or perform any independent analysis in connection with any of the product information contained herein. Publisher does not assume, and expressly disclaims, any obligation to obtain and include information other than that provided to it by the manufacturer. The reader is expressly warned to consider and adopt all safety precautions that might be indicated by the activities herein and to avoid all potential hazards. By following the instructions contained herein, the reader willingly assumes all risks in connection with such instructions.

The Publisher makes no representation or warranties of any kind, including but not limited to, the warranties of fitness for particular purpose or merchantability, nor are any such representations implied with respect to the material set forth herein, and the publisher takes no responsibility with respect to such material. The publisher shall not be liable for any special, consequential, or exemplary damages resulting, in whole or part, from the readers' use of, or reliance upon, this material.

Delmar Staff
Publisher: Susan Simpfenderfer
Acquisitions Editor: Marlene McHugh Pratt
Developmental Editor: Melissa Riveglia
Production Manager: Linda Helfrich
Art and Design Coordinator: Rich Killar
Project Editor: William Trudell

Printed in the United States of America
3 4 5 6 7 8 9 10 XXX 05 04 03 02 01 00

For more information, contact Delmar, 3 Columbia Circle, PO Box 15015, Albany, NY 12212-0515; or find us on the World Wide Web at http://www.delmar.com

International Division List

Japan:
Thomson Learning
Palaceside Building 5F
1-1-1 Hitotsubashi,
Chiyoda-ku
Tokyo 100 0003 Japan
Tel: 813 5218 6544
Fax: 813 5218 6551

Australia/New Zealand
Nelson/Thomson
Learning
102 Dodds Street
South Melbourne,
Victoria 3205
Australia
Tel: 61 39 685 4111
Fax: 61 39 685 4199

UK/Europe/Middle East:
Thomson Learning
Berkshire House
168-173 High Holborn
London
WC1V 7AA United
Kingdom
Tel: 44 171 497 1422
Fax: 44 171 497 1426

Latin America:
Thomson Learning
Seneca, 53
Colonia Polanco
11560 Mexico D.F.
Mexico
Tel: 525-281-2906
Fax: 525-281-2656

Canada:
Nelson/Thomson
Learning
1120 Birchmount Road
Scarborough, Ontario
Canada M1K 5G4
Tel: 416-752-9100
Fax: 416-752-8102

Asia:
Thomson Learning
60 Albert Street, #15-01
Albert Complex
Singapore 189969
Tel: 65 336 6411
Fax: 65 336 7411

Spain:
Thomson Learning
Calle Magallanes, 25
28015-MADRID
ESPANA
Tel: 34 91 446 33 50
Fax: 34 91 445 62 18

Library of Congress Cataloging-in-Publication Data:
Delmar's principles of radiographic positioning and procedures pocket
guide / Richard R. Carlton…[et al.].
p. cm.
Includes index.
ISBN 0-8273-6372-9
1. Radiography, Medical—Positioning—Handbooks, manuals, etc.
I. Carlton, Richard R. II. Title: Principles of radiographic positioning
and procedures pocket guide.
RC78.4.D435 1999
616.07'572—cd21
98-43726
CIP

This pocket guide is dedicated to our colleagues who have taught and inspired us through their unstinting professionalism—and

Marion Frank, Middlesex Hospital, London
Terry West, International Society of
Radiographers and Radiologic Technologists
Barry Burns, University of North Carolina
Bonnie Wold, American Healthcare Radiology
Administrators and the Association of Educators
in Radiological Sciences
Eugene Frank, The Mayo Clinic
Phil Ballinger, The Ohio State University
Edith Applegate, Kettering College of Medical Arts
Susan Hanrahan, Ray Winters, Lyn Hubbard, & Jeannean Hall,
Arkansas State University

Rick Carlton

All the radiologic technology students I've had the privilege of teaching . . . I learned something from each of them.

Joanne Greathouse

Don, Meredith, & Katie

Arlene Adler

Meta, Megan & Jared. . . . . you are my reason for living.

Ray Winters

Contents

Preface

We believe there is a need for a comprehensive and complete pocket guide for radiography that includes not only a quick reference to appropriate positioning procedures, radiation protection standards, and space for recording technical exposure factors, but also a practical technique system guide.

Delmar's Principles of Radiographic Positioning and Procedures Pocket Guide meets these needs for both experienced radiographers and students in an admirable fashion. We have attempted to provide on a single pair of pages, all the information necessary to remind the radiographer of the basic procedural details, typical technical considerations, and appropriate modifications for 165 common procedures.

The pocket guide directly references the contents of two popular textbooks: Greathouse's *Delmar's Radiographic Positioning and Procedures, Volume I: Basic Positioning and Procedures* and Carlton and Adler's *Principles of Radiographic Imaging: An Art and a Science.*

We recommend that technical factors always be written in pencil to permit updating due to normal fluctuations in radiation output (such as those caused by tube aging, kVp and mA station drift, and processor variation). It is especially important to record **film-screen combination relative speed**, **generator type** and **grid ratio** to permit quick and easy modification of technical factors to accommodate any new clinical situation.

Rick Carlton, Jonesboro, Arkansas
Joanne Greathouse, Chicago, Illinois
Arlene Adler, Gary, Indiana
Ray Winters, Jonesboro, Arkansas

How to Use This Pocket Guide

Technical Considerations
All the necessary elements for a competent examination are provided:

- film-screen speed
- grid
- kVp range
- SID

There are also four icons to quickly remind you of:

- film size, position, and lead blocker placement
- radiation protection
- AEC (phototiming) cell
- AEC density settings

Patient Position
Concise positioning instructions are consistent with the Greathouse textbook.

Part Position
The fastest and easiest method of placing the part into position is listed.

Central Ray
CR direction and angle are given.

Patient Instructions
Breathing and other important patient information is cited.

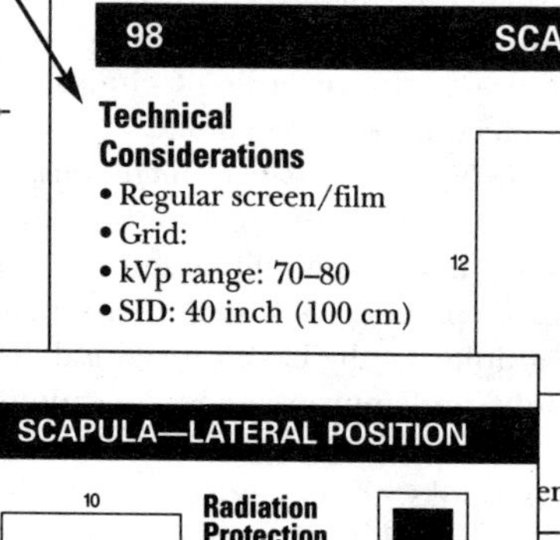
98 SCA

Technical Considerations
- Regular screen/film
- Grid:
- kVp range: 70–80
- SID: 40 inch (100 cm)

SCAPULA—LATERAL POSITION

• kVp range: 70–80
• SID: 40 inch (100 cm)

Patient Position
Recumbent or upright, depending on patient condition; all potential artifacts removed fror

Part Position Start from the supine positior reach across the chest and grasp the unaffect patient 30° away from the affected side (LPO right side and RPO for injuries to the left sid obliquity to place the scapula perpendicular t the film is placed 1 to 2 inches above the acr

Central Ray Perpendicular to the midscapu or to the coracoid process.

Breathing Instructions Suspend on inspirat

Example Exposure Techniques
Space for exposure techniques is provided with the routine part sizes indicated. The charts on p.xix are designed to help you set up a personal technique system.

Example Exposure Techn						
Measure at CR and Use Cha						
Room	cm	kVp	mAs	mA	Sec	Bean
	10					
	11					
	12					
	13					
	14					

Evaluation Criteria
Primary checkpoints for an acceptable image are given.

Exam Rationale
The reasons for performing the examination are provided to assist in gathering an appropriate history for the physician.

Tips
Useful hints provide variations of basic positioning.

Basic Radiographic Exposure
The best positioning skills will be useless without the selection of appropriate technical factors that make it possible to visualize the image on film. Optimal radiographic quality requires a thorough knowledge of the principles of radiation exposure as well as familiarity with an institution's specific equipment. Manipulation of the three exposure factors—kilovoltage (kV), milliamperage (mA), and time—or appropriate selection of phototiming parameters must be combined with an understanding

SCAPULA—LATERAL POSITION

Evaluation Criteria
- Entire scapula should be demonstrated free of superimposition from ribs.
- Coracoid process should be projected anteriorly.
- Acromion process should be projected posteriorly.
- Unlike the scapular Y projection, which has similar positioning, the shaft of the humerus should not be superimposed on the body of the scapula on the lateral scapula radiograph.

Exam Rationale The lateral is one of two routine positions of the scapula. Structures demonstrated on the radiograph include the coracoid process, acromion process, and the body of the scapula in a lateral perspective, free from superimposing rib and lung anatomy.

Tip If patient condition allows, anterior obliques may be done on the upright to achieve less object-film distance. With the patient facing the film, rotate the patient into a 60° oblique

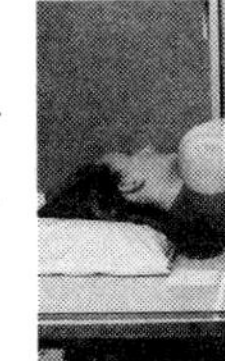

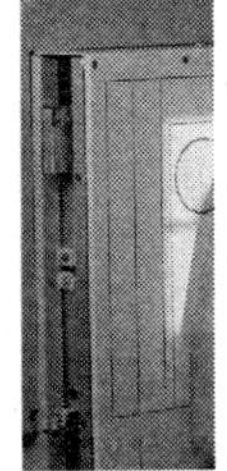

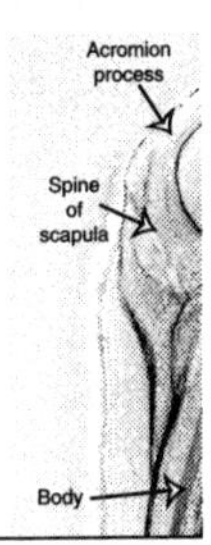

of the primary image quality factors of density, contrast, recorded detail, and distortion to produce an optimally diagnostic image.

In this text, suggested kVp ranges have been provided for each of the positions/procedures. These are only a guide. The actual kVp selection should be based on the equipment, imaging systems, department protocol, and physician preference at your institution.

Recommendations are also provided for the use of automatic exposure control (AEC), commonly referred to as "phototiming." AECs produce a mid-range diagnostic level density for the structures placed between the ion cell and the x-ray tube. In other words, the art of phototiming is the art of positioning. Whatever is placed over the activated ion cells will be imaged in the middle of the diagnostic range of densities. Thus, a selective determination must be made regarding which AEC cells should be activated and then the anatomical area of interest must be placed over these cells.

The following icon is provided for positions/projections where AEC is an appropriate consideration.

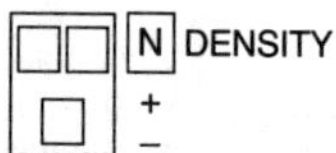

The 3 cells located in the large square represent the location of the ion chambers in the x-ray equipment. In keeping with common practice, the cell(s) which are to be activated for a given position/projection are blackened to indicate they are on. The small box with the N represents the film density control. The "N" represents "normal" density. When special conditions make it desirable to increase or decrease the average density, a "+" or "–", respectively, is used beneath the density control box.

Principles of Radiation Protection

As a form of electromagnetic radiation, x-rays have the potential to cause harmful effects on living cells. Every effort must be made to protect the patient, operator, and others from unnecessary radiation exposure; the radiographer is bound by the Code of Ethics to do so. A thorough understanding of the principles of radiation protection is essential to achieving this goal.

Because the developing embryo or fetus is especially sensitive to radiation, women of childbearing age must be asked about the possibility of pregnancy. Many women are unaware of pregnancy in its early stages, so the patient history should include questions about when the last menstrual period occurred. Some facilities prefer that abdominal x-rays of females of reproductive age be done during the first 10 days following the onset of menstruation because it is less likely that a patient would be pregnant at this time (often referred to as the 10-day rule).

Patient radiation exposure can be limited with the use of appropriate exposure factors used in conjunction with appropriate imaging systems, use of appropriate beam-limiting devices (including collimation), proper filtration, and proper immobilization. Attention to minimizing patient radiation exposure must also include gonadal shielding whenever possible without compromising the radiographic examination. In this text, an icon is used to identify those situations in which gonadal shields should be used.

 contact shield 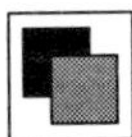 shadow shield

Particular care must be taken when radiographing children. Because the rapidly dividing cells of children are more sensitive to radiation than those of adults, the principles of radiation protection warrant even more careful attention in pediatric work.

Radiographers also have a responsibility to protect themselves and others from unnecessary exposure. All radiographers should be familiar with the three primary principles of radiation protection:

1. Keep time of exposure to radiation to a minimum.
2. Maintain the maximum distance possible between the radiation source and the operator.
3. Use protective shielding (e.g., lead aprons and gloves) between the source and radiographer.

Although radiation monitoring devices such as film badges and dosimeters do not afford protection from exposure, they are an essential component of radiation control and should be worn whenever the radiographer is in a radiation area.

An important, but often overlooked, factor in minimizing radiation exposure to both the patient and the radiographer is limiting the number of repeat exposures. It is in the patient's and the radiographer's best interests for the radiographer to position the patient and tube carefully and otherwise work conscientiously so that, whenever possible, the first film is adequate and repeat exposures to correct avoidable mistakes are strictly limited.

How to Set Up a Personal Exposure Technique System

We recommend that technical factors always be written in pencil to permit updating due to normal fluctuations in radiation output (such as those caused by tube aging, kVp and mA station drift, and processor variation).

It is especially important to record the following in order to permit quick and easy modification of technical factors to accommodate any new clinical situation:

- **part size**
- **film-screen combination relative speed**
- **generator type (1 phase or multi phase)**
- **grid ratio**

The following technique chart is provided for each position/projection in this pocket guide.

Example Exposure Techniques **Measure at CR and Use Chart (p.6)**									
Room	**cm**	**kVp**	**mAs**	**mA**	**Sec**	**Beam**	**Film**	**Grid**	**1Ø3Ø**

MASTER CHARTS

You can greatly simplify your technique system by developing master charts from the following projections:

- **PA Chest** — **CHEST Master Chart**
- **PA Hand** — **EXTREMITIES Master Chart**
- **AP Abdomen** — **ABDOMEN Master Chart**
- **AP Cervical Spine** — **SPINE Master Chart**
- **Skull** — **HEAD Master Chart**
- **RAO Upper GI** — **GI Master Chart**

It then becomes easy to refer back to these charts for all other positions/projections. For example, an 8 cm AP elbow can be exposed using the technical factor settings on the Extremity Master Chart (PA Hand).

The pages with these master charts are easily identified by a black strip that is visible at the right side when your pocket guide is closed.

> See Chapter 31/Developing Exposure Charts in Carlton and Adler's *Principles of Radiographic Imaging.*

If you follow the suggested steps below, you can create a functional personal exposure technique system that will produce diagnostic quality images in nearly all situations.

Follow an accepted process for establishing a technique chart:

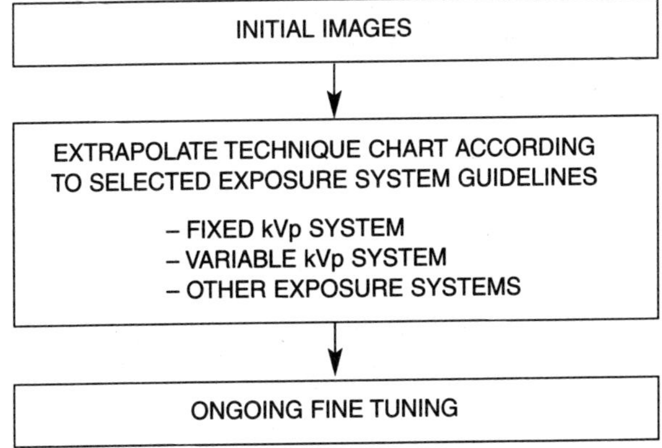

Initial Images

To start a chart in a facility that does not have one, it is mandatory to use a phantom body part to establish the first acceptable images. (Try borrowing from a school or large hospital.)

To establish a personal chart, simply observe images that meet your own quality standards and record the part size and other factors. (This is a great opportunity to compliment colleagues on high-quality work.)

Extrapolate Technique Chart

Select a technique system from the section "Technique System Theories" (see page xxiii). Then use the rules given under the section "Technique Rules" to extrapolate (or fill in) missing lines in the charts (see page xxii). Although an entire chart can be extrapolated from the factors for a single fine image, it is advised that a minimum of two observed or phantom images be used for each of the master charts.

Ongoing Fine Tuning

It is important that a system of ongoing fine tuning be established as a quality control monitoring method. Whenever a technique chart produces an unacceptable image, it should be noted. Since all technical factors are written in pencil, they are easy to modify as system changes become obvious. X-ray tubes and cassette intensifying screens age, processor function varies, and a myriad of other factors can also affect the accuracy of technique selections. **A good technique chart is constantly being modified for current conditions.**

Acceptance Limits

> See Chapter 31/Establishing Imaging Standards in Carlton and Adler's *Principles of Radiographic Imaging.*

All images should be produced with a goal of perfection in mind. Clinical reality dictates however, that a process is necessary for times when perfection is not achieved. The process that assists in obtaining quality diagnostic images can be thought of as an **acceptance limit**, as illustrated below:

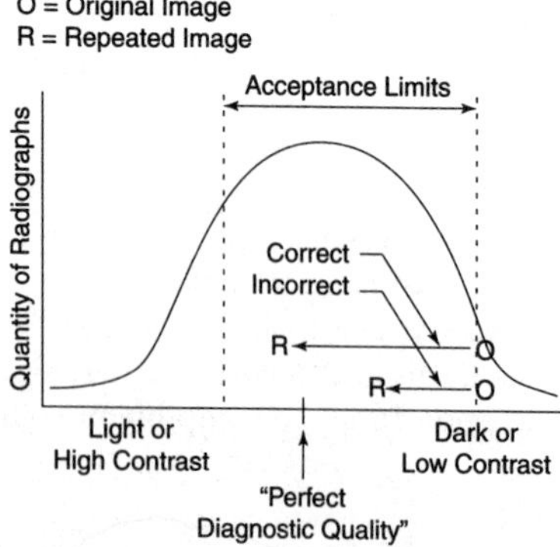

When a less than perfect image is produced, the goal is to repeat the image so it meets the definition of "perfect." Of course, this is much easier said than done. If the image is conceived as "perfect" within 1 visible density, it is possible to establish actual technical factor standards for clinical situations.

The concept of one visible density can be understood by recalling the definition of a visible density change as:

- 25-33% change in mAs

OR

- 3-5% change in kVp

Nearly all radiologic professionals can justify submitting an image that is 1 or 2 visible density values too dark or 1 visible density value too light. The rationale is that the image quality, while not perfect, is within the acceptable range for diagnosis and not poor enough quality to justify repeating the image (which doubles the exposure to the patient). Depending on conditions, some professionals will also justify submitting an image that is 3 visible density values too dark or 2 visible density values too light. This essentially creates a normal "acceptance limit" from -2 to +3 visible densities, as shown below:

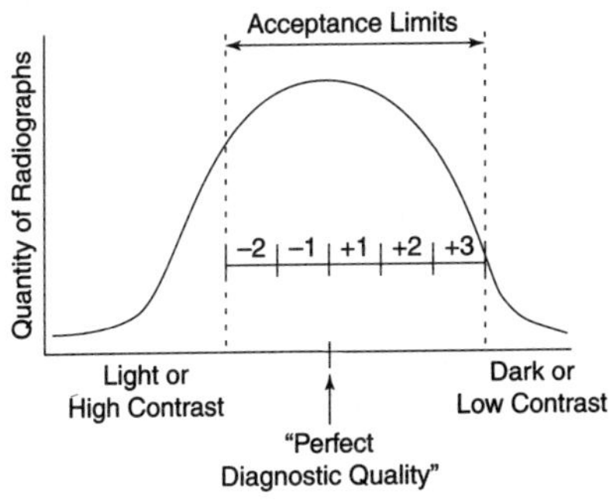

If each visible density value is considered to be a 33% mAs change, the "acceptance limit" for the mAs that would achieve a "perfect" image is -50% to +100%. This means that anything from half to double the required mAs will produce an acceptable image. (A similar argument can be made for contrast and kVp changes from -10% to +15%.) While this range definitely does not produce a satisfactory daily operating procedure, it does permit the establishment of an initial exposure technique chart that will produce diagnostic quality images. **It is critical to constantly fine tune any technique chart from this liberal interpretation of a diagnostic quality image.**

The importance of this concept of acceptance limits is that it permits a complete exposure technique chart to be extrapolated from a very few initial technical factors. The following section of this pocket guide details how to do this.

TECHNIQUE RULES

See Chapter 36/Exposure Conversion Problems in Carlton and Adler's *Principles of Radiographic Imaging.*

All these rules help **maintain the same density.**

• 2 KVP/CM RULE

Variable kVp Theory
Maintains density by changing kVp for different part sizes.
Change by 2 kVp for every cm of part size.
EXAMPLE: 60 kVp for 10 cm = 64 kVp for 12 cm

• 4-5 CM RULE

Fixed kVp Theory
Maintains density by changing mAs for different part sizes.
Double or halve mAs for every 4-5 cm part size.
EXAMPLE: 10 mAs for 20 cm = 20 mAs for 24 cm

• 15% RULE

Variable and Fixed kVp Theory
Maintains density when kVp is changed.
Increase kVp 15% AND Decrease mAs to half
EXAMPLE: 60 kVp and 10 mAs = 69 kVp and 5 mAs
Decrease kVp 15% AND Increase mAs double
EXAMPLE: 60 kVp and 10 mAs = 51 kVp and 20 mAs

Disclaimer: The above rules are not "Laws of Exposure" by any means. They are simply rules of thumb that have proven useful for generations of radiographers. The actual physical processes that determine exact exposure rates and image quality factors are extremely complex and vary not only from one radiographic unit to another, but over time with the same unit. **These rules may be considered useful within a range of 1-2 densities for part sizes from 10-20 cm and kVp ranges of 60-80.** However, they are often close enough to produce diagnostically useful images throughout the diagnostic radiography range of body part sizes and kVp levels.

See Appendix B

See Chapter 25/Density and Chapter 26/Contrast in Carlton and Adler's *Principles of Radiographic Imaging.*

Technique System Theories

See Chapter 32/Fixed Kilovoltage Systems and Chapter 32/Variable Kilovoltage Systems in Carlton and Adler's *Principles of Radiographic Imaging.*

There are two generally accepted technique theories (systems) in common use: fixed kVp and variable kVp. There are pros and cons to both:

	Fixed kVp Systems	Variable kVp Systems
Advantages	• decreased patient exposure • uniform contrast • longer exposure latitude • extends x-ray tube life • may decrease patient motion	• permits small incremental changes • higher overall contrast

Continued

Continued	**Fixed kVp Systems**	**Variable kVp Systems**
Disadvantages	• small incremental changes may be difficult • lower overall contrast	• increased patient exposure • erratic contrast between images • shorter exposure latitude • decreases x-ray tube life • may increase patient motion

Fixed kVp Systems

The concept is to **fix an optimal kVp and vary the mAs depending on measured body part thickness.**

Fixed kVp uses an optimal kVp for each procedure (i.e., hand, chest, hip). The kVp is not fixed for all examinations, only for a range of procedures with similar tissue properties (i.e., hand, finger, wrist, forearm, elbow). The optimal kVp is selected by each person or facility. It should be the **highest kVp and lowest contrast that is within acceptable limits** as determined by the physicians responsible for interpreting the images. Here is a chart of common optimal kVp ranges:

Common Optimal kVp Ranges For The Major Body Regions

Region	Optimal kVp Range
Small extremities	50 – 60
Iodine-based contrast media studies	68
Large extremities	70
Skull	80
Abdomen and ribs	80
AP vertebral column	80
Lateral vertebral column	90
Chest	120
Barium-based contrast media studies	120

Here is an example of a fixed kVp chart that was extrapolated using the concepts of optimal kVp and the 4-5 cm rule:

Fixed kVp Technique Chart

Blank Chart with Phantom Technique			**Extrapolation of Additional mAs Values**	**Fine Tuning of Extrapolated mAs Values**	**Extrapolation of Final mAs Values**
		Step 1	Step 2	Step 3	Step 4
cm	*kVp*	*mAs*			
16	68				30
17	68				35
18	68				40
19	68				45
20	68	50	50	50	50
21	68				60
22	68				70
23	68				80
24	68				90
25	68		100	100	100
26	68				115
27	68				130
28	68				145
29	68				160
30	68		200	180	180
31	68				215
32	68				250
33	68				285
34	68				320
35	68		400	360	360

Variable kVp Systems

The concept is to **vary the kilovoltage depending on measured body part thickness while maintaining relatively the same mAs.**

To assure adequate penetration of the body part, variable kVp charts use a variation of the 2 kVp/cm rule:

2 kVp/cm + constant

The constant is determined by the user to establish a kVp level equal to an acceptable level of contrast. This is a subjective opinion and should be confirmed by asking others involved in the diagnostic process (quality control technologists, radiologists, etc.) Common constants are 30, 40, or 50 kVp, as shown in these charts:

Variable Kilovoltage Scale

A 2 kVp/cm + 30		B 2 kVp/cm + 40		C 2 kVp/cm + 50	
cm	kVp	cm	kVp	cm	kVp
2	34	2	44	2	54
3	36	3	46	3	56
4	38	4	48	4	58
5	40	5	50	5	60
6	42	6	52	6	62
7	44	7	54	7	64
8	46	8	56	8	66
9	48	9	58	9	68
10	50	10	60	10	70
11	52	11	62	11	72
12	54	12	64	12	74
13	56	13	66	13	76
14	58	14	68	14	78
15	60	15	70	15	80
16	62	16	72	16	82
17	64	17	74	17	84
18	66	18	76	18	86
19	68	19	78	19	88
20	70	20	80	20	90
21	72	21	82	21	92
22	74	22	84	22	94
23	76	23	86	23	96
24	78	24	88	24	98
25	80	25	90	25	100
26	82	26	92	26	102
27	84	27	94	27	104
28	86	28	96	28	106
29	88	29	98	29	108
30	90	30	100	30	110
31	92	31	102	31	112
32	94	32	104	32	114
33	96	33	106	33	116
34	98	34	108	34	118
35	100	35	110	35	120
36	102	36	112	36	122

It is also common to use a stepped variable kvp chart. This type of chart solves three major fixed kVp system problems:

- kVp settings must provide contrast acceptable to interpreting physicians
- kVp for small parts must provide adequate penetration
- kVp for large parts must avoid excessive scatter radiation fog

There is a three step process that assures a properly stepped variable kVp chart. It is demonstrated in the following table (page xxvii).

Stepped Variable kVp Technique Chart

2 kVp/cm + 40

	Establishing a Limited Variable kVp Scale Step 1			Extrapolating kVp Steps Step 2		Fine Tuning of Extrapolated kVp Values Step 3	
cm	*kVp*	*mAs*	*evaluation*	*kVp*	*mAs*	*kVp*	*mAs*
4	54	20	reject	70	5	70	5
6	56	20	reject	72	5	72	5
8	58	20	reject	74	5	74	5
10	60	20	reject	76	5	76	5
11	62	20	reject	78	5	70	10
12	64	20	reject	80	5	72	10
13	66	20	reject	82	5	74	10
14	68	20	reject	84	5	76	10
15	70	20	acceptable	70	20	70	20
16	72	20	acceptable	72	20	72	20
17	74	20	acceptable	74	20	74	20
18	76	20	acceptable	76	20	76	20
19	78	20	acceptable	78	20	78	20
20	80	20	acceptable	80	20	80	20
21	82	20	acceptable	82	20	82	20
22	84	20	acceptable	84	20	84	20
23	86	20	reject	70	80	78	40
24	88	20	reject	72	80	80	40
25	90	20	reject	74	80	82	40
26	92	20	reject	76	80	84	40
27	94	20	reject	78	80	78	80
28	96	20	reject	80	80	80	80
29	98	20	reject	82	80	82	80
30	100	20	reject	84	80	84	80
31	102	20	reject	70	320	78	160
32	104	20	reject	72	320	80	160
33	106	20	reject	74	320	82	160
34	108	20	reject	76	320	84	160
35	110	20	reject	78	320	78	320
36	112	20	reject	80	320	80	320
37	114	20	reject	82	320	82	320
38	118	20	reject	84	320	84	320

TYPICAL SURFACE LANDMARKS

Corresponding Vertebrae	Landmark
C1	Mastoid tip
C2, C3	Gonion
C5	Thyroid cartilage
C7	Vertebra prominens
T1	Approximately 2 inches superior to sternal (manubrial) notch
T2, T3	Level of sternal notch
	Superior margin of scapulae
T4, T5	Level of sternal angle
T7	Level of inferior angle of scapulae
T10	Level of xiphoid tip
L3	Costal margin
L3, L4	Level of umbilicus
L4	Level of most superior aspect of iliac crest
S1	Level of anterior superior iliac spine
Coccyx	Level of pubic symphysis and greater trochanter

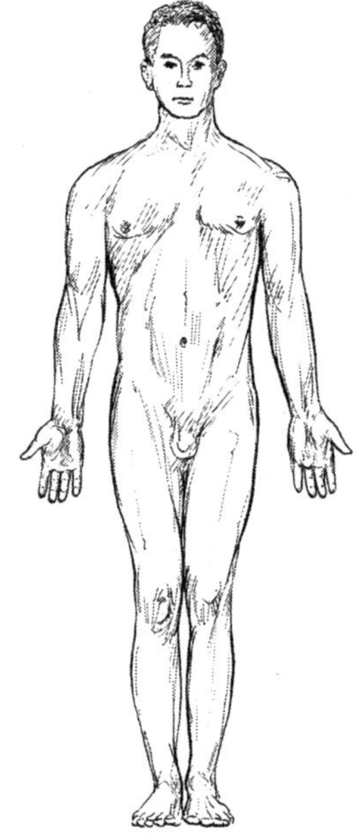

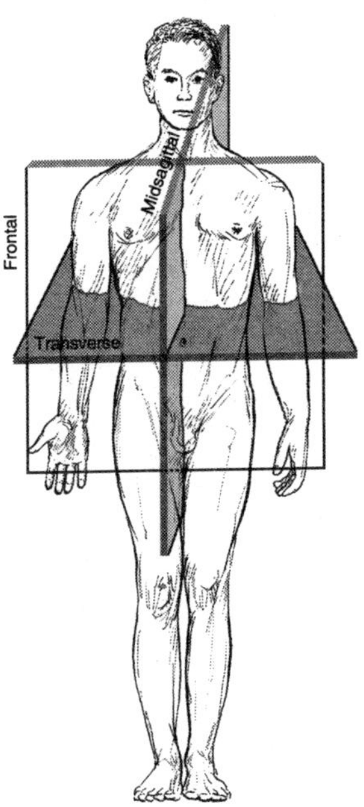

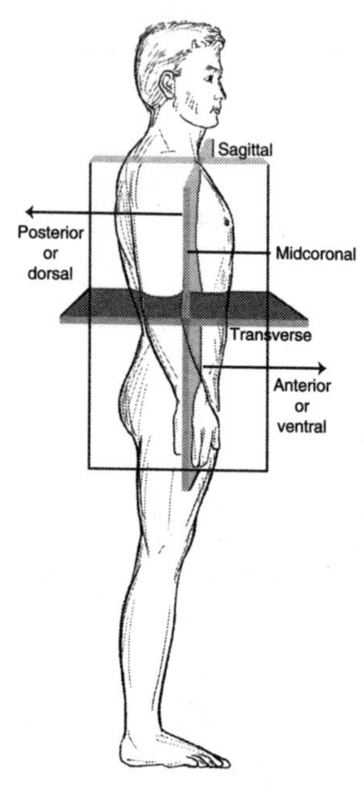
Sagittal
Posterior
or
dorsal
Midcoronal
Transverse
Anterior
or
ventral

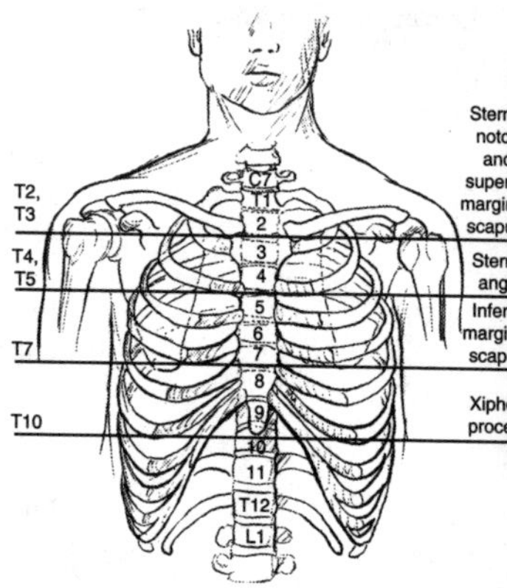
T2,
T3
T4,
T5
T7
T10
C7
T1
2
3
4
5
6
7
8
9
10
11
T12
L1

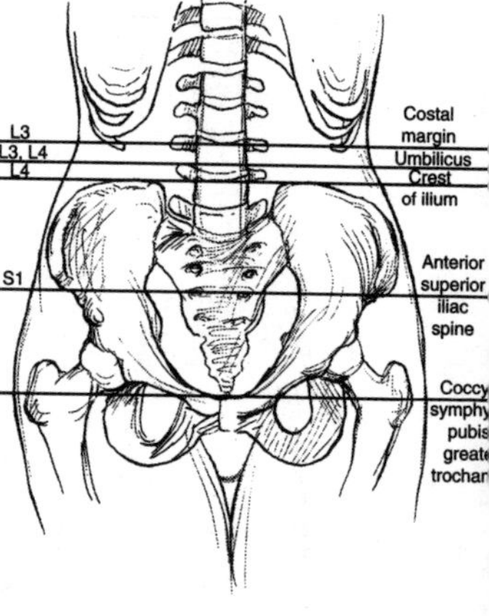
L3
L3, L4
L4
S1
Costal
margin
Umbilicus
Crest
of ilium
Anterior
superior
iliac
spine

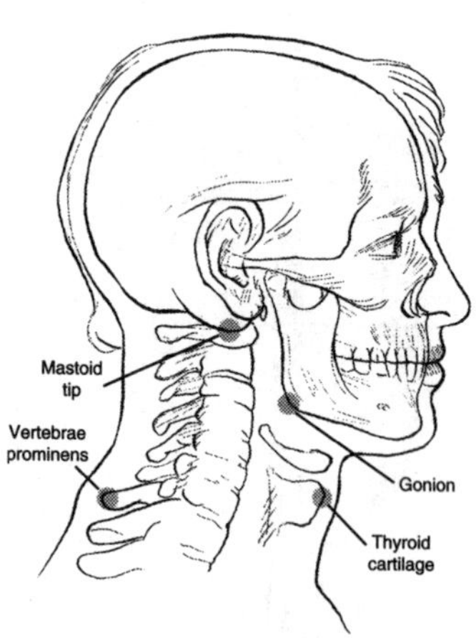
Mastoid
tip
Vertebrae
prominens
Gonion
Thyroid
cartilage

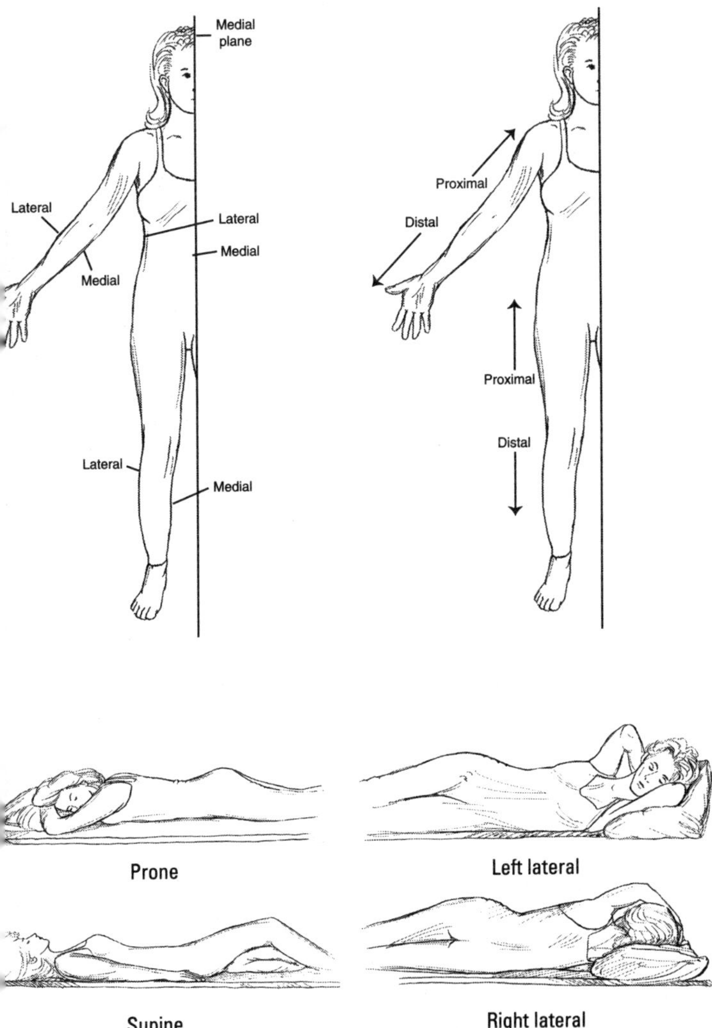

Prone

Left lateral

Supine

Right lateral

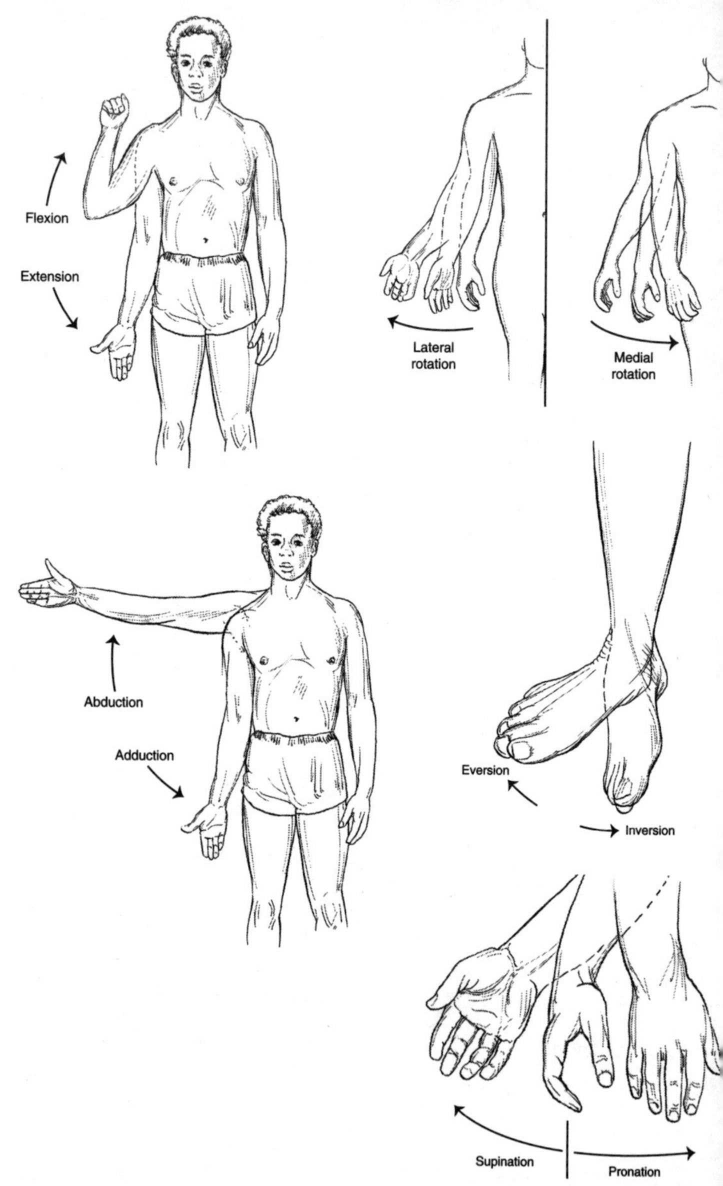
Flexion
Extension
Lateral rotation
Medial rotation
Abduction
Adduction
Eversion
Inversion
Supination
Pronation

ROUTINE AND ALTERNATIVE POSITIONS/PROJECTIONS

Part	Routine	Page	Alternative	Page
Chest	PA	6	PA (stretcher/stool)	10
			Supine/semi-erect AP	14
			Lateral decubitus	16
			AP lordotic	18
	Lateral	8	Oblique (LAO/RAO)	20
			Lateral (stretcher/stool)	12

Patient Preparation In adition to having the patient disrobe from the waist up, the patient should be instructed to remove all potential artifacts from the thoracic and neck regions (e.g., necklace or other jewelry). Long hair, especially wet hair, braids, or pony tails, should be pulled to the side. Any patient tubing (e.g., nasogastric tubes, oxygen tubes) that can be moved should also be carefully placed to one side.

To best demonstrate fluid in the lungs, patients must be in the upright, semi-upright, or decubitus position for a minimum of 10 minutes. This allows the fluid in the lungs or the pleural spaces to settle in the lowest level.

Upright Position Chest radiography should be performed with the patient in an upright postion, whether the examination is performed in the radiography department or at the bedside. Three important considerations for the upright chest radiograph are:

- The diaphragm is permitted to move to the lowest possible position.
- Engorgement of the pulmonary vessels is prevented, which minimizes distortion of these vessels.
- Air/fluid levels can be demonstrated.

Long SID To prevent magnification of the heart shadow, a 72-inch (180 cm) or 120-inch (300 cm) SID is used. The longer SID uses the more vertical portion of the x-ray beam, which minimizes distortion and allows for a more accurate diagnosis of cardiac enlargement.

Technical Considerations

- Regular screen/film
- Grid
- kVp range: 100–120
- SID: 72 inch (180 cm)

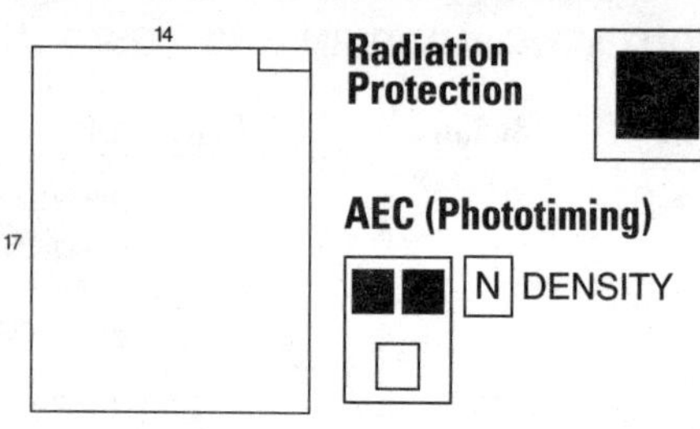

Patient Position

Erect with weight equally distributed on both feet; top of film 1 1/2 to 2 inches (4–5 cm) above shoulders and centered to film T6–T7.

Part Position Hands low on hips, palms facing outward; shoulders relaxed; scapulae rotated forward; chin elevated.

Central Ray Perpendicular to the film holder.

Breathing Instructions Suspend at end of 2nd inspiration.

Evaluation Criteria

- Sternoclavicular joints should be equidistant from the vertebral column.

Example Exposure Techniques **Measure at CR and Use this Chart**									
Room	**cm**	**kVp**	**mAs**	**mA**	**Sec**	**Beam**	**Film**	**Grid**	**1Ø3Ø**
	14								
	16								
	18								
	20								
	22								
	24								
	26								
	28								
	30								
	32								

- Distance between the vertebral column and the outer margin of the rib cage should be equal on each side.
- Entire apices should be demonstrated 1 inch above the clavicles.
- Both costophrenic angles should be included on the film.
- Scapulae should be rotated outside the lung field.
- Mandible should not be superimposed over the lung field.
- A minimum of ten posterior ribs should be demonstrated.

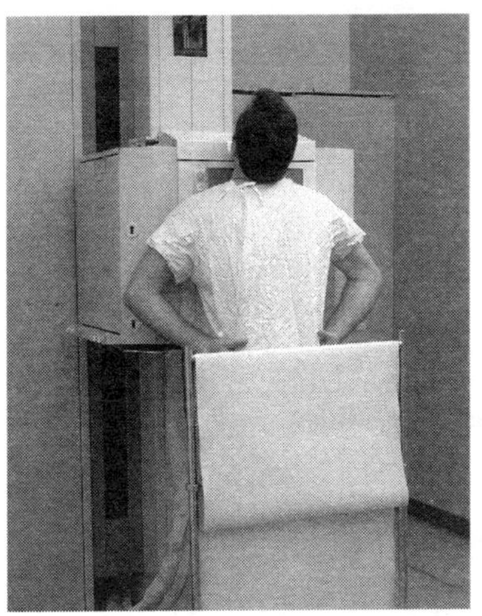

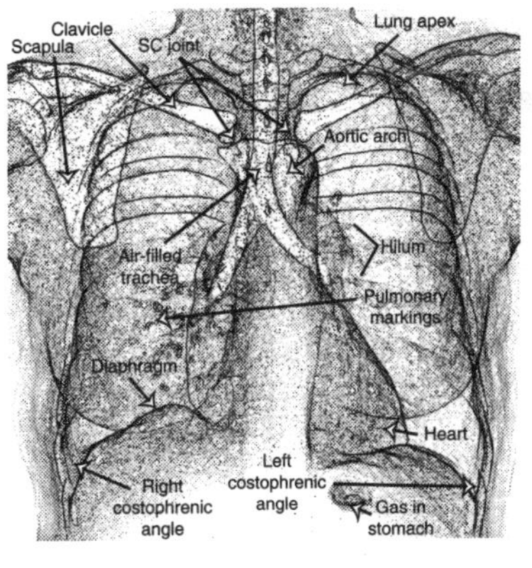

Exam Rationale The PA chest is performed to outline the anatomy of the lungs, heart, great vessels, and mediastinal structures to detect the presence of chest lesions.

Tips

1. The film should be turned crosswise for patients with a wide chest.
2. To remove overlapping breast shadows, women with large pendulous breasts should be asked to lift their breasts and pull them to the side holding them in place while leaning forward to the film holder.
3. To demonstrate a pneumothorax, an inhalation and exhalation chest radiograph should be performed. The exhalation chest enhances the pneumothorax.

Technical Considerations

- Regular screen/film
- Grid
- kVp range: 100–120
- SID: 72 inch (180 cm)

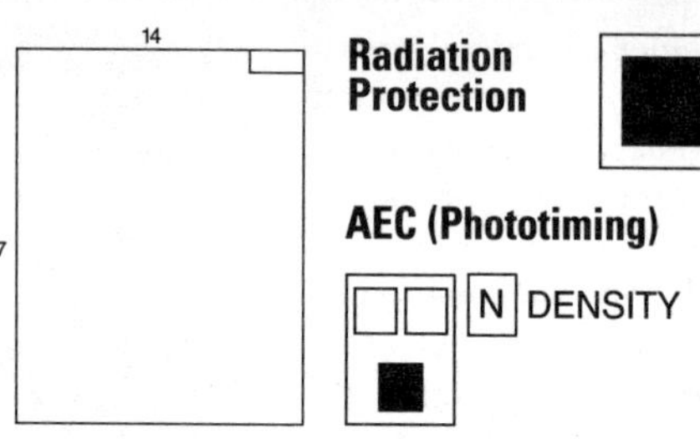

Patient Position

Erect; with weight equally distributed on both feet; top of film 1 1/2 to 2 inches (4–5 cm) above shoulders; center x-ray tube to film (T6–T7).

Part Position Feet, hips, and shoulders in true lateral position; arms raised over the head with each hand grasping opposite elbow (Figure 2.13); or grasp bar positioned in front of and over patient's head underhanded; chin elevated; midcoronal plane centered to the film holder.

Central Ray Perpendicular to the film holder.

Breathing Instructions Suspend at end of 2nd inspiration.

Example Exposure Techniques
Measure at CR and Use Chart (p.6)

Room	cm	kVp	mAs	mA	Sec	Beam	Film	Grid	1Ø3Ø
	20								
	22								
	24								
	26								
	28								
	30								
	32								
	34								
	36								
	38								

Evaluation Criteria

- Posterior aspect of the ribs and lungs should be superimposed.
- Intervertebral joint spaces of the thoracic vertebra should be clearly visible.
- Sternum should be in lateral position.
- Apices and costophrenic angles should be included on the film.
- Hilum should be near the center of the film.
- Midsagittal plane of the patient should be vertical—the patient should not be leaning forward or backward.

Exam Rationale The lateral chest demonstrates the anatomy of the lungs, heart, great vessels, and mediastinum structures 90° from the PA to detect the presence of chest lesions.

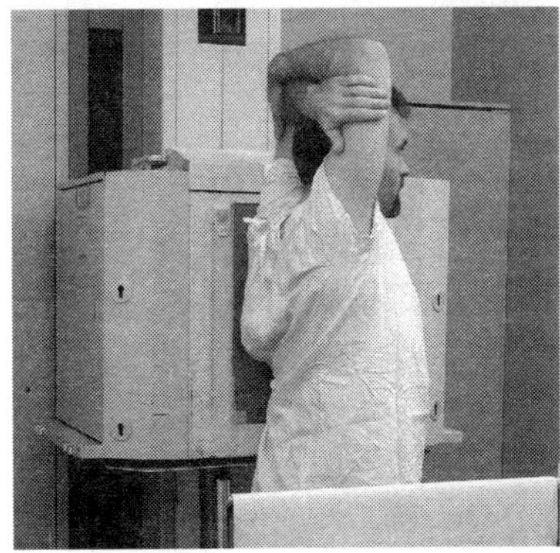

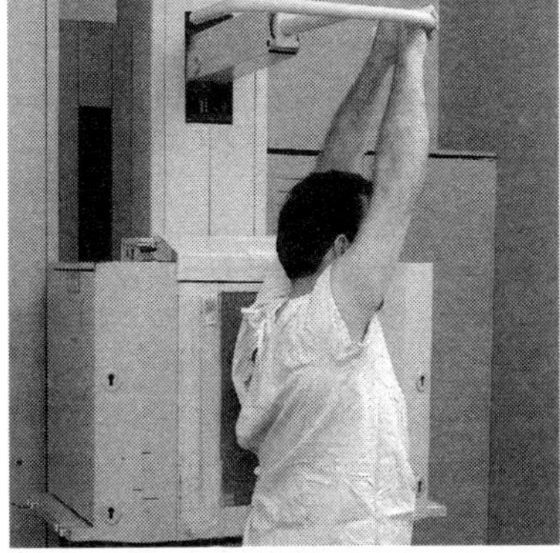

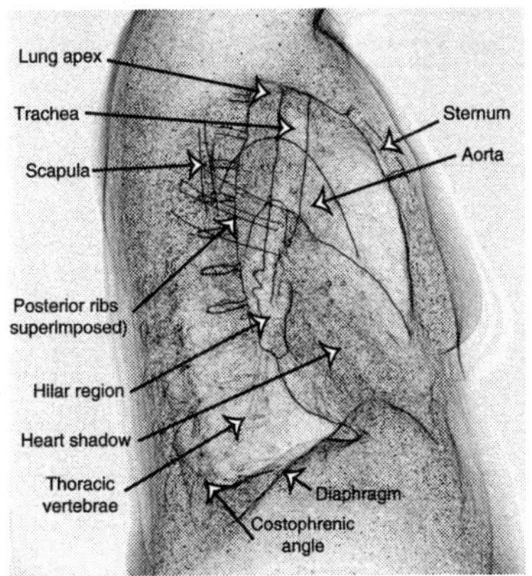

Technical Considerations

- Regular screen/film
- Grid
- kVp range: 100–120
- SID: 72 inch (180 cm)

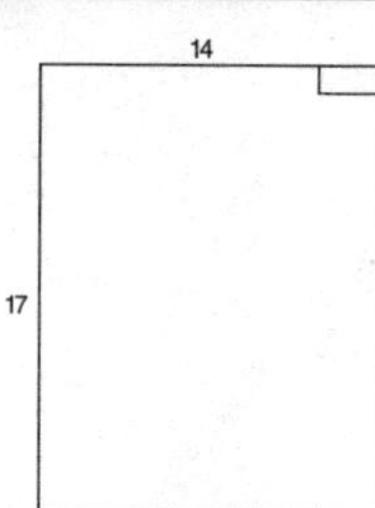

Radiation Protection

AEC (Phototiming)

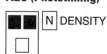

Patient Position

Erect; weight equally distributed on the ischial tuberosities; legs dangling off side of stretcher; top of film 1 1/2 to 2 inches (4–5 cm) above shoulders centered to T6–T7.

Part Position Hands low on hips, palms facing outward; shoulders relaxed; scapulae rotated forward; chin elevated.

Central Ray Perpendicular to the film holder.

Breathing Instructions Suspend at end of 2nd inspiration.

Example Exposure Techniques **Measure at CR and Use Chart (p.6)**									
Room	cm	kVp	mAs	mA	Sec	Beam	Film	Grid	1Ø3Ø
	14								
	16								
	18								
	20								
	22								
	24								
	26								
	28								
	30								
	32								

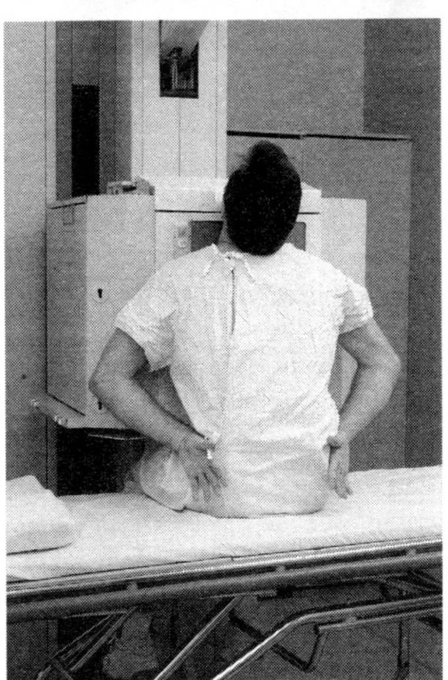

Evaluation Criteria Same as for routine PA chest.

Exam Rationale The PA chest is performed to outline the anatomy of the lungs, heart, great vessels, and mediastinum structures to detect the presence of chest lesions.

Tips

1. Lock stool or stretcher in place to prevent movement during the exposure.
2. Center the patient on the stretcher to maintain balance of the stretcher.
3. If the patient is unable to dangle the legs off the stretcher, have him hold the cassette in place.

Technical Considerations

- Regular screen/film
- Grid
- kVp range: 100–120
- SID: 72 inch (180 cm)

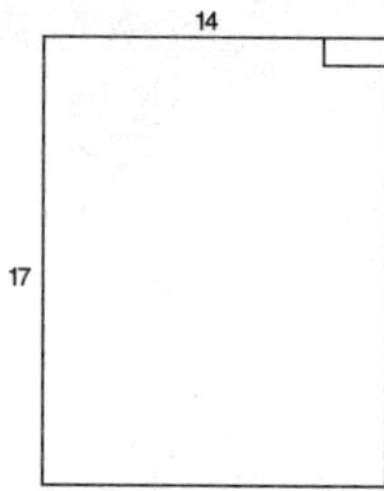

Radiation Protection

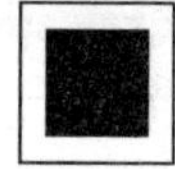

AEC (Phototiming)

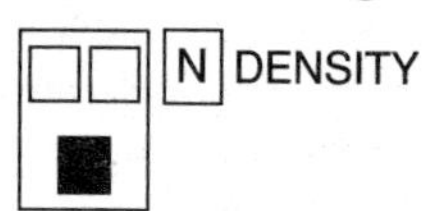

Patient Position

Erect; sitting on a stretcher with legs extended or seated upright on a stool with weight equally distributed on the ischial tuberosities; top of film 1 1/2 to 2 inches (4–5 cm) above shoulders centered to T6–T7.

Part Position Hips and shoulders in true lateral position; arms raised over the head with each hand grasping the opposite elbow; or, grasp bar positioned in front of and over patient's head underhanded; chin elevated; midcoronal plane centered to film holder.

Central Ray Perpendicular to the film holder.

Example Exposure Techniques **Measure at CR and Use Chart (p.6)**									
Room	**cm**	**kVp**	**mAs**	**mA**	**Sec**	**Beam**	**Film**	**Grid**	**1Ø3Ø**
	20								
	22								
	24								
	26								
	28								
	30								
	32								
	34								
	36								
	38								

Breathing Instructions
Suspend at end of 2nd inspiration.

Evaluation Criteria Same as for routine lateral chest.

Exam Rationale The lateral chest demonstrates the anatomy of the lungs, heart, and mediastinal structures 90° from the PA to detect the presence of chest lesions for patients unable to stand.

Tip If the patient is unable to sit upright without the aid of a support, a wheelchair or stretcher with the head of the stretcher raised should be used. A radiolucent support is placed behind the patient's back to prevent superimposition of the posterior aspect of the chest and the wheelchair or stretcher.

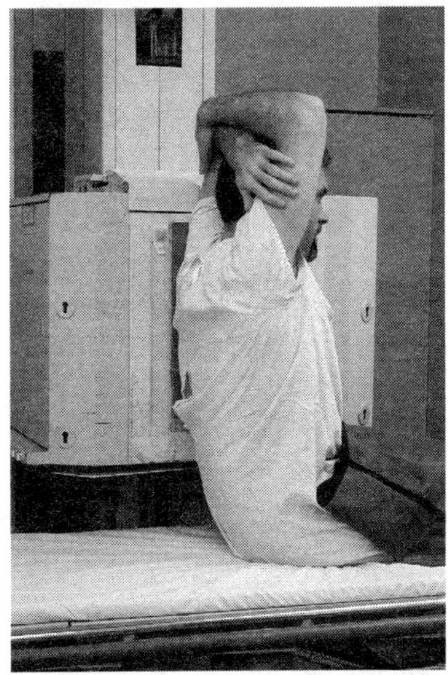

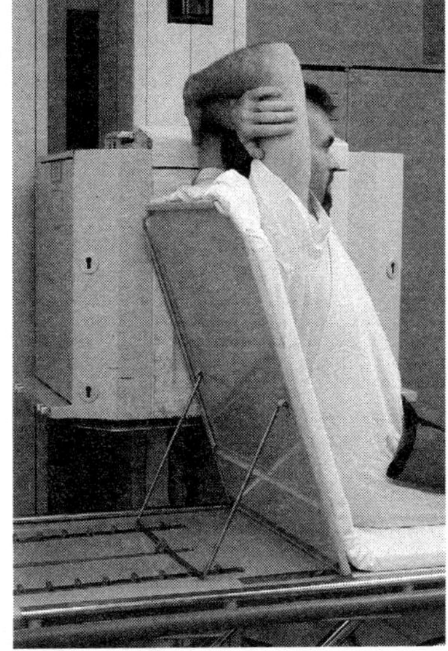

Technical Considerations

- Regular screen/film
- Grid
- kVp range: 100–120 (Note: if grid is not used, the kVp range is 75–90.)
- SID: Minimum 40 inch (100 cm)

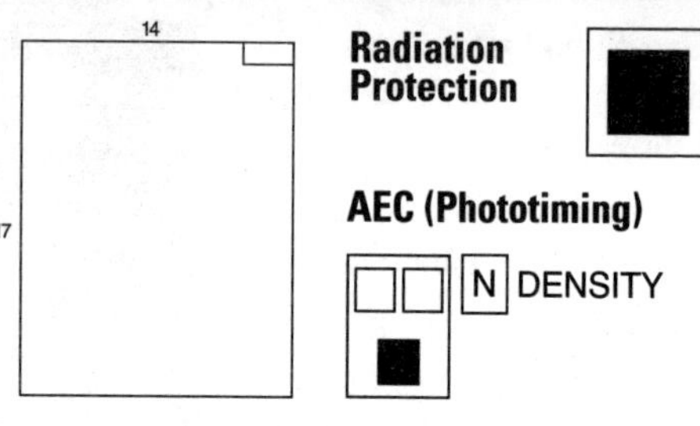

Patient Position Supine or semi-erect on the stretcher or bed; top of film holder 1 1/2 to 2 inches (4–5 cm) above shoulders.

Part Position Hands are pronated and elbows bent and brought out to the side, rotate scapulae forward away from the lung field; midsagittal plane centered to the film holder.

Central Ray Perpendicular to the sternum and centered to the film holder (level of T7 or 3–4 inches (8–10 cm) inferior to suprasternal notch).

Example Exposure Techniques
Measure at CR and Use Chart (p.6)

Room	cm	kVp	mAs	mA	Sec	Beam	Film	Grid	1Ø3Ø
	14								
	16								
	18								
	20								
	22								
	24								
	26								
	28								
	30								
	32								

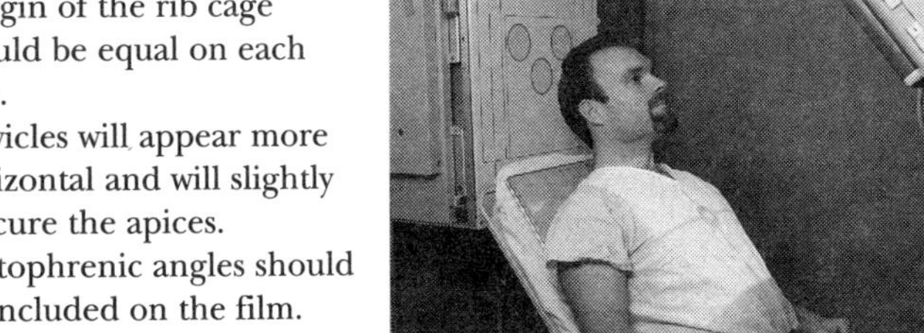

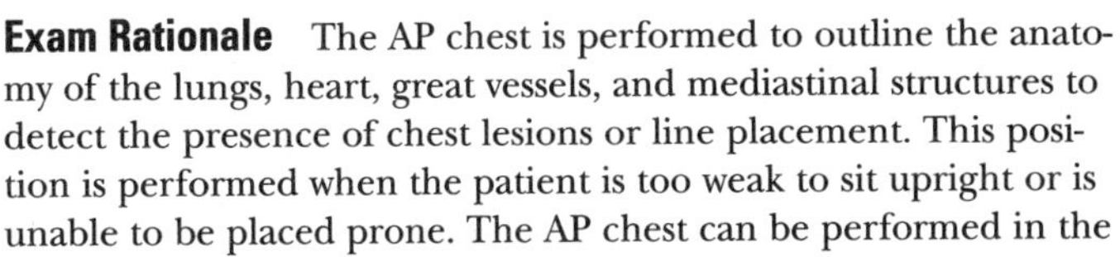

Breathing Instructions

Suspend at end of 2nd inspiration.

Evaluation Criteria

- Sternoclavicular joints should be equidistant from the vertebral column.
- Distance between the vertebral column and the outer margin of the rib cage should be equal on each side.
- Clavicles will appear more horizontal and will slightly obscure the apices.
- Costophrenic angles should be included on the film.
- Scapula should be rotated outside the lung field.
- Seven to nine posterior ribs should be demonstrated.

Exam Rationale The AP chest is performed to outline the anatomy of the lungs, heart, great vessels, and mediastinal structures to detect the presence of chest lesions or line placement. This position is performed when the patient is too weak to sit upright or is unable to be placed prone. The AP chest can be performed in the radiography department or as bedside radiography.

Tips

1. To minimize enlargement of the heart in the supine or semi-erect AP chest, use the maximum distance achievable.
2. If possible, the head of the bed or stretcher should be elevated to achieve a semi-erect position.
3. In the supine or semi-erect position, the diaphragm is elevated and full inhalation will be difficult for the patient to obtain.
4. If the patient is on a respirator, make the exposure after the respirator has completed the full inspiration.

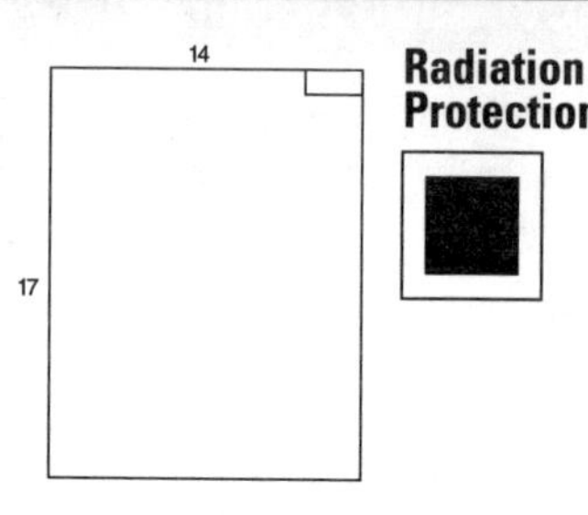

Technical Considerations
- Regular screen/film
- Grid
- kVp range: 100–120
- SID: 72 inch (180 cm)

Patient Position
Lateral recumbent position; both arms raised over patient's head; ankles and knees on top of one another and the knees flexed for support.

Part Position Adjust pelvis and shoulders parallel to the film holder; adjust the center of the film holder to the midsagittal plane and place the top of the film 2 inches (5 cm) above the shoulders.

Central Ray Perpendicular to the film holder; center x-ray tube to film (T6–T7).

Breathing Instructions Suspend at end of 2nd inspiration.

Example Exposure Techniques **Measure at CR and Use Chart (p.6)**									
Room	**cm**	**kVp**	**mAs**	**mA**	**Sec**	**Beam**	**Film**	**Grid**	**1Ø3Ø**
	14								
	16								
	18								
	20								
	22								
	24								
	26								
	28								
	30								
	32								

Evaluation Criteria

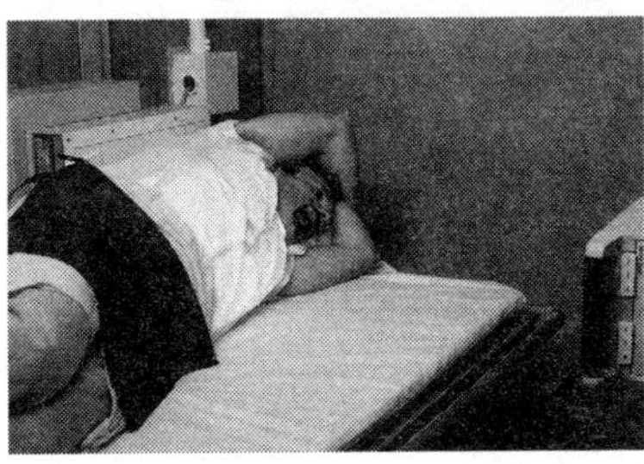

- Sternoclavicular joints should be equidistant from the vertebral column.
- Distance between the vertebral column and the outer margin of the rib cage should be equal on each side.
- Apices and both costophrenic angles should be included on the film.
- Affected side must be included on the film.
- Affected side should not be superimposed by the support.
- Patient's arms should not superimpose the upper lung region.

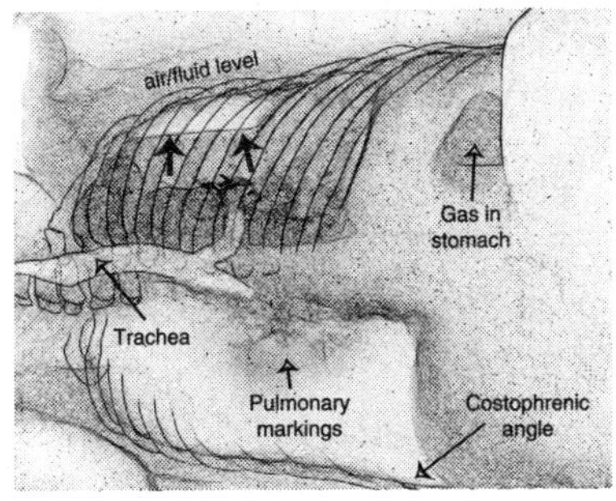

Exam Rationale This position is used to demonstrate small amounts of fluid in the pleural cavity, which would be demonstrated with the patient lying on the affected side, or small amounts of air in the pleural cavity, which would be demonstrated with the patient lying on the unaffected side.

Tips

1. Marker placement is important. A left or right marker can be used but must be placed on the correct side of the patient.
2. If demonstrating fluid levels, the patient should be placed on a radiolucent support to elevate the dependent side enough for the entire side to be demonstrated on the film.

Technical Considerations

- Regular screen/film
- Grid
- kVp range: 100–120
- SID: 72 inch (180 cm)

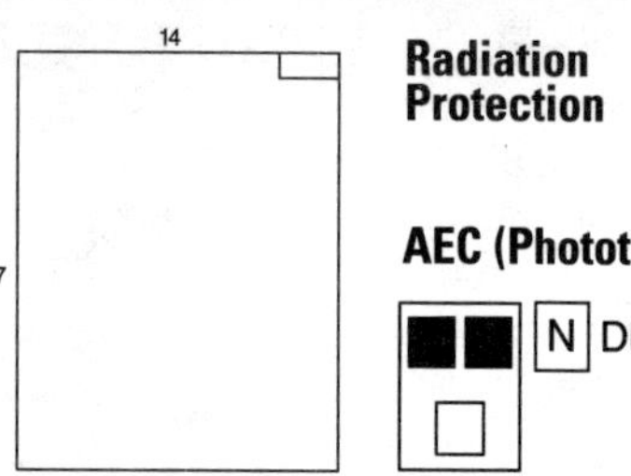

Radiation Protection

AEC (Phototiming)

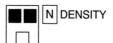

Patient Position

Erect; top of the film approximately 3–4 inches (8–10 cm) above the shoulders.

Part Position Standing approximately 1 foot from the film holder, facing forward and leaning back so the top of the shoulder, neck, and head are against the film holder; hands on hips and shoulders rotated forward; midsagittal plane centered to the film holder.

Central Ray Perpendicular to the film holder and centered mid-sternum. (3–4 inches (8–10 cm) inferior to suprasternal notch).

Breathing Instructions Suspend at end of 2nd inspiration.

Example Exposure Techniques **Measure at CR and Use Chart (p.6)**									
Room	**cm**	**kVp**	**mAs**	**mA**	**Sec**	**Beam**	**Film**	**Grid**	**1Ø3Ø**
	14								
	16								
	18								
	20								
	22								
	24								
	26								
	28								
	30								
	32								

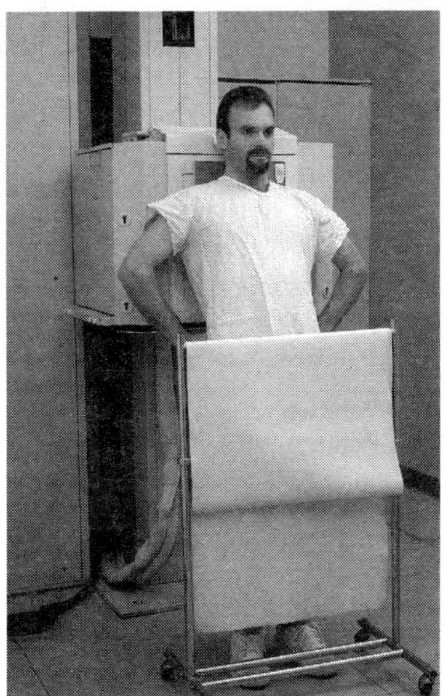

Evaluation Criteria

- Clavicles will appear horizontal above the apices.
- Sternoclavicular joints should be equidistant from the vertebral column.
- Distance between the vertebral column and the outer margin of the rib cage should be equal on each side.
- Proper exposure factors will demonstrate lung markings throughout the lung field, especially in the apices.
- Ribs will appear distorted with the anterior and posterior ribs somewhat superimposed.

Exam Rationale This position is used to demonstrate the apices free from superimposition of the clavicles or to demonstrate a right middle lobe pneumothorax.

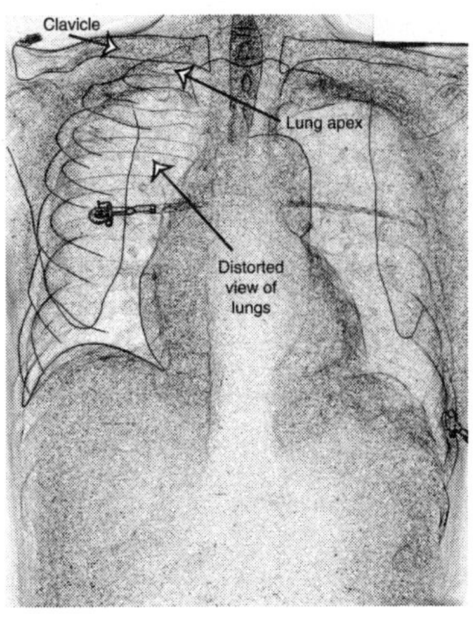

Tips

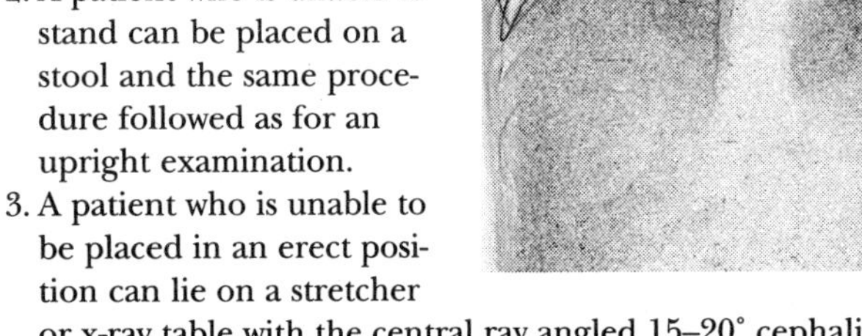

1. Always assist the patient out of this position.
2. A patient who is unable to stand can be placed on a stool and the same procedure followed as for an upright examination.
3. A patient who is unable to be placed in an erect position can lie on a stretcher or x-ray table with the central ray angled 15–20° cephalic to the midsternum.

Technical Considerations

- Regular screen/film
- Grid
- kVp range: 100–120
- SID: 72 inch (180 cm)

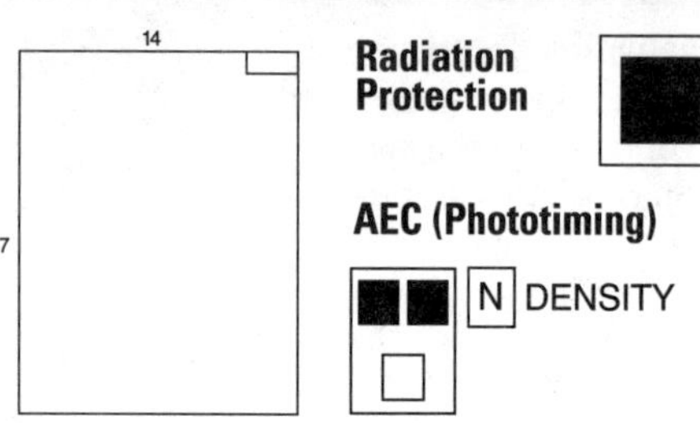

Patient Position Erect; weight equally distributed on both feet; top of film 1 1/2 to 2 inches (4–5 cm) above shoulders centered to T6–T7.

Part Position Rotate patient 45° from the straight PA with either the left (LAO) or right (RAO) shoulder and chest against film holder; the hand closest to the film is on the waist and the opposite hand raised over patient's head resting on the film holder; chin elevated. Patient adjusted so both sides are included.

Central Ray Perpendicular to the film holder.

Breathing Instructions Suspend at end of 2nd inspiration.

Example Exposure Techniques
Measure at CR and Use Chart (p.6)

Room	cm	kVp	mAs	mA	Sec	Beam	Film	Grid	1Ø3Ø
	20								
	22								
	24								
	26								
	28								
	30								
	32								
	34								
	36								
	38								

Evaluation Criteria

- Side furthest from the film holder should be approximately twice the size as the side closest to the film holder.
- Apices and both costophrenic angles should be included on the film.

Exam Rationale This position is used to demonstrate the trachea, right and left bronchial trees, heart, and aorta free from superimposition of the vertebral column. Either a right or left oblique position or both may be indicated. The side furthest from the film is demonstrated, so the LAO will demonstrate the right lung and the RAO will demonstrate the left lung.

Tips

1. The degree of rotation may vary according to patient pathology.
2. A 60° LAO may be used to separate the aorta from the thoracic spine.
3. AP obliques can be performed if the patient is unable to stand upright or lie prone. AP obliques demonstrate the side down. The RPO will demonstrate the same structures as the LAO, and the LPO will demonstrate the same structures as the RAO.

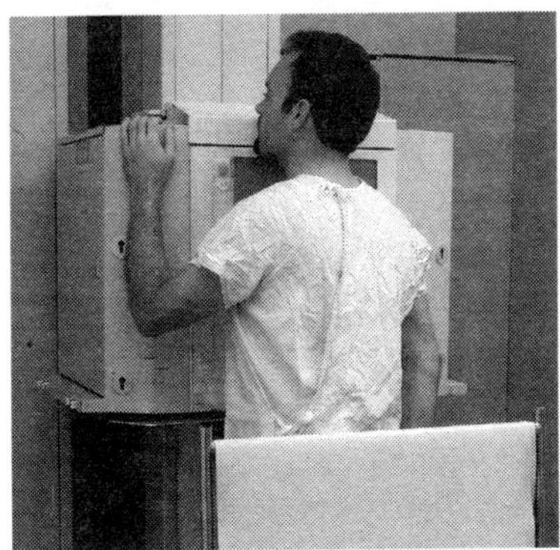

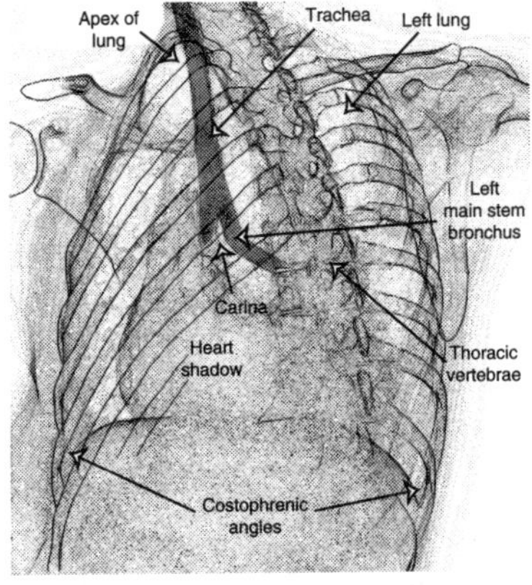

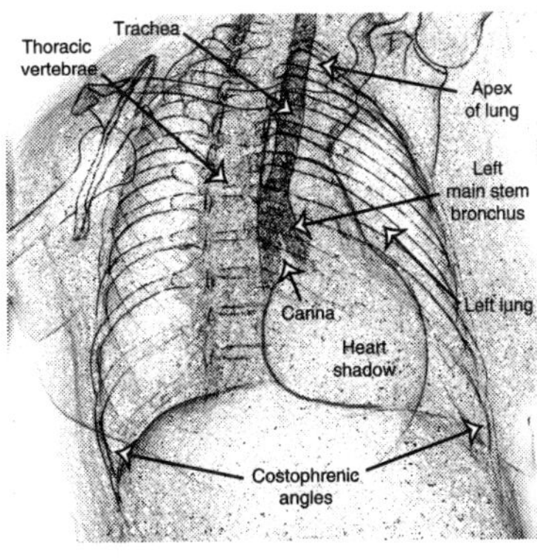

Pediatric Considerations Chest radiography for the pediatric patient can be extremely challenging, but quality chest radiographs are important. If the pediatric patient is able to hold up his or her head, the patient can be placed in a Pigg-o-Stat or other immobilization device. The Pigg-o-Stat immobilization device provides the necessary radiolucent restraining device, protective lead shield, markers, and cassette holder.

If the pediatric patient is unable to hold up his or her head, then AP and lateral recumbent chest radiographs need to be performed. If a guardian (not pregnant and properly shielded) is available, he or she should hold the patient's arms over the head and the patient's legs should be extended. For the lateral position, have the guardian hold the patient on the left side with the arms over the head and the legs extended. Place a small radiolucent sponge under the patient's head for support and comfort. If a guardian is unavailable, immobilization techniques need to be used. A heavy sandbag can be placed across each arm and the legs for the AP projection. For the lateral projection, position the patient on the left side, place a heavy sandbag over each arm and one across the patient's waist. Place a small radiolucent sponge under the patient's head for support and comfort. For both situations, a protective lead shield is placed across the patient's waist.

Pediatric chest radiography should always be performed non-grid using a screen/film combination. The kVp for pediatric chest radiography will vary depending on the patient's age but should range between 65 and 80. The mA should be high and the exposure time low to prevent artifacts from heart motion or patient motion. A minimum 40 inch (100 cm) SID should be used and a longer SID used when possible.

ABDOMEN

ROUTINE AND ALTERNATIVE POSITIONS/PROJECTIONS

Part	Routine	Page	Alternative	Page
Abdomen	Supine/KUB	24		
	AP upright	26	Lateral decubitus	30
	Acute abdomen series	23		
			Lateral	28

Patient Preparation For abdominal radiography, the patient should disrobe from the waist down and don a patient gown. Any tubing (e.g., nasogastric) should be carefully removed from the radiographic field.

ACUTE ABDOMEN SERIES

Exam Rationale A primary indication for an acute abdominal series is abdomen pain. This series includes the following three views with modifications as noted.

1. Supine abdomen: refer to page 24; no modification.
2. Upright abdomen: refer to page 26. The central ray should be at the level of the iliac crests. A portion of symphysis pubis should be evident at bottom of film.
3. PA chest: refer to page 6; no modification.

Technical Considerations

- Regular screen/film
- Grid
- kVp range: 70–80
- SID: 40 inch (100 cm)

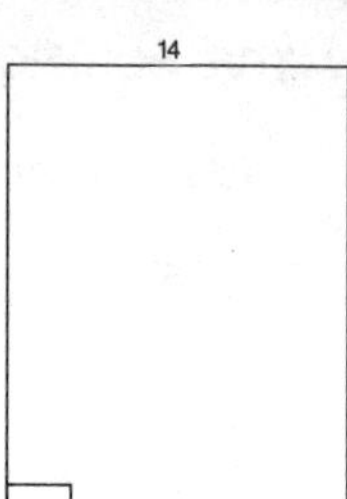

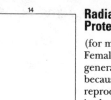

Radiation Protection

(for males). Females are generally not shielded because the female reproductive organs lie in the area of interest.

Patient Position

Supine on the table.

AEC (Phototiming)

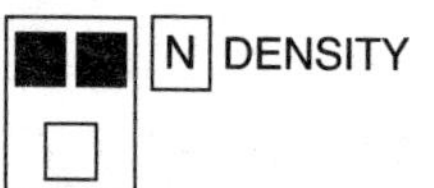

Part Position

Midsagittal plane of the body is centered to the midline of the table; the shoulders adjusted to lie in the same transverse plane laying at the patient's side, away from the body; the pelvis adjusted so that it is not rotated (distance from anterior superior iliac spine and table top is the same on both sides); the knees may be flexed for patient comfort.

Central Ray Cassette should be positioned so that its lower border is at the level of the greater trochanter (symphysis pubis); central ray perpendicular to midpoint of the film (centered at level of iliac crests).

Example Exposure Techniques **Measure at CR and Use this Chart**									
Room	**cm**	**kVp**	**mAs**	**mA**	**Sec**	**Beam**	**Film**	**Grid**	**1Ø3Ø**
	10								
	14								
	18								
	22								
	26								
	30								
	34								
	38								
	42								
	46								

Breathing Instructions
Suspend on expiration.

Evaluation Criteria

- Pelvis and abdomen should not be rotated as evidenced by:
  —symmetrical iliac alae
  —spinous processes in center of vertebral bodies
- Vertebral column is in center of radiograph.
- A portion of the symphysis pubis must be included at the bottom portion of the radiograph.
- Density should be sufficient to demonstrate bony anatomy of pelvis and soft tissue structures of the abdomen.

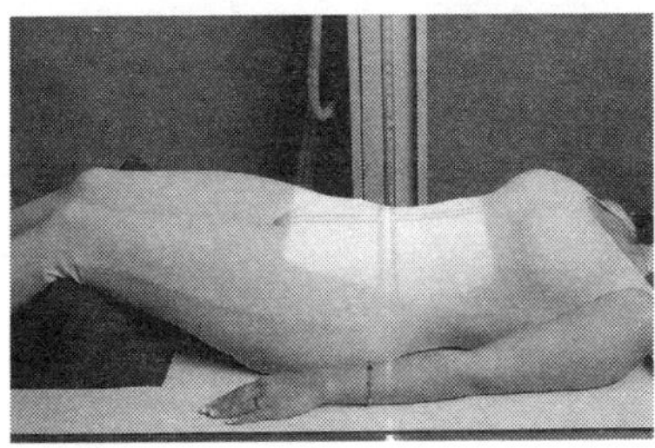

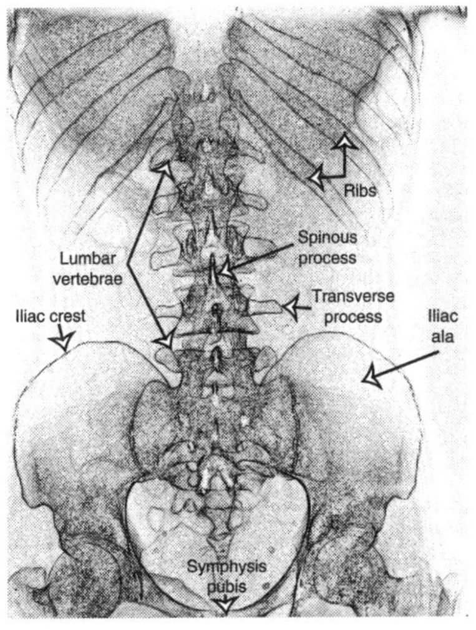

Exam Rationale This projection often serves as a scout view for various radiologic exams (e.g., GI, GU). It is valuable for visualizing abdominal masses, calcifications, foreign bodies, and intestinal obstruction. The projection also provides a general survey of the abdominal gas pattern, soft tissue shadows, organ configuration, and skeletal structures.

Tip If radiographing a hypersthenic patient, two 14 × 17 cassettes placed crosswise should be used to cover the entire abdominal field.

Technical Considerations

- Regular screen/film
- Grid
- kVp range: 75–85
- SID: 40 inch (100 cm)

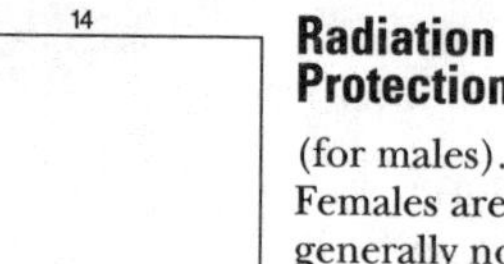

Patient Position Erect with back against Bucky or other film holder.

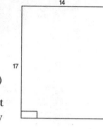

Radiation Protection

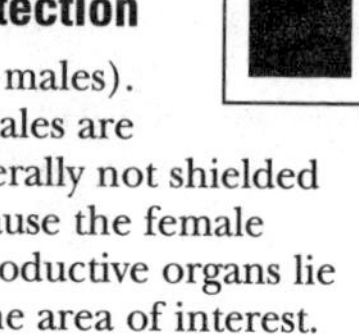

(for males). Females are generally not shielded because the female reproductive organs lie in the area of interest.

AEC (Phototiming)

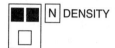

Part Position The midsagittal plane of the body should be centered to the midline of the upright Bucky or film holder; weight equally distributed on both feet.

Central Ray To include diaphragm center 2 to 3 inches (5–8 cm) above level of iliac crests; central ray perpendicular to the midpoint of the film.

Breathing Instructions Suspend on expiration.

Evaluation Criteria

- Patient should be standing straight as evidenced by spine vertically aligned on radiograph.

Example Exposure Techniques
Measure at CR and Use Chart (p.24)

Room	cm	kVp	mAs	mA	Sec	Beam	Film	Grid	1Ø3Ø
	10								
	14								
	18								
	22								
	26								
	30								
	34								
	38								
	42								
	46								

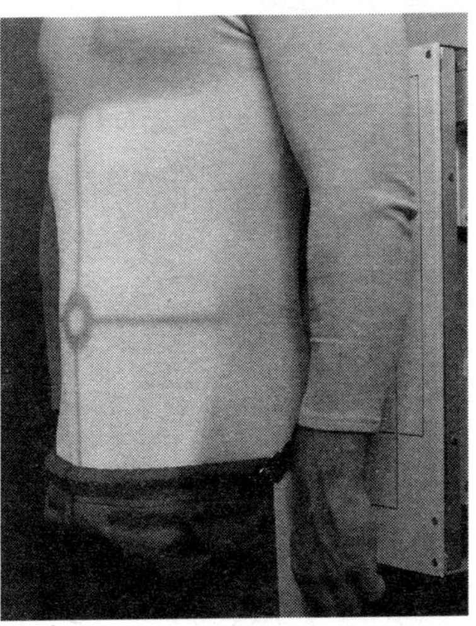

- Pelvis and abdomen should not be rotated as evidenced by:
  —symmetrical iliac alae
  — spinous processes in center of vertebral bodies
- Diaphragm should be included at top of radiograph and demonstrate no motion.
- Density should be sufficient to demonstrate bony anatomy of pelvis and soft tissue structures of the abdomen.

Exam Rationale This projection is most valuable for demonstrating free intraperitoneal air and air/fluid levels. It is also good for visualization of soft tissue structures, bowel gas patterns, and skeletal structures.

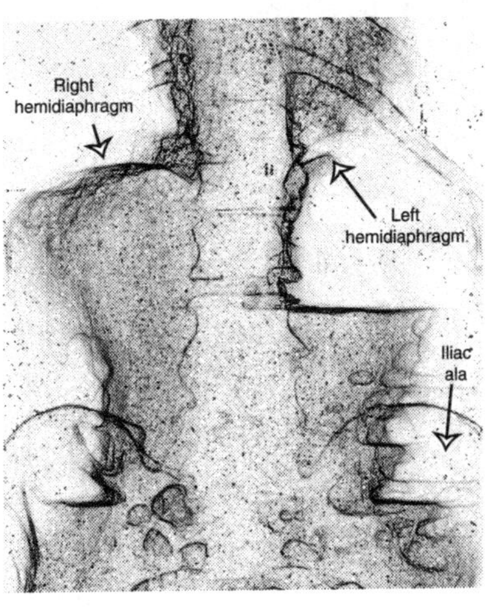

Tips

1. The patient should be erect a minimum of 5 minutes before exposure.
2. Mark the film as upright with appropriate marker.
3. If a PA or AP chest is performed, centering for the abdomen examination is at the level of the iliac crest.
4. If using a radiographic table, the table may be tilted if the patient has difficulty standing. Compression bands on the chest and legs may also be used for support. The central ray remains horizontal.
5. This projection may be replaced by the left lateral decubitus if the patient has difficulty standing.

Technical Considerations

- Regular screen/film
- Grid
- kVp range: 75–85
- SID: 40 inch (100 cm)

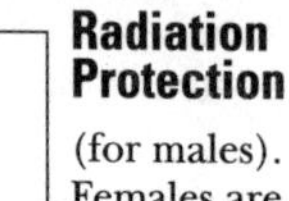

Radiation Protection

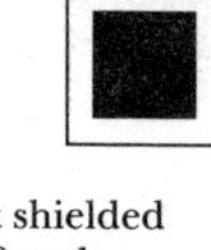

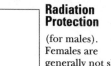

(for males). Females are generally not shielded because the female reproductive organs lie in the area of interest.

AEC (Phototiming)

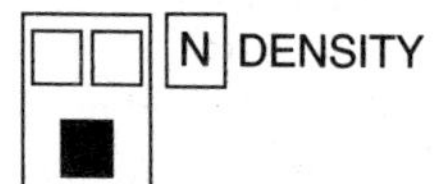

Patient Position

Patient lying on left side.

Part Position Knees may be bent for patient support; arms and elbows moved toward head so that they are not in the area of interest; shoulders and pelvis should be in true lateral position.

Central Ray Perpendicular to the midpoint of the film at the level of the iliac crests approximately 2 inches (5 cm) anterior to the midaxillary plane.

Breathing Instructions Suspend on expiration.

Example Exposure Techniques **Measure at CR and Use Chart (p.24)**									
Room	**cm**	**kVp**	**mAs**	**mA**	**Sec**	**Beam**	**Film**	**Grid**	**1Ø3Ø**
	26								
	28								
	30								
	32								
	34								
	36								
	38								
	40								
	42								
	44								

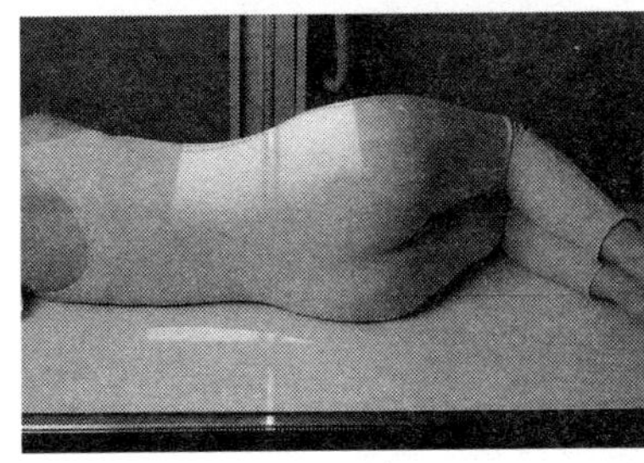

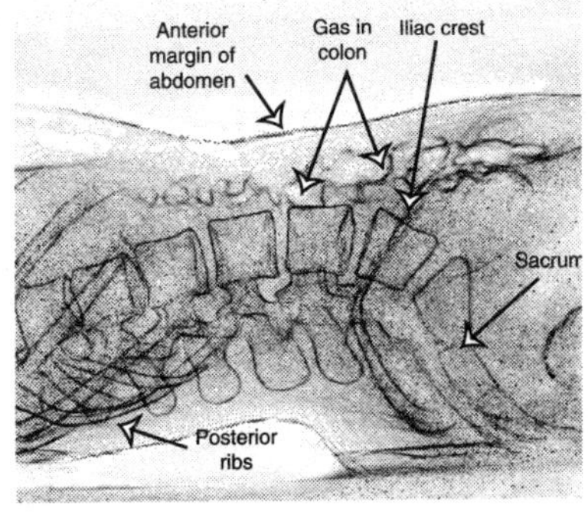

Evaluation Criteria

- Pelvis and lumbar vertebrae are not rotated.
- Density is sufficient to demonstrate soft tissue structures of abdomen.
- Anterior portion of abdomen is demonstrated.

Exam Rationale This position is useful for demonstration of calcification of the aorta and blood vessels and aneurysms.

Tip The centering light should extend to anterior margin of abdomen.

Technical Considerations

- Regular screen/film
- Grid
- kVp range: 70–80
- SID: 40 inch (100 cm)

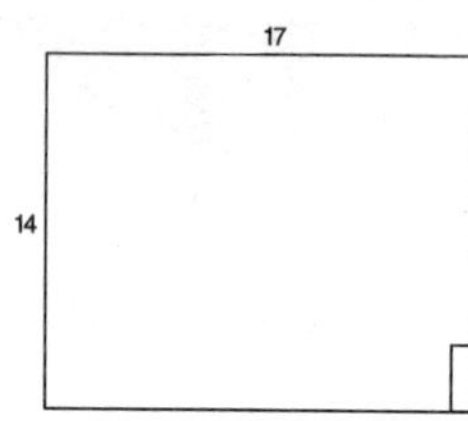

Radiation Protection

(for males). Females are generally not shielded because the female reproductive organs lie in the area of interest.

AEC (Phototiming)

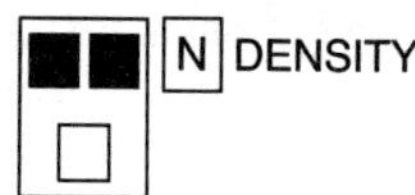

Patient Position

Patient lying on left side on top of radiolucent sponge.

Part Position Knees slightly flexed for patient support; arms and elbows moved toward head so that they are not in the area of interest; shoulders and pelvis should be in true lateral position. (If patient is on a radiolucent pad, move the cassette below the level of the pad to include both sides. If both sides cannot be imaged, include the elevated side [in cases of free air] or the dependent side [for fluid visualization]).

Example Exposure Techniques
Measure at CR and Use Chart (p.24)

Room	cm	kVp	mAs	mA	Sec	Beam	Film	Grid	1Ø3Ø
	12								
	16								
	20								
	24								
	28								
	32								
	36								
	40								
	44								
	48								

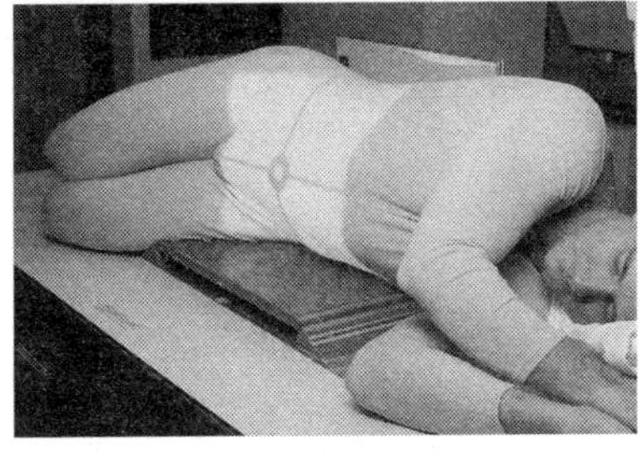

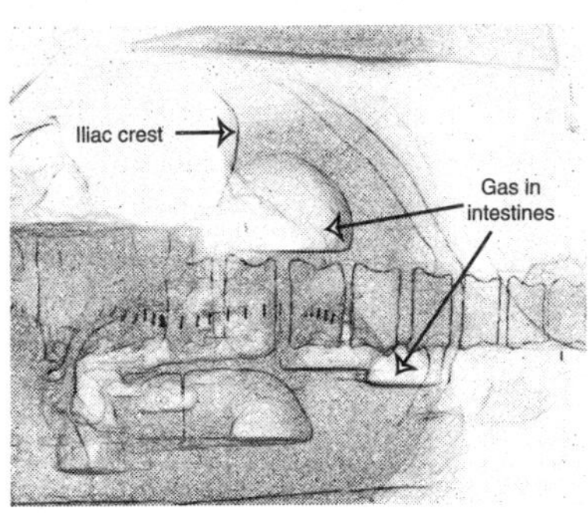

Central Ray Horizontal beam, perpendicular to the midpoint of the film centered 2 to 3 inches (5–8 cm) above level of iliac crests and aligned to midsagittal plane of patient.

Breathing Instructions
Suspend on expiration.

Evaluation Criteria
- Pelvis and abdomen should not be rotated as evidenced by:
  —symmetrical iliac alae
  —spinous processes in center of vertebral bodies
- Density should be slightly less than for supine abdomen to enable visualization of air/fluid levels and any free intra-abdominal air.
- Diaphragm should be included and demonstrate no motion.

Exam Rationale This position is useful for demonstrating air/fluid level or free intraperitoneal air in cases of bowel obstruction or perforated viscus. It also demonstrates abdominal masses and soft tissue structures of the abdomen.

Tips
1. This projection may be performed in either the AP or PA position.
2. Mark the radiograph appropriately to demonstrate the side up.

Pediatric Considerations When radiographing the abdomen of pediatric patients, the biggest challenge often comes from flailing arms, legs, and movement of the abdomen. Although immobilization may be a time-consuming process and is not always well received by the patient or parents, immobilization of a patient unable or unwilling to cooperate by holding still is highly preferable to repeating radiographs due to motion artifacts.

Infant immobilization is important because abdomen radiographs are often a preliminary film for such examinations as barium enemas, upper GI series, and the like. It is vital that the patient be immobile yet able to assume the necessary positions during the procedure. For a conventional abdomen radiograph, an effective method of immobilization is to mummify the infant. Care should be taken to ensure the arms are not in the area of interest. Sandbags are an additional aid for immobilization. As always, gonadal shielding is critical when radiographing pediatric patients.

UPPER LIMB AND SHOULDER GIRDLE

ROUTINE AND ALTERNATIVE POSITIONS/PROJECTIONS

Technical Considerations

- Extremity screen/film
- Non-grid
- kVp range: 55–60
- SID: 40 inch (100 cm)

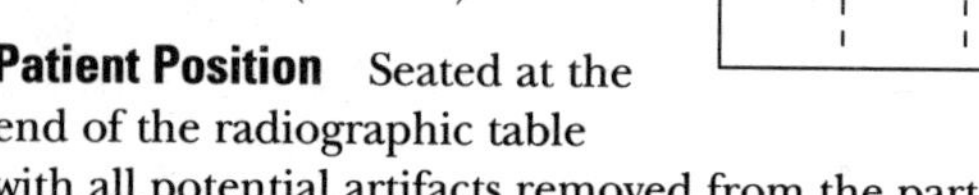

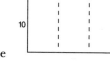

Radiation Protection

Patient Position Seated at the end of the radiographic table with all potential artifacts removed from the part.

Part Position Pronate the hand and wrist to place them flat on cassette with fingers slightly spread.

Central Ray Perpendicular to the metacarpophalangeal joint of the affected finger.

Breathing Instructions Normal respiration.

Evaluation Criteria

- Phalanges should not be rotated.
- Distal, middle, and proximal phalanges should be included.
- Distal end of the metacarpal should be included.

Example Exposure Techniques

Measure at CR and Use Chart (p.42)

Room	cm	kVp	mAs	mA	Sec	Beam	Film	Grid	1Ø3Ø
	1.0								
	2.0								
	3.0								
	4.0								

Exam Rationale The most common indication for finger examinations is trauma. Joint diseases such as arthritis or gout may also be visualized on finger radiographs. Structures demonstrated on the radiograph include all three phalanges and most or all of the metacarpal of the affected finger.

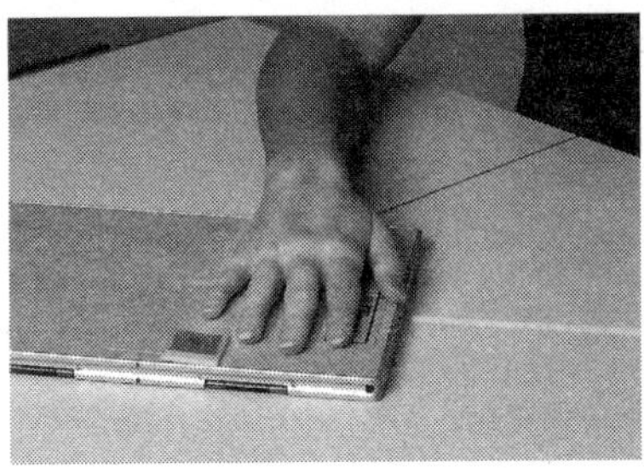

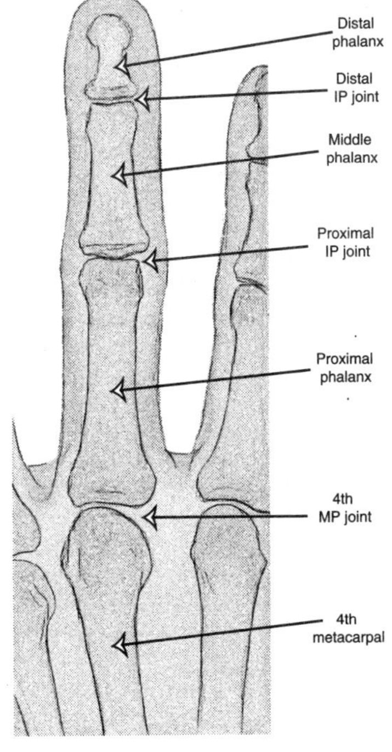

Tips

1. This same position of the hand and wrist gives an oblique view of the thumb.
2. Some department protocols require that the entire metacarpal be included.
3. In cases of trauma where a PA would not yield a satisfactory radiograph, the fingers can be radiographed in the AP position.
4. If only the distal end of the finger is affected and it is not necessary to demonstrate the entire metacarpal, the central ray may be directed to the proximal interphalangeal joint.

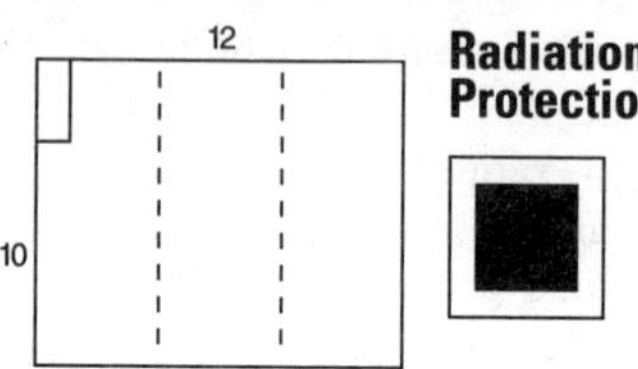

Technical Considerations

- Extremity screen/film
- Non-grid
- kVp range: 55–60
- SID: 40 inch (100 cm)

Patient Position Seated at the end of the radiographic table with all potential artifacts removed from the part.

Part Position Begin with the hand pronated and rotate the finger 45°; fingers should be spread slightly to avoid superimposition with other fingers.

Central Ray Perpendicular to the metacarpophalangeal joint of the affected finger.

Breathing Instructions Normal respiration.

Evaluation Criteria

- Affected finger must not be superimposed on other fingers.
- Distal, middle, and proximal phalanges should be included.
- Distal end of the metacarpal should be visualized.

Example Exposure Techniques **Measure at CR and Use Chart (p.42)**									
Room	**cm**	**kVp**	**mAs**	**mA**	**Sec**	**Beam**	**Film**	**Grid**	**1Ø3Ø**
	1.0								
	2.0								
	3.0								
	4.0								

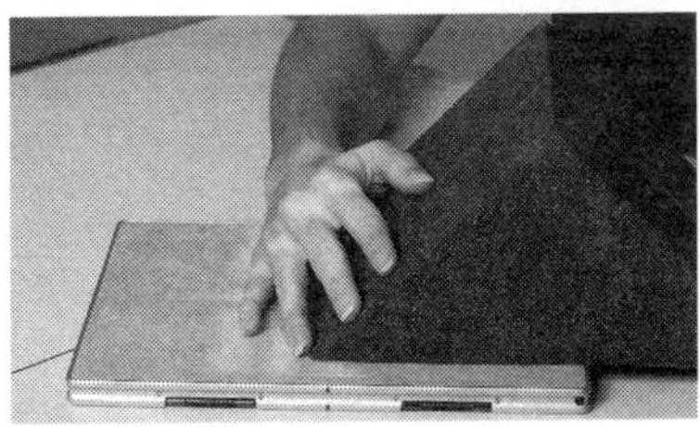

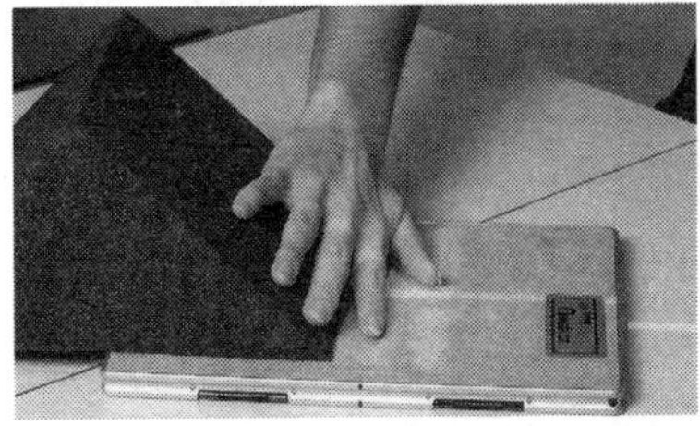

Exam Rationale The oblique is a routine position of the finger that gives a different perspective from the PA, that of a 45° oblique. Structures demonstrated on the radiograph include all three phalanges and most or all of the metacarpal of the affected finger.

Tips

1. A 45° foam wedge is helpful in maintaining the finger parallel to the film at the correct angle.
2. For the second finger, a reduced object film distance may be obtained by rotating the digit medially instead of laterally.
3. Like the PA finger, if only the distal end of the finger is affected, the central ray may be directed to the proximal interphalangeal joint.

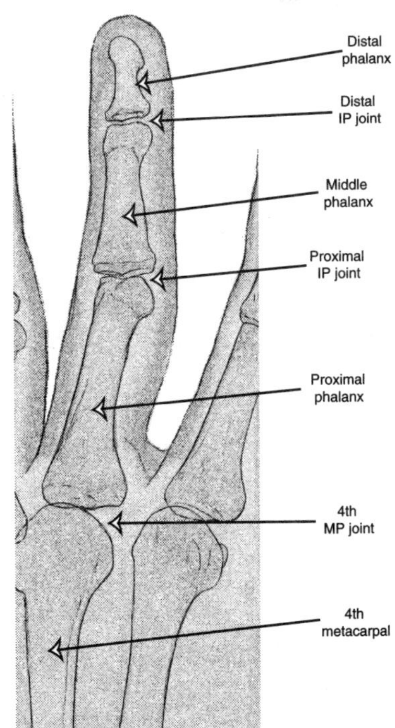

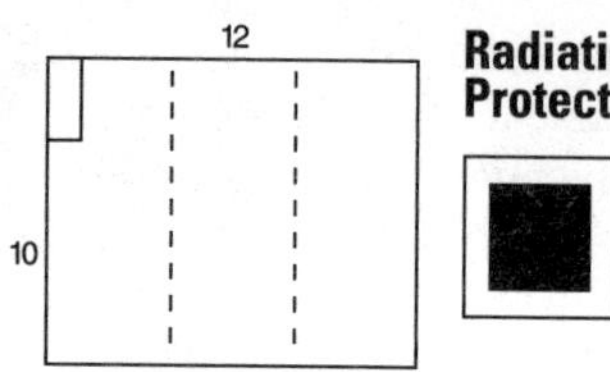

Technical Considerations
- Extremity screen/film
- Nop-grid
- kVP range: 55–60
- SID: 40 inch (100 cm)

Patient Position Seated at the end of the radiographic table with all potential artifacts removed from the part.

Part Position Place the hand at a 90° angle to the film, ulnar side down, with the affected finger in a fully extended lateral position, parallel to the film; flex all remaining fingers.

Central Ray Perpendicular to the proximal interphalangeal joint.

Breathing Instructions Normal respiration.

Evaluation Criteria
- Phalanx of interest should be seen in profile.
- Distal, middle, and proximal phalanges should be included.
- Metacarpals will not be completely visualized due to superimposition.

Example Exposure Techniques **Measure at CR and Use Chart (p.42)**									
Room	**cm**	**kVp**	**mAs**	**mA**	**Sec**	**Beam**	**Film**	**Grid**	**1Ø3Ø**
	1.0								
	2.0								
	3.0								
	4.0								

Exam Rationale The lateral, taken at 90° to the PA, is used to demonstrate anterior or posterior displacements of the bony structures and to localize foreign bodies. Structures demonstrated on the radiograph include all three phalanges of the affected finger.

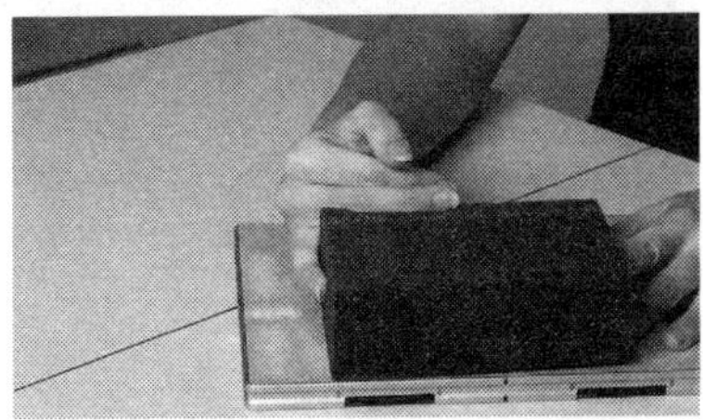

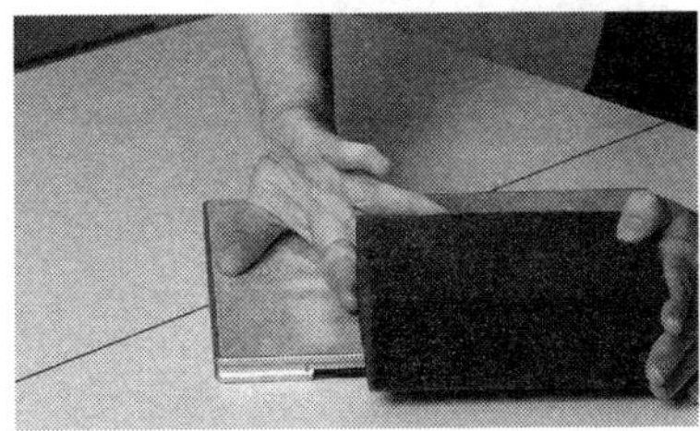

Tips

1. Immobilization is highly recommended.
2. For the second finger, a reduced object film distance may be obtained by placing the radial side of the hand closest to the film.

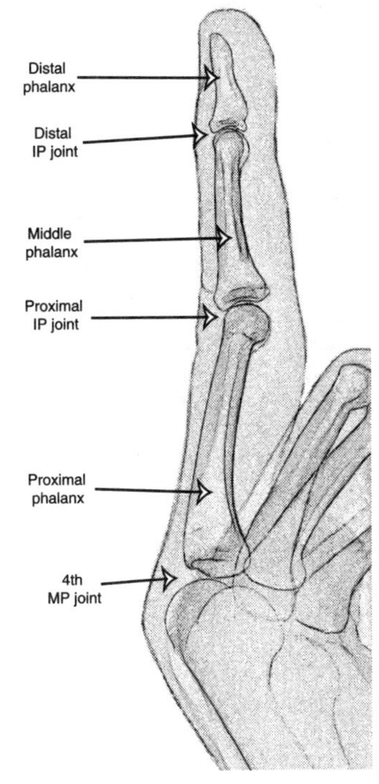

Technical Considerations

- Extremity screen/film
- Non-grid
- kVp range: 55–60
- SID: 40 inch (100 cm)

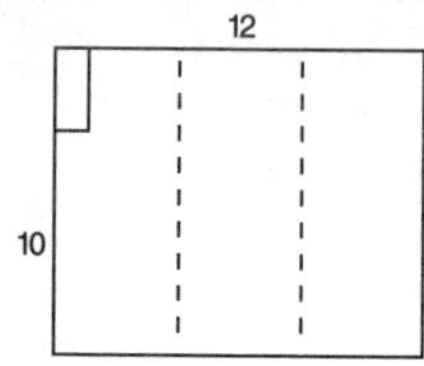

Radiation Protection

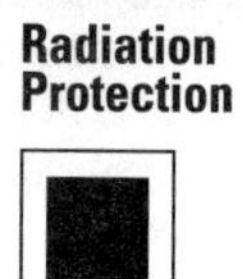

Patient Position Seated at the end of the radiographic table with all potential artifacts removed from the part.

Part Position

- AP: rotate the hand internally until the posterior surface of the thumb is flat on the cassette.
- Oblique: pronate the hand and place the hand and thumb flat on the cassette (same as PA hand).
- Lateral: begin with the hand pronated and rotate the thumb toward the radial side until the digit is in a true lateral position.

Central Ray Perpendicular to the first metacarpophalangeal joint.

Breathing Instructions Normal respiration.

Example Exposure Techniques
Measure at CR and Use Chart (p.42)

Room	cm	kVp	mAs	mA	Sec	Beam	Film	Grid	1Ø3Ø
	1.0								
	2.0								
	3.0								
	4.0								
	5.0								

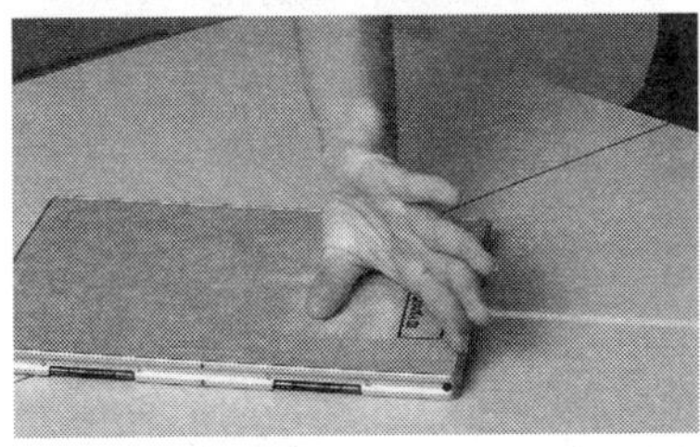

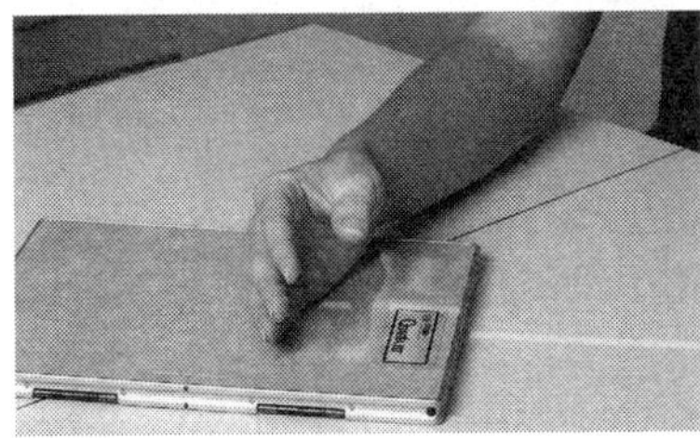

Evaluation Criteria

- Distal and proximal phalanges should be included.
- Distal end of the first metacarpal should be visualized.
- Some department protocols require that the entire metacarpal be included.

Exam Rationale The most common indication for thumb examinations is trauma. Although its routine positions are the same as other fingers, the thumb has several unique features that require modifications in positioning. Structures demonstrated on the radiograph include both phalanges and most or all of the first metacarpal.

Tip When only the tip of the distal phalanx is injured, the PA thumb is sometimes substituted for the AP.

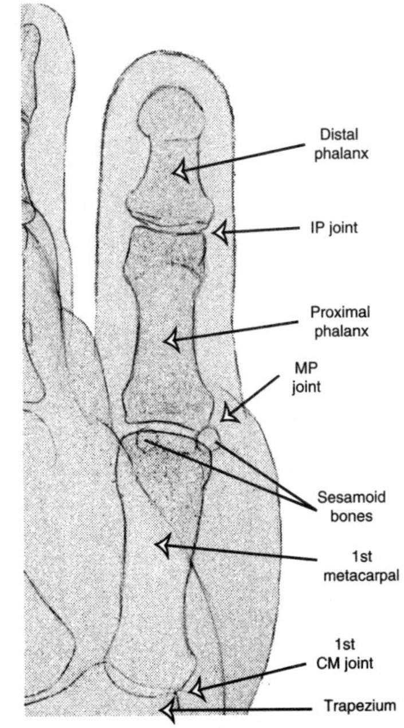

Technical Considerations

- Extremity screen/film
- Non-grid
- kVp range: 55–60
- SID 40 inch (100 cm)

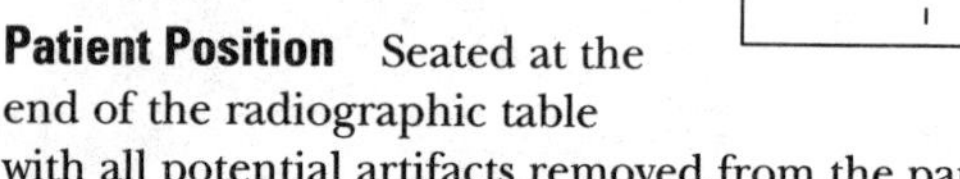

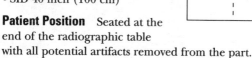

Radiation Protection

Patient Position Seated at the end of the radiographic table with all potential artifacts removed from the part.

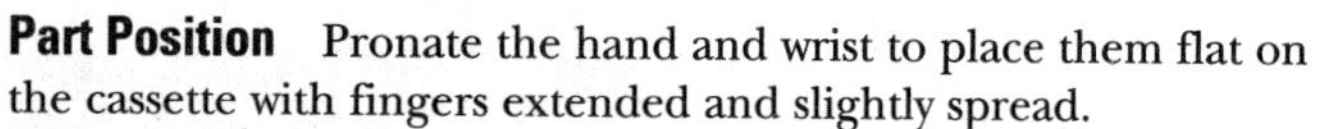

Part Position Pronate the hand and wrist to place them flat on the cassette with fingers extended and slightly spread.

Central Ray Perpendicular to the third metacarpophalangeal joint.

Breathing Instructions Normal respiration.

Evaluation Criteria

- All phalanges, metacarpals, and carpals should be included.
- Phalanges and metacarpals should not be rotated.
- Joint spaces of the hand should be open.
- Thumb should be in an oblique view.

Example Exposure Techniques **Measure at CR and Use this Chart**									
Room	**cm**	**kVp**	**mAs**	**mA**	**Sec**	**Beam**	**Film**	**Grid**	**1Ø3Ø**
	2.0								
	3.0								
	4.0								
	5.0								
	6.0								

- One-half to 1 inch (1–3 cm) of the distal radius/ulna should be visualized.

Exam Rationale The most common indications for hand examinations are trauma and joint diseases such as arthritis or gout. Structures demonstrated on the radiograph include all of the phalanges, the metacarpals, the carpals, and joints of the hand and wrist.

Tips

1. The part should be immobilized with tape or sandbags if motion is a potential problem.
2. An AP projection may be substituted if the hand cannot be flattened or the fingers extended because the diverging x-ray beam will assist in opening the joint spaces.
3. An AP projection better demonstrates the bases of the metacarpals.

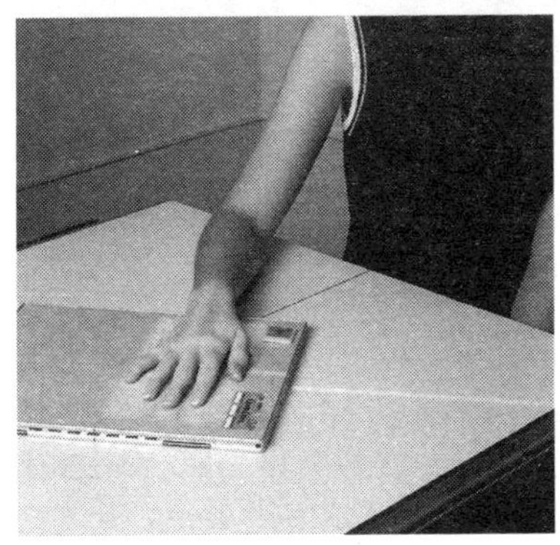

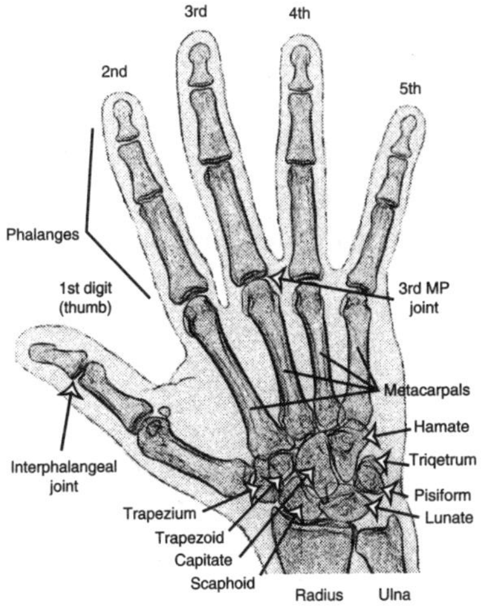

Technical Considerations
- Extremity screen/film
- Non-grid
- kVp range: 55–60
- SID: 40 inch (100 cm)

12

10

Radiation Protection

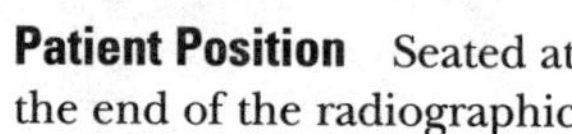

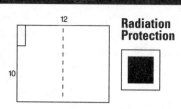

Patient Position Seated at the end of the radiographic table with all potential artifacts removed from the part.

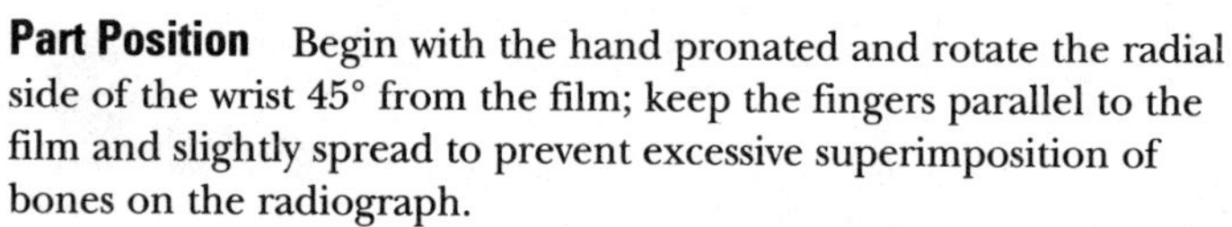

Part Position Begin with the hand pronated and rotate the radial side of the wrist 45° from the film; keep the fingers parallel to the film and slightly spread to prevent excessive superimposition of bones on the radiograph.

Central Ray Perpendicular to the third metacarpophalangeal joint.

Breathing Instructions Normal respiration.

Evaluation Criteria
- All phalanges, metacarpals, and carpals should be included.
- Thumb should be in an oblique view.

Example Exposure Techniques
Measure at CR and Use Chart (p.42)

Room	cm	kVp	mAs	mA	Sec	Beam	Film	Grid	1Ø3Ø
	3.0								
	4.0								
	5.0								
	6.0								
	7.0								

- One-half to 1 inch (1–3 cm) of the distal radius/ulna should be visualized.
- Little or no overlap of the metacarpals should be evident on the radiograph.

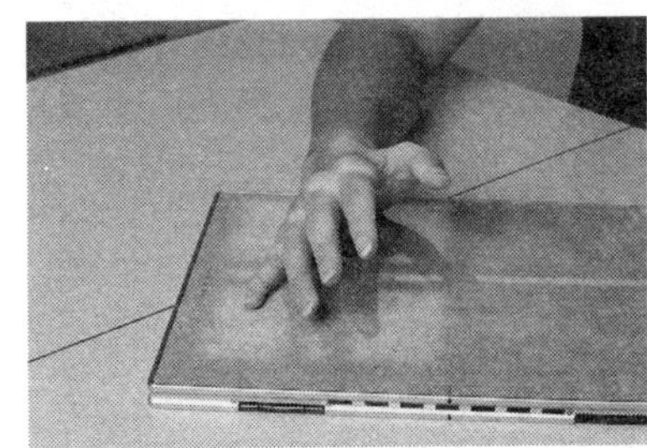

Exam Rationale The oblique is a routine position of the hand, which gives a different perspective from the PA, that of a 45° oblique. Structures demonstrated on the radiograph include all phalanges, metacarpals, carpals, and joints of the hand and wrist.

Tip A 45° angle sponge may be used to support the hand and to obtain the correct part angle.

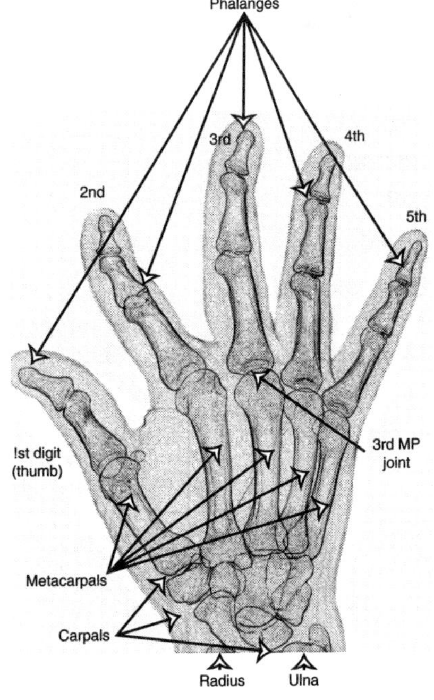

Technical Considerations
- Extremity screen/film
- Non-grid
- kVp range: 60–65 (5 more than the PA)
- SID: 40 inch (100 cm)

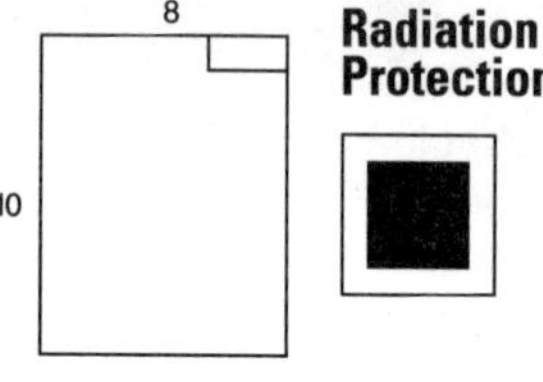

Patient Position Seated at the end of the radiographic table with all potential artifacts removed from the part.

Part Position Place the hand and wrist at a 90° angle to the film, ulnar side down; fingers should be spread in a fan-like manner; thumb should be projecting away from the palm and parallel to the film.

Central Ray Perpendicular to the second metacarpophalangeal joint.

Breathing Instructions Normal respiration.

Evaluation Criteria
- Metacarpals should be superimposed on each other.
- Fingers two through five should be seen in profile.

Example Exposure Techniques **Measure at CR and Use Chart (p.42)**									
Room	**cm**	**kVp**	**mAs**	**mA**	**Sec**	**Beam**	**Film**	**Grid**	**1Ø3Ø**
	6.0								
	7.0								
	8.0								
	9.0								
	10.0								

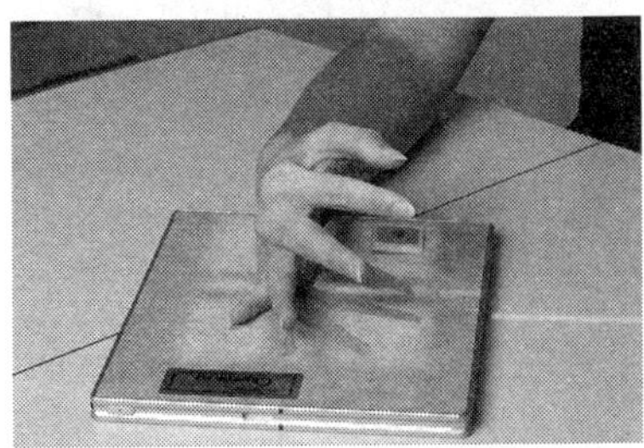

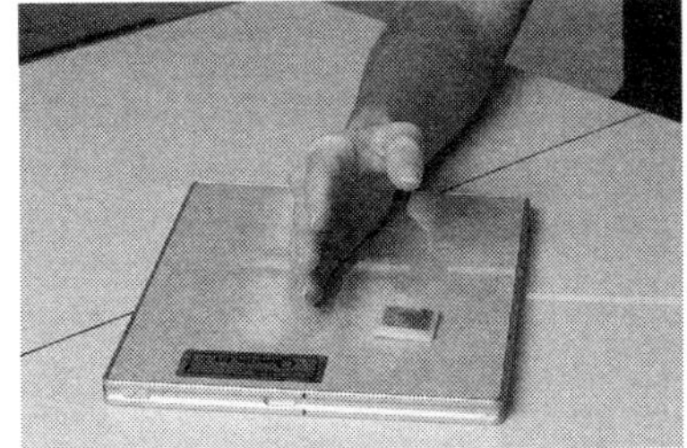

- Carpals and distal radius/ulna should be in true lateral position.
- Thumb should be in PA position.

Exam Rationale The lateral, taken at 90° to the PA, is used to demonstrate anterior or posterior displacements of the bony structures and to localize foreign bodies. Structures demonstrated on the radiograph include all phalanges, metacarpals, carpals, and joints of the hand and wrist.

Tips

1. Patient motion is very common on this position, so immobilization of the part is recommended.
2. Some department protocols require the fingers to be fully extended and superimposed.

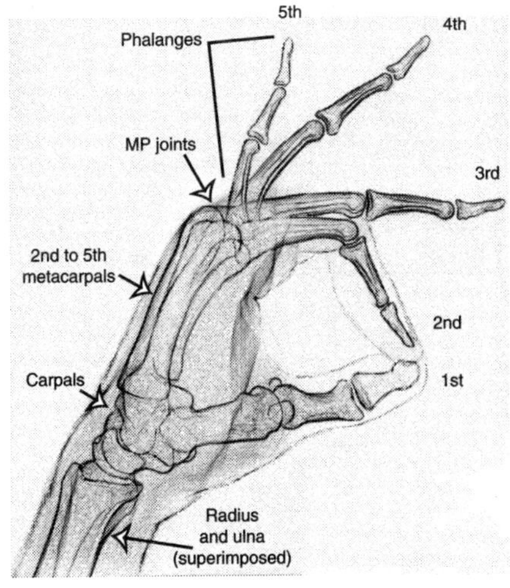

Technical Considerations

- Extremity screen/film
- Non-grid
- kVp range: 55–60
- SID: 40 inch (100 cm)

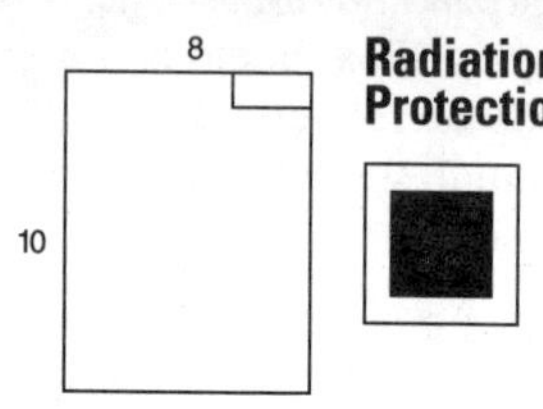

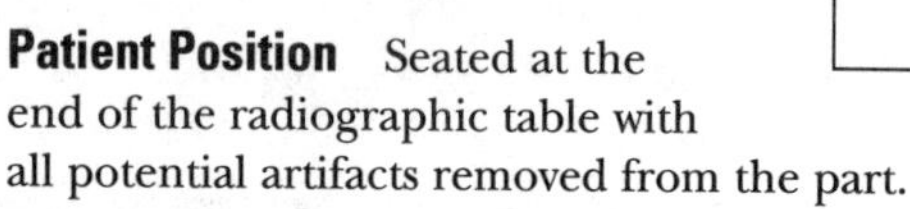

Patient Position Seated at the end of the radiographic table with all potential artifacts removed from the part.

Part Position Begin with the hand pronated and flat on the cassette; hyperextend the hand and wrist; rotate the hand to place the thumb parallel to the cassette.

Central Ray Directed to the first carpometacarpal joint at a 45° angle toward the forearm.

Breathing Instructions Normal respiration.

Evaluation Criteria

- First carpometacarpal joint space should be opened.
- Trapezium should be visualized.

Example Exposure Techniques
Measure at CR and Use Chart (p.42)

Room	cm	kVp	mAs	mA	Sec	Beam	Film	Grid	1Ø3Ø
	1.0								
	2.0								
	3.0								
	4.0								

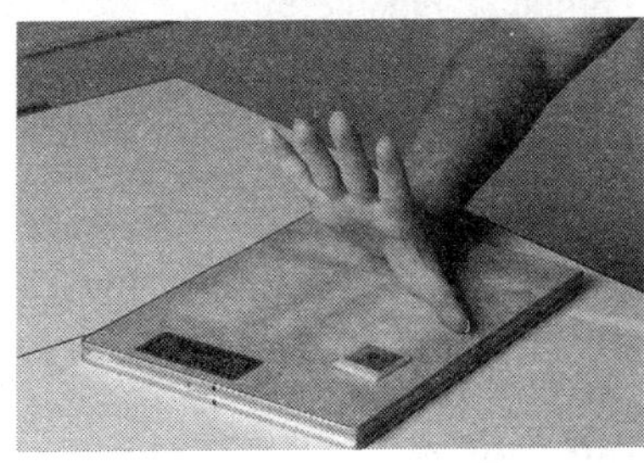

Exam Rationale This projection is used to demonstrate trauma to the first carpometacarpal joint. Although the resultant image is distorted, the joint space is better demonstrated than on PA hand or AP wrist projections.

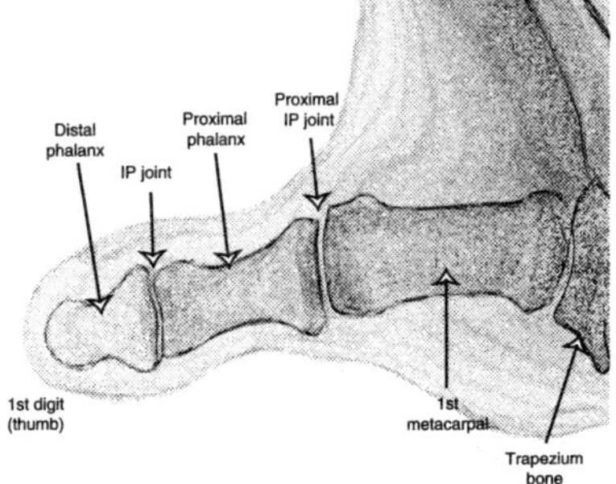

Tips

1. Tape or a bandage may assist the patient in obtaining and maintaining adequate hyperextension of the fingers.
2. This position is difficult to obtain because many patients cannot tolerate hyperextension of the hand; it should not be performed when there has been severe trauma.

Technical Considerations

- Extremity screen/film
- Non-grid
- kVp range: 55–60
- SID: 40 inch (100 cm)

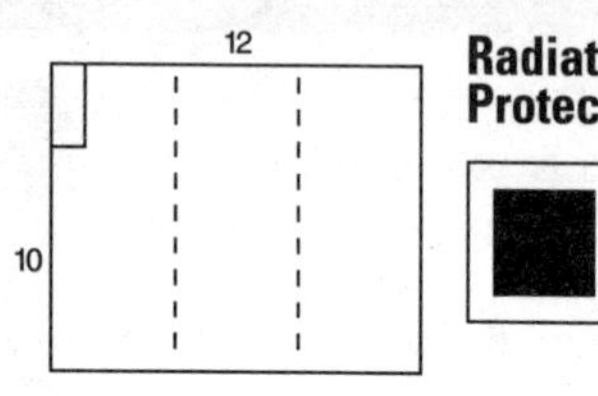

Patient Position Seated at the end of the radiographic table with all potential artifacts removed from the part.

Part Position Pronate the hand and wrist to place them flat on the cassette; flex the fingers by curling them into a fist, to place the carpals parallel to the film.

Central Ray Perpendicular to the midcarpals.

Breathing Instructions Normal respiration.

Example Exposure Techniques **Measure at CR and Use Chart (p.42)**									
Room	**cm**	**kVp**	**mAs**	**mA**	**Sec**	**Beam**	**Film**	**Grid**	**1Ø3Ø**
	2.0								
	3.0								
	4.0								
	5.0								
	6.0								

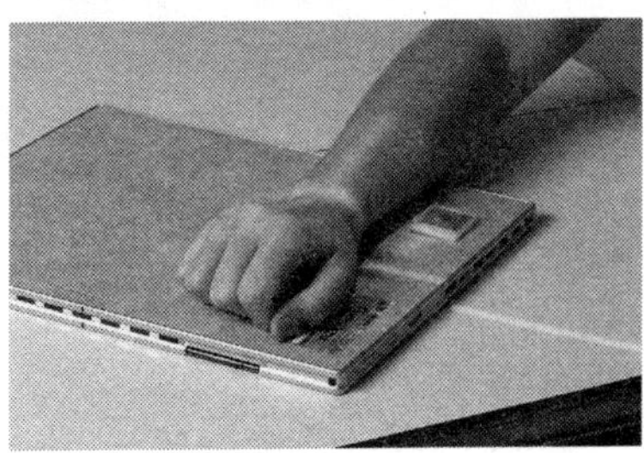

Evaluation Criteria

- All eight carpals should be included.
- One to 2 inches (3–5 cm) distal radius/ulna should be included.

Exam Rationale The most common indication for wrist examinations is trauma. Structures demonstrated on the radiograph include all eight carpals and portions of the proximal metacarpals and distal radius/ulna.

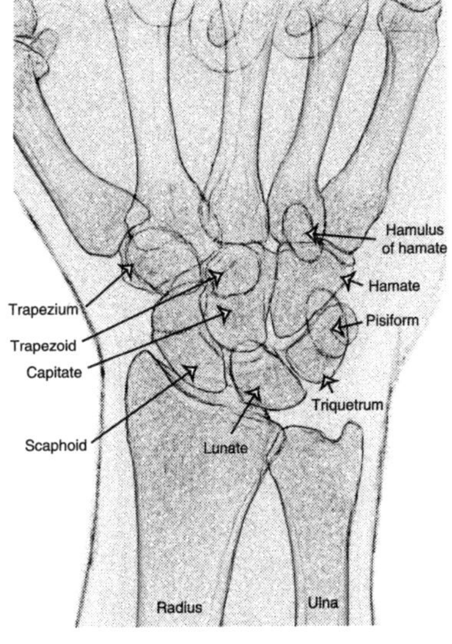

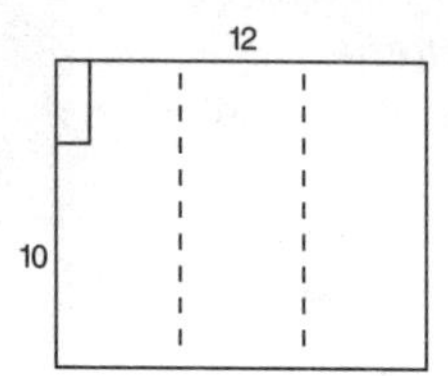

Radiation Protection

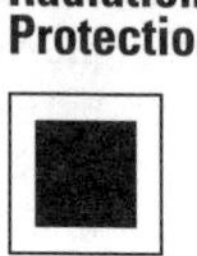

Technical Considerations
- Extremity screen/film
- Non-grid
- kVp range: 55–60
- SID: 40 inch (100 cm)

Patient Position Seated at the end of the radiographic table with all potential artifacts removed from the part.

Part Position Begin with the hand pronated and rotate the radial side of the wrist 45° from the film; the fingers and wrist are extended.

Central Ray Perpendicular to the midcarpals.

Breathing Instructions Normal respiration.

Evaluation Criteria
- All eight carpals should be included.
- One to 2 inches (3–5 cm) of the metacarpals and distal radius/ulna should be included.
- Scaphoid and trapezium should be well demonstrated.

Example Exposure Techniques
Measure at CR and Use Chart (p.42)

Room	cm	kVp	mAs	mA	Sec	Beam	Film	Grid	1Ø3Ø
	3.0								
	4.0								
	5.0								
	6.0								
	7.0								

Exam Rationale The oblique is a routine position of the wrist, which gives a different perspective from the PA, that of a 45° oblique. Structures demonstrated on the radiograph include all eight carpals and portions of the proximal metacarpals and distal radius/ulna.

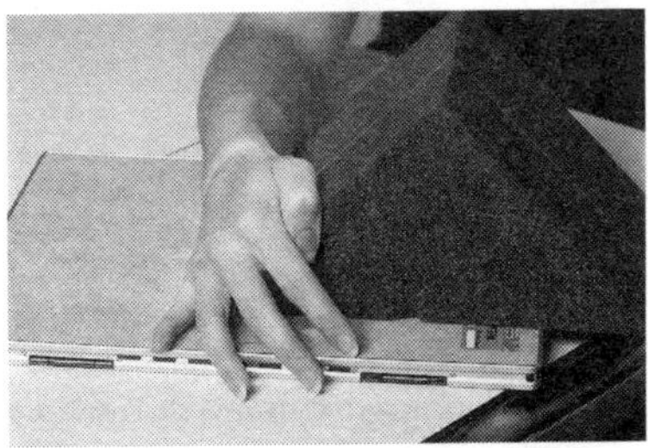

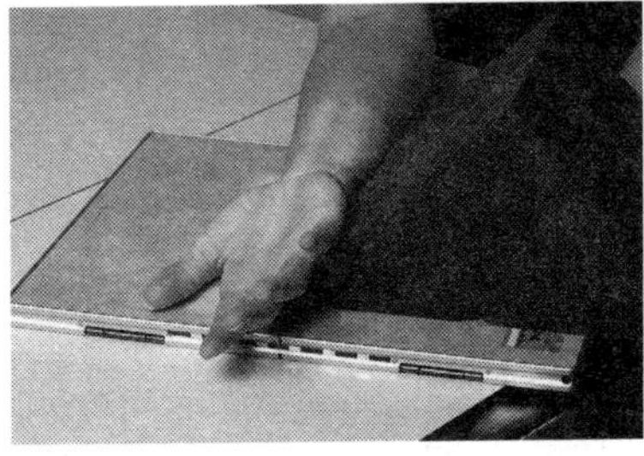

Tips

1. A 45° angle sponge may be used to support the wrist and to obtain the correct part angle.
2. The less common semi-supination oblique position is sometimes taken to better demonstrate the pisiform, hamate, and triquetrum.

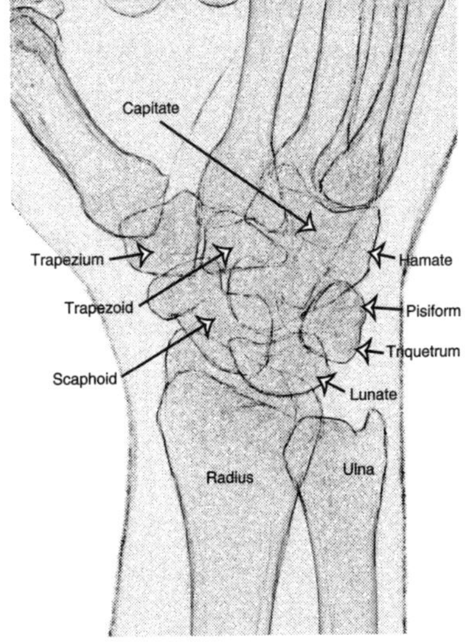

Technical Considerations

- Extremity screen/film
- Non-grid
- kVp range: 60–65
- SID: 40 inch (100 cm)

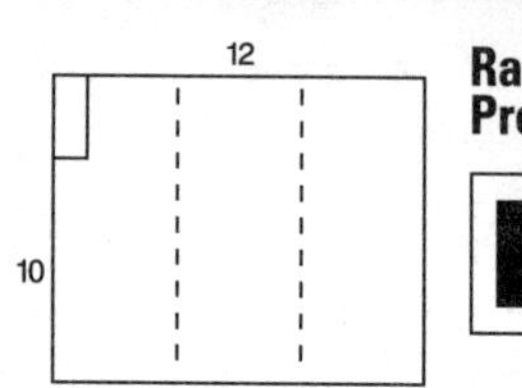

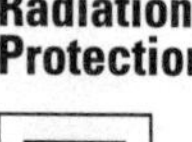

Radiation Protection

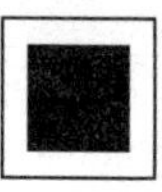

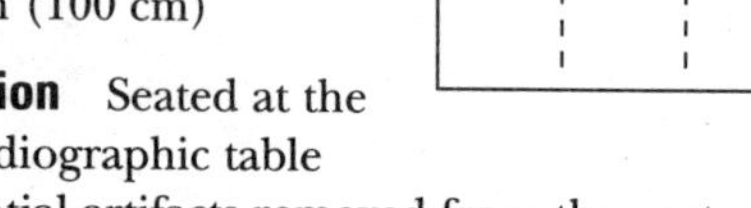

Patient Position Seated at the end of the radiographic table with all potential artifacts removed from the part.

Part Position Extend the fingers and place the hand and wrist at a 90° angle to the film, ulnar side down. The elbow should be flexed 90°.

Central Ray Perpendicular to the midcarpals.

Breathing Instructions Normal respiration.

Evaluation Criteria

- Carpals should be mostly superimposed on each other.
- Distal radius and ulna should be superimposed.
- Scaphoid should be projected anteriorly.

Example Exposure Techniques **Measure at CR and Use Chart (p.42)**									
Room	**cm**	**kVp**	**mAs**	**mA**	**Sec**	**Beam**	**Film**	**Grid**	**1Ø3Ø**
	4.0								
	5.0								
	6.0								
	7.0								
	8.0								

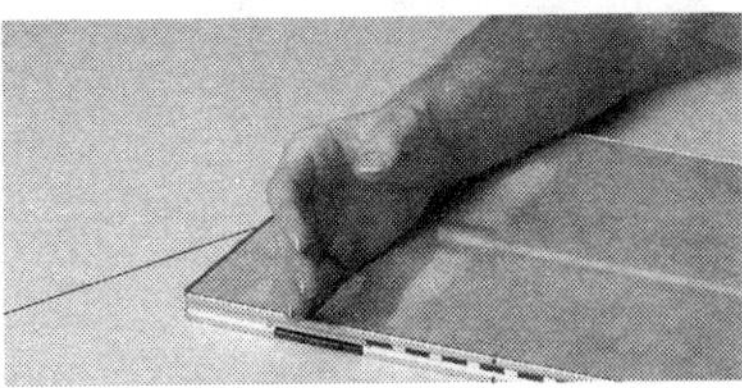

Exam Rationale The lateral, taken at 90° to the PA, is used to demonstrate anterior or posterior displacements of the bony structures. Although all eight carpals are demonstrated on the radiograph, they are substantially superimposed. Also demonstrated are portions of the proximal metacarpals and distal radius/ulna.

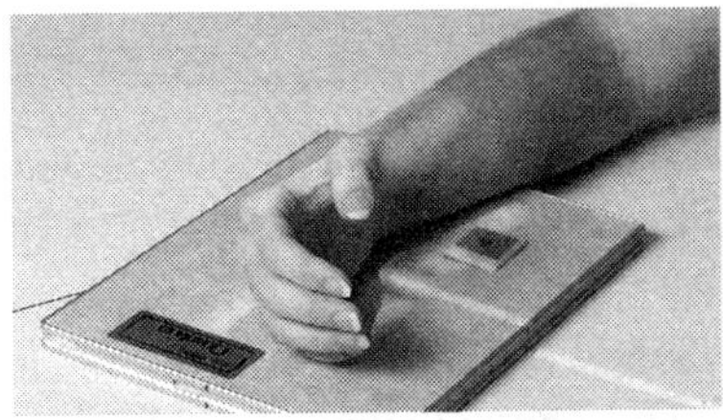

Tip This position may also be used to demonstrate widening of the wrist joint due to fracture or dislocation by taking two films—one with the wrist in maximum flexion and one with the wrist in hyper-extension.

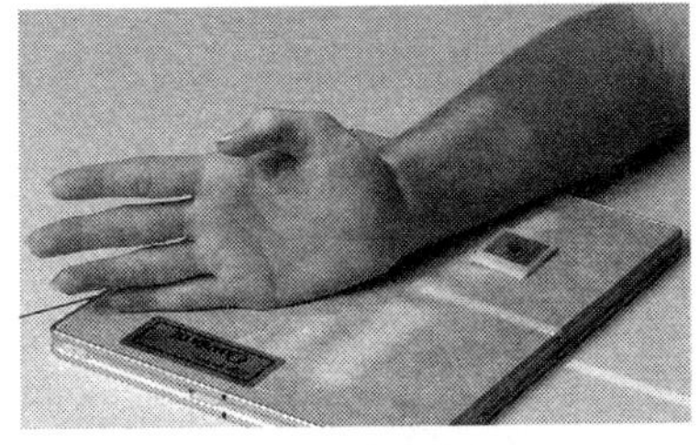

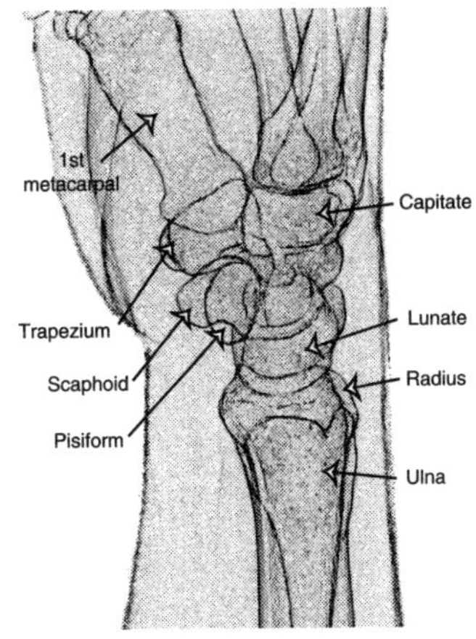

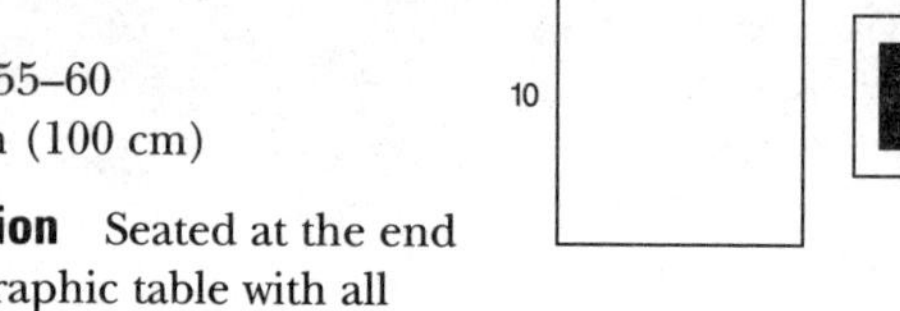

Technical Considerations
- Extremity screen/film
- Non-grid
- kVp range: 55–60
- SID: 40 inch (100 cm)

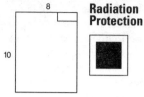

Patient Position Seated at the end of the radiographic table with all potential artifacts removed from the part.

Part Position Pronate the hand and wrist to place them flat on the cassette, as in a PA hand projection; evert (externally flex) the wrist as much as possible.

Central Ray Directed toward the forearm at a 15° to 20° angle and centered to the scaphoid.

Breathing Instructions Normal respiration.

Evaluation Criteria
- Scaphoid should be elongated and projected free from superimposition from other carpals.

Example Exposure Techniques **Measure at CR and Use Chart (p.42)**									
Room	**cm**	**kVp**	**mAs**	**mA**	**Sec**	**Beam**	**Film**	**Grid**	**1Ø3Ø**
	2.0								
	3.0								
	4.0								
	5.0								
	6.0								

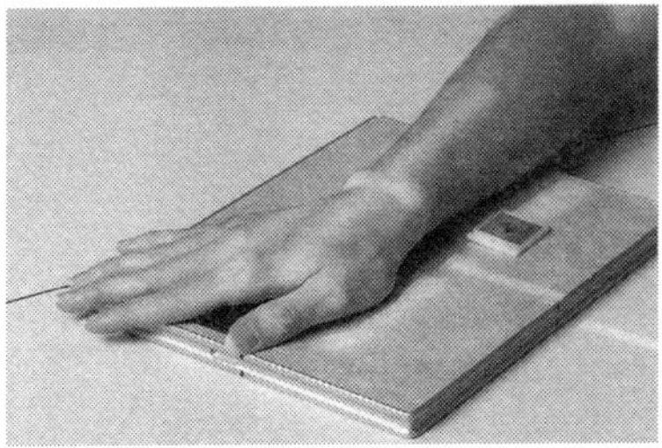

Exam Rationale The primary purpose of the ulnar flexion position is to obtain an elongated view of the scaphoid, free from superimposition. The scaphoid is the carpal most frequently fractured. Structures demonstrated on the radiograph include the scaphoid and usually the other carpals and portions of the proximal metacarpals and distal radius/ulna.

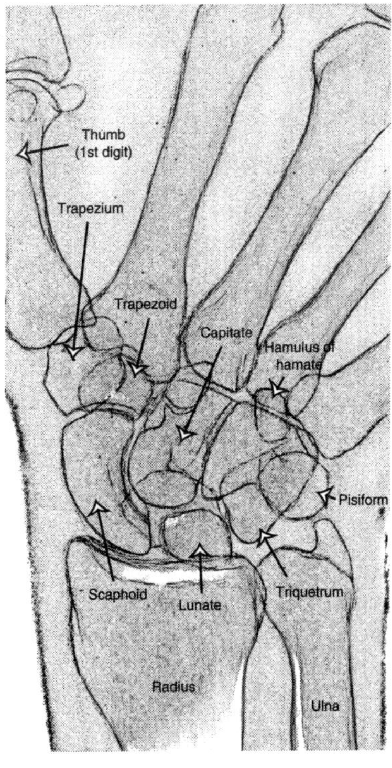

Tips

1. Ulnar flexion is sometimes called radial deviation.
2. Do not attempt to flex the wrist of patients with severe trauma.
3. Many department protocols require that all carpals, proximal metacarpals, and the distal radius/ulna also be included on the radiograph.
4. Some department protocols use a perpendicular central ray.
5. Some department protocols call for the central ray to be directed to the midcarpal area.

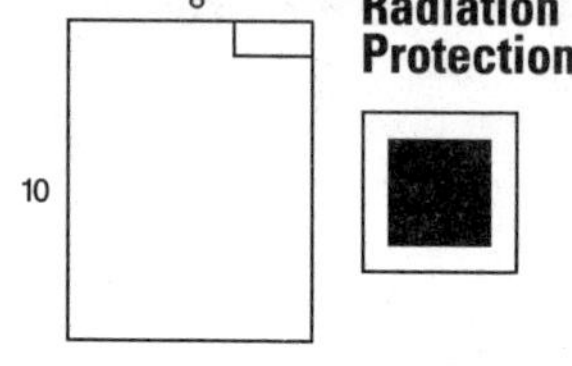

Technical Considerations

- Extremity screen/film
- Non-grid
- kVp range: 55–60
- SID: 40 inch (100 cm)

Patient Position Seated at the end of the radiographic table with all potential artifacts removed from the part.

Part Position Pronate the hand and wrist to place them flat on the cassette, as in a PA hand projection; invert (flex internally) the wrist as much as possible.

Central Ray Perpendicular to the midcarpals.

Breathing Instructions Normal respiration.

Evaluation Criteria

- Capitate, hamate, and triquetrum should be well visualized.
- Pisiform remains mostly superimposed on triquetrum.
- Joint spaces of the medial carpals should be opened to a greater degree than is seen on the PA wrist.

Example Exposure Techniques **Measure at CR and Use Chart (p.42)**									
Room	**cm**	**kVp**	**mAs**	**mA**	**Sec**	**Beam**	**Film**	**Grid**	**1Ø3Ø**
	2.0								
	3.0								
	4.0								
	5.0								
	6.0								

Exam Rationale The primary purpose of the radial flexion position is to open joint spaces between the carpals on the medial side of the wrist, including the capitate, hamate, triquetrum, and pisiform.

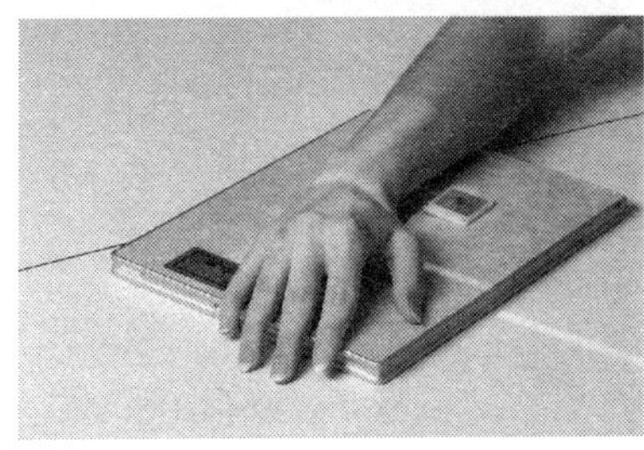

Tips

1. Radial flexion is sometimes called ulnar deviation.
2. Do not attempt to flex the wrist of patients with severe trauma.

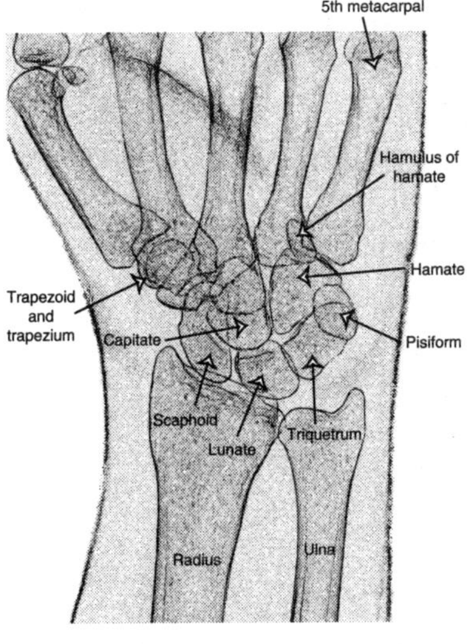

Technical Considerations

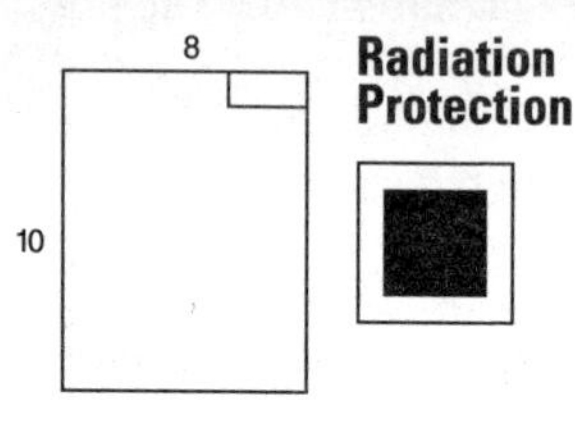

- Extremity screen/film
- Non-grid
- kVp range: 55–60
- SID: 40 inch (100 cm)

Patient Position Seated at the end of the radiographic table with all potential artifacts removed from the part.

Part Position Pronate the hand and wrist to place them flat on the cassette. Without allowing forearm to move, evert hand (toward ulnar side) as much as patient can tolerate.

Central Ray Directed toward the forearm at a 20° angle and centered to the scaphoid.

Breathing Instructions Normal respiration.

Evaluation Criteria

- Scaphoid should be elongated and projected free from superimposition from other carpals.

Example Exposure Techniques
Measure at CR and Use Chart (p.42)

Room	cm	kVp	mAs	mA	Sec	Beam	Film	Grid	1Ø3Ø
	2.0								
	3.0								
	4.0								
	5.0								
	6.0								

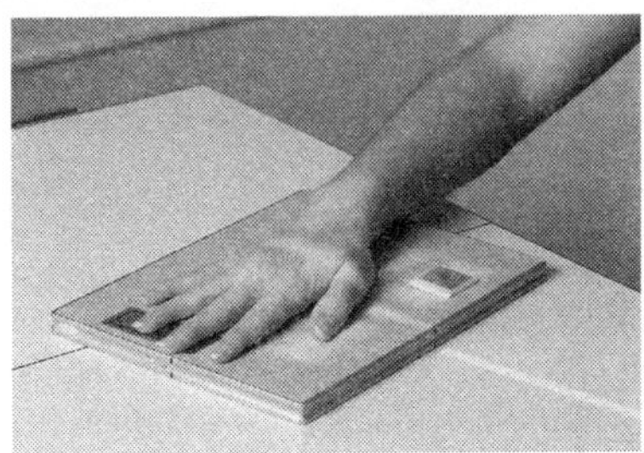

- Many department protocols require that all carpals, proximal metacarpals, and the distal radius/ulna also be included on the radiograph.

Exam Rationale The primary purpose of this position is to obtain an elongated view of the scaphoid, free from superimposition. The scaphoid is the carpal most frequently fractured. Structures demonstrated on the radiograph include the scaphoid and usually the other carpals and portions of the proximal meta-carpals and distal radius/ulna.

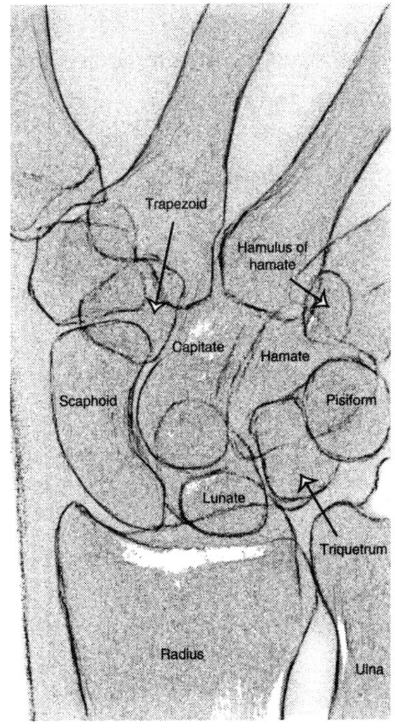

Tips

1. As originally described by Stecher, the wrist may be placed on a 20° angle sponge and the central ray directed perpendicular.
2. Some department protocols call for the central ray to be placed in the mid-carpal area.

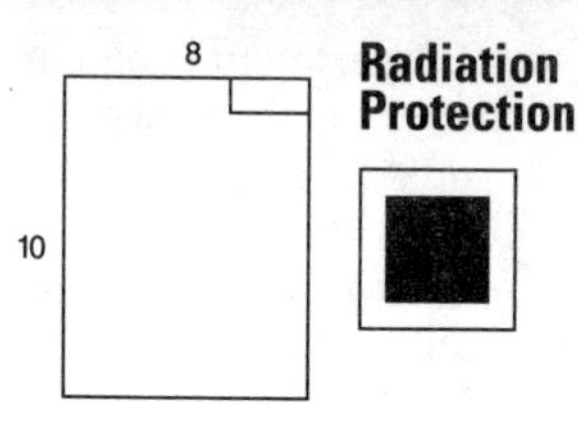

Technical Considerations
- Extremity screen/film
- Non-grid
- kVp range: 60–65
- SID: 40 inch (100 cm)

Patient Position Seated at the end of the radiographic table with all potential artifacts removed from the part.

Part Position Begin with the hand pronated and flat on the cassette, hyperextending the wrist as much as possible; patient should/may hold hand back.

Central Ray Directed to the midcarpals at a 25–30° angle toward the forearm.

Breathing Instructions Normal respiration.

Evaluation Criteria
- Concave arch of the carpal canal should be clearly demonstrated.
- Scaphoid, pisiform, trapezium, and the hamulus of the hamate should be visualized.

Example Exposure Techniques
Measure at CR and Use Chart (p.42)

Room	cm	kVp	mAs	mA	Sec	Beam	Film	Grid	1Ø3Ø
	5.0								
	6.0								
	7.0								
	8.0								
	9.0								

WRIST—TANGENTIAL PROJECTION: CARPAL CANAL (GAYNOR-HART METHOD)

Exam Rationale This position of the wrist is taken to visualize the palmar aspect of the carpals known as the carpal canal or tunnel. Carpals best demonstrated on the radiograph include the scaphoid, pisiform, trapezium, and hamate.

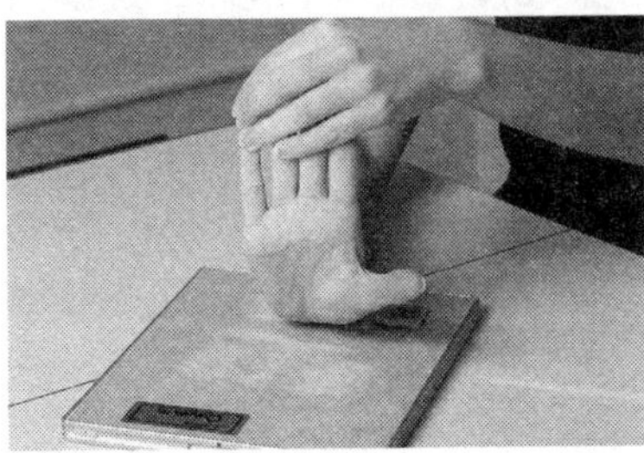

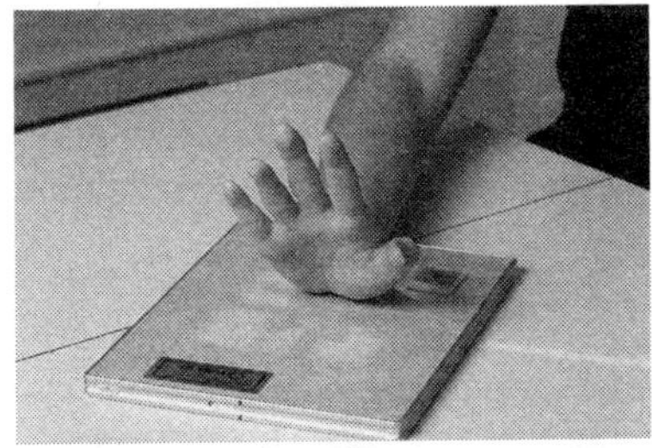

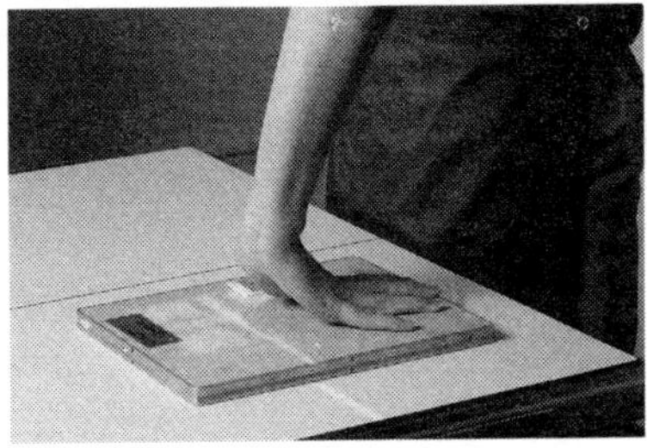

Tips

1. Tape or a bandage may assist the patient in obtaining and maintaining this hyperextension.
2. This position is difficult to obtain because many patients cannot tolerate hyperextension of the hand. The following variations are sometimes performed:

- Place the fingers at a 75° angle to the film and angle the tube 40°.
- A superoinferior projection may also be substituted. With the patient standing and the palmar surface of the hand on the cassette, the central ray is angled according to the amount of hyperextension obtained to maintain an approximate 45° angle between the palmar surface of the hand and the central ray.

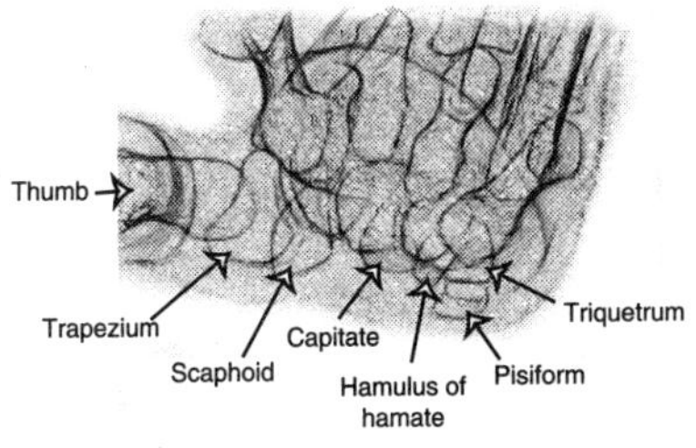

Technical Considerations

- Extremity screen/film
- Non-grid
- kVp range: 60–65
- SID: 40 inch (100 cm)

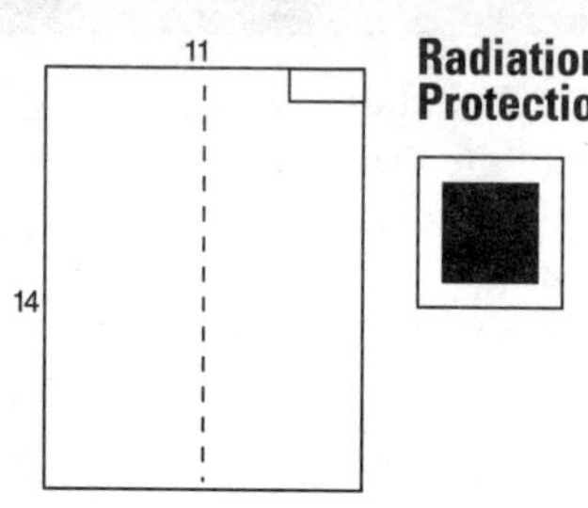

Patient Position Seated at the end of the radiographic table with all potential artifacts removed from the part.

Part Position With the hand supinated, center the long axis of the forearm to the film and attempt to get both the wrist and elbow flat on the cassette; the entire upper limb from the shoulder to the hand should lie in the same horizontal plane, parallel to the cassette.

Central Ray Perpendicular to the mid-forearm.

Breathing Instructions Normal respiration.

Example Exposure Techniques **Measure at CR and Use Chart (p.42)**									
Room	**cm**	**kVp**	**mAs**	**mA**	**Sec**	**Beam**	**Film**	**Grid**	**1Ø3Ø**
	4.0								
	5.0								
	6.0								
	7.0								
	8.0								

Evaluation Criteria

- Both wrist and elbow joints should be included.
- Radius and ulna should have only slight superimposition at both the proximal and distal ends.

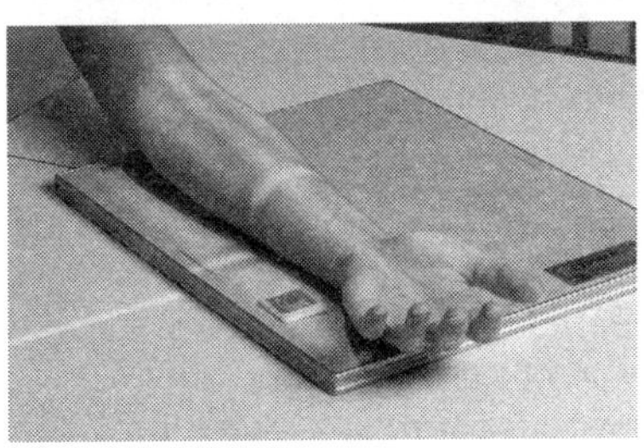

Exam Rationale The most common indication for forearm examinations is trauma. Structures demonstrated on the radiograph include the entire radius and ulna, including portions of the wrist and elbow joints.

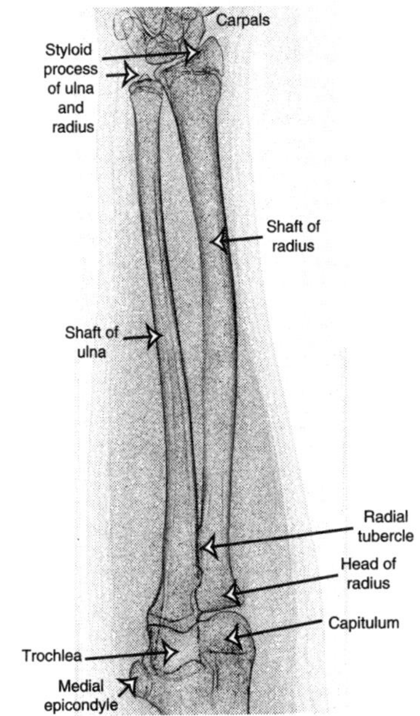

Tips

1. The PA projection is never performed because the radius and ulna cross over each other.
2. If both elbow and wrist joints cannot be demonstrated on a single film, a separate AP of one joint should be done.

Technical Considerations
- Extremity screen/film
- Non-grid
- kVp range: 60–65
- SID: 40 inch (100 cm)

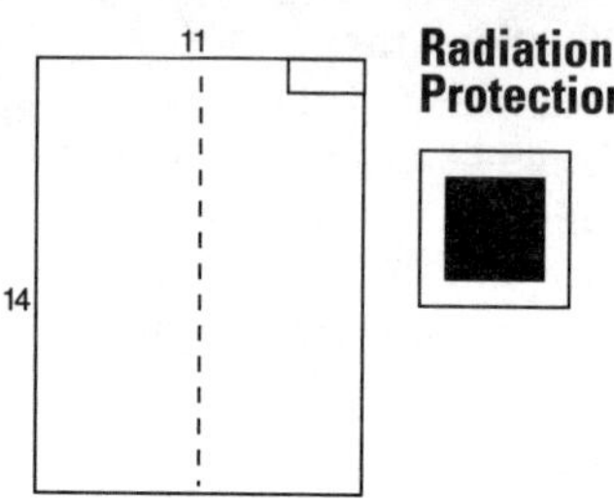

Patient Position Seated at the end of the radiographic table with all potential artifacts removed from the part.

Part Position Flex the elbow 90° and place the hand, wrist, and elbow in a true lateral position, resting on the ulnar surface; the patient may need to lean forward to place the entire upper limb in the same plane.

Central Ray Perpendicular to the mid-forearm.

Breathing Instructions Normal respiration.

Example Exposure Techniques **Measure at CR and Use Chart (p.42)**									
Room	**cm**	**kVp**	**mAs**	**mA**	**Sec**	**Beam**	**Film**	**Grid**	**1Ø3Ø**
	5.0								
	6.0								
	7.0								
	8.0								
	9.0								

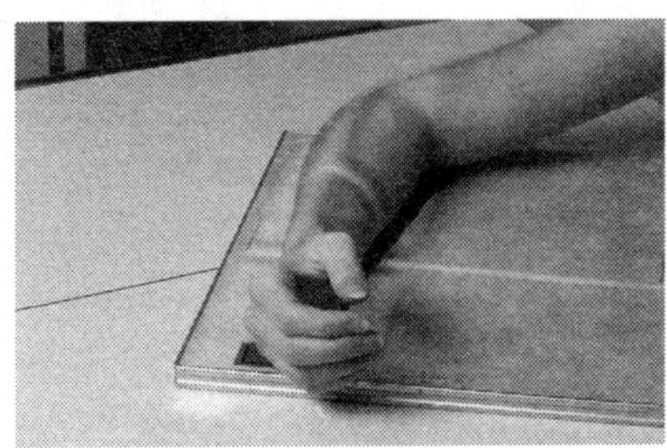

Evaluation Criteria

- Radius and ulna should be mostly superimposed.
- Both wrist and elbow joints should be included.

Exam Rationale The lateral is the second of two basic positions of the forearm. Structures demonstrated on the radiograph include the entire radius and ulna, including portions of the wrist and elbow joints.

Tip If both elbow and wrist joints cannot be demonstrated on a single film, a separate lateral of one joint should be done.

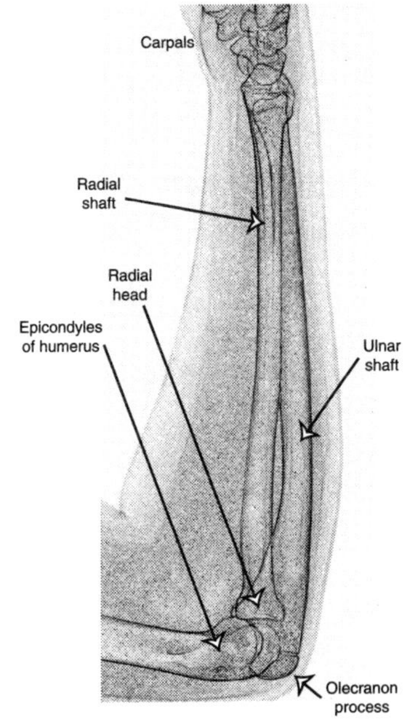

Technical Considerations

- Extremity screen/film
- Non-grid
- kVp range: 65–70
- SID: 40 inch (100 cm)

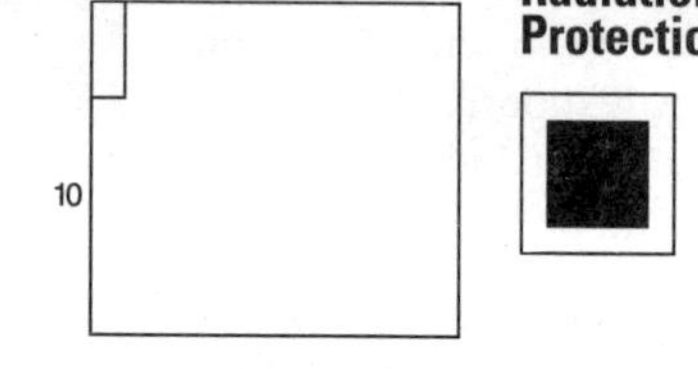

Patient Position Seated at the end of the radiographic table with all potential artifacts removed from the part.

Part Position Place both the humerus and forearm flat on the film, parallel to the cassette; with the hand supinated, fully extend the elbow and place the epicondylar line parallel to the film.

Central Ray Perpendicular to the elbow joint.

Breathing Instructions Normal respiration.

Evaluation Criteria

- Joint space should be open and centered to the film.
- Radius and ulna should be slightly superimposed near the radial tuberosity.
- Epicondyles should not be rotated.

Example Exposure Techniques **Measure at CR and Use Chart (p.42)**									
Room	**cm**	**kVp**	**mAs**	**mA**	**Sec**	**Beam**	**Film**	**Grid**	**1Ø3Ø**
	4.0								
	5.0								
	6.0								
	7.0								
	8.0								

Exam Rationale The most common indication for elbow examinations is trauma. Structures demonstrated on the radiograph include the elbow joint space, proximal radius/ulna, and distal humerus.

Tip For patients who are unable to fully extend their arm, the trauma AP projection should be substituted.

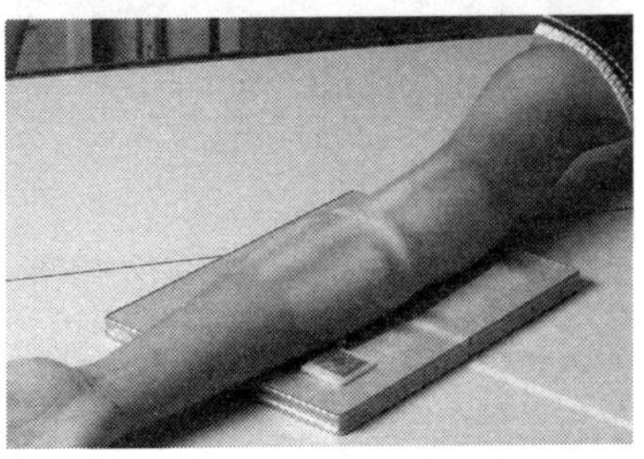

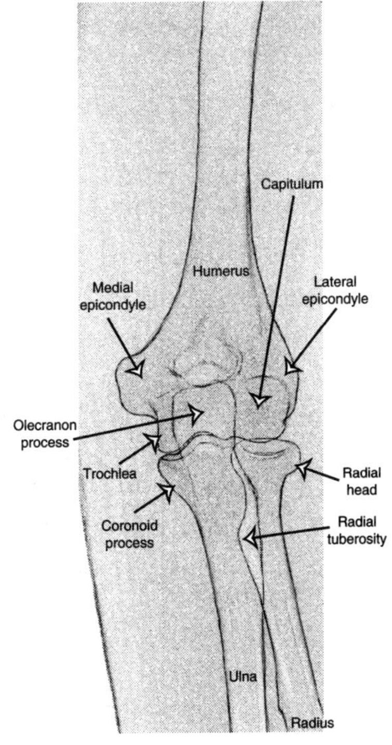

Technical Considerations

- Extremity screen/film
- Non-grid
- kVp range: 65–70
- SID: 40 inch (100 cm)

12

10

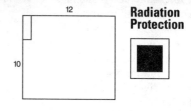

Radiation Protection

Patient Position Seated at the end of the radiographic table with all potential artifacts removed from the part.

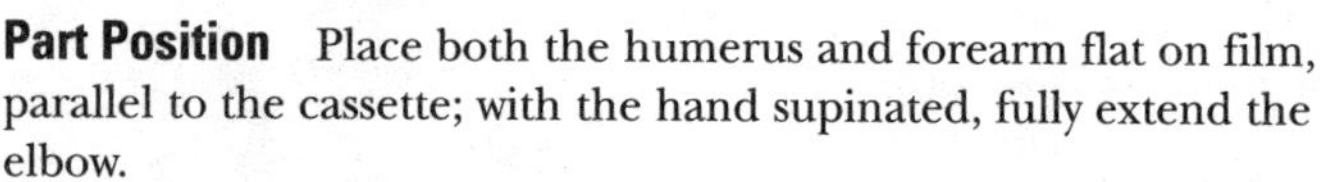

Part Position Place both the humerus and forearm flat on film, parallel to the cassette; with the hand supinated, fully extend the elbow.

- Medial (internal) oblique: pronate the hand until the elbow joint is rotated medially 45° .
- Lateral (external) oblique: supinate the hand until the elbow joint is rotated laterally 45°.

Central Ray Perpendicular to the elbow joint.

Breathing Instructions Normal respiration.

Example Exposure Techniques **Measure at CR and Use Chart (p.42)**									
Room	**cm**	**kVp**	**mAs**	**mA**	**Sec**	**Beam**	**Film**	**Grid**	**1Ø3Ø**
	4.0								
	5.0								
	6.0								
	7.0								
	8.0								

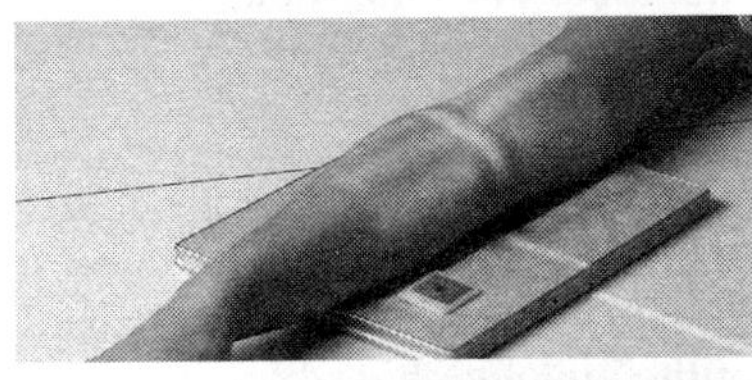

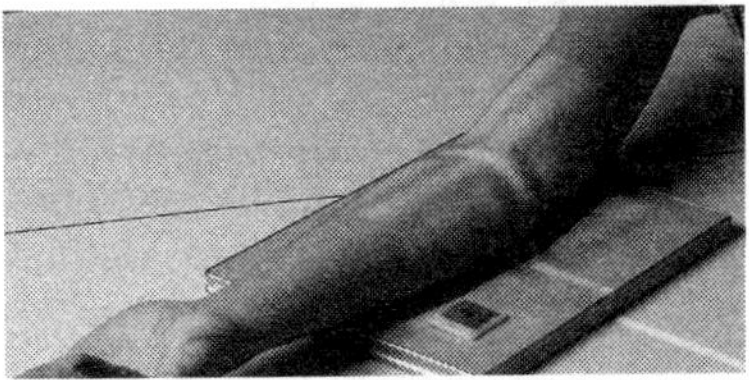

Evaluation Criteria

- Internal oblique: radius and ulna should be substantially superimposed with the coronoid process visualized in profile.
- External oblique: radius and ulna should be free from superimposition of each other with the radial tuberosity, head, and neck clearly demonstrated.

Exam Rationale Although the obliques demonstrate anatomy similar to what is demonstrated on the AP, they are essential to better visualize certain specific structures. The medial (internal) oblique demonstrates the coronoid process in profile, whereas the lateral (external) oblique demonstrates the radial tuberosity, head, and neck free of superimposition.

Tip In cases of acute injury, trauma obliques should be substituted.

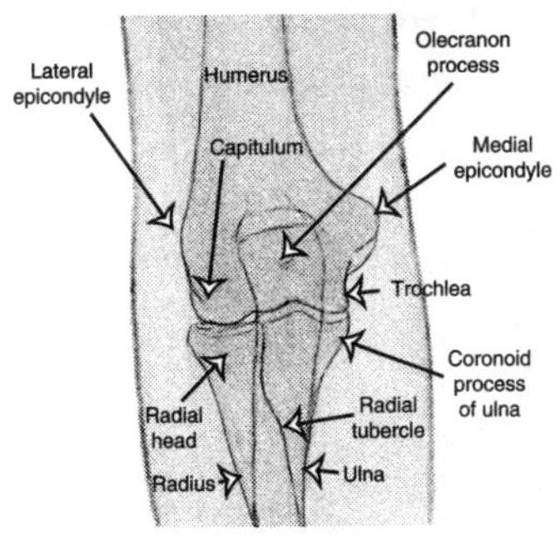

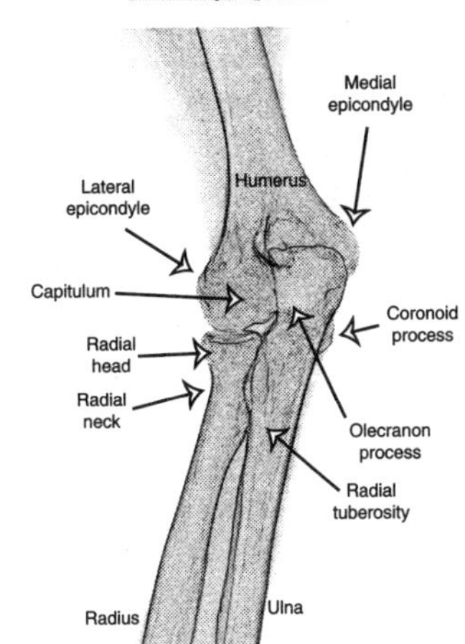

Technical Considerations

- Extremity screen/film
- Non-grid
- kVp range: 65–70
- SID: 40 inch (100 cm)

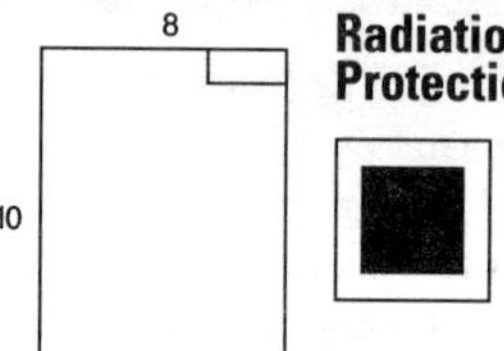

Radiation Protection

Patient Position Seated at the end of the radiographic table with all potential artifacts removed from the part.

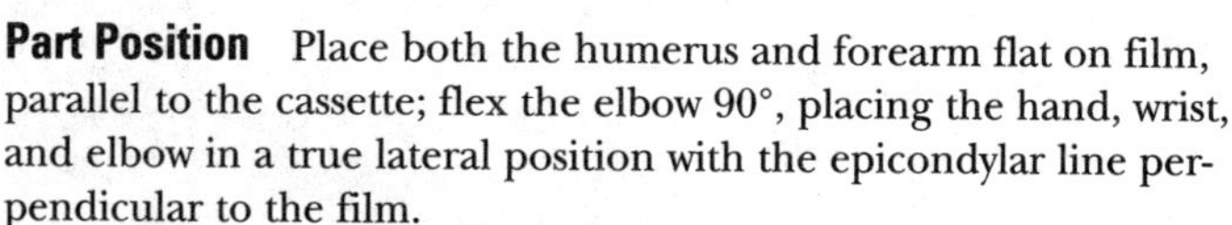

Part Position Place both the humerus and forearm flat on film, parallel to the cassette; flex the elbow 90°, placing the hand, wrist, and elbow in a true lateral position with the epicondylar line perpendicular to the film.

Central Ray Perpendicular to the elbow joint.

Breathing Instructions Normal respiration.

Evaluation Criteria

- Humerus and radius/ulna should form a 90° angle.
- Epicondyles should be superimposed.

Example Exposure Techniques
Measure at CR and Use Chart (p.42)

Room	cm	kVp	mAs	mA	Sec	Beam	Film	Grid	1Ø3Ø
	5.0								
	6.0								
	7.0								
	8.0								

Exam Rationale The lateral is a routine position of the elbow that demonstrates the elbow joint space, proximal radius/ulna, and distal humerus. Of the routine elbow positions, the lateral gives the best visualization of the olecranon process.

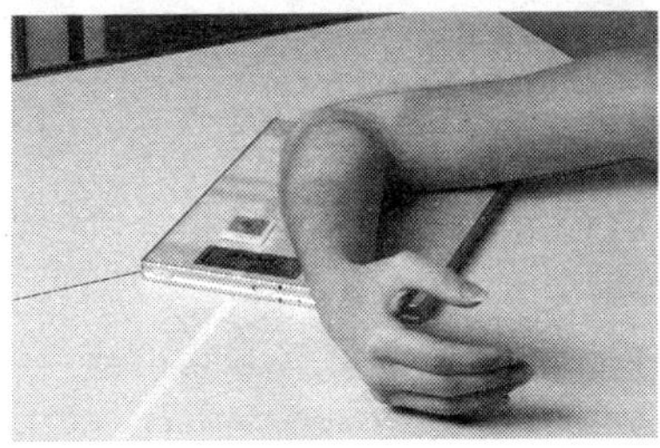

Tip It is essential that the elbow be flexed 90° because this gives the best visualization of fat pads, which offer clues to possible elbow fractures.

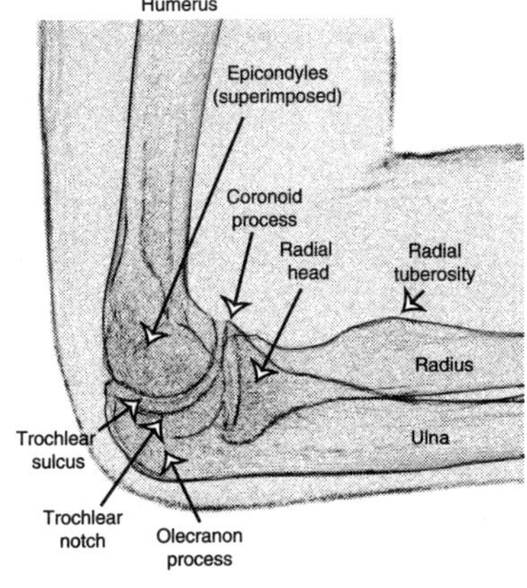

Technical Considerations

- Extremity screen/film
- Non-grid
- kVp range: 65–70
- SID: 40 inch (100 cm)

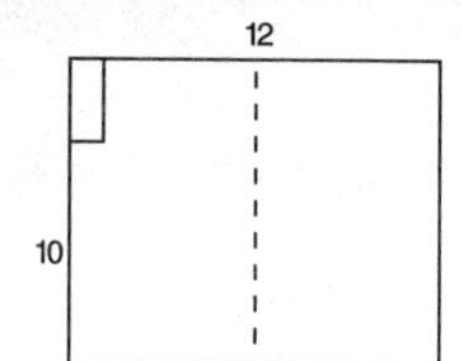

Radiation Protection

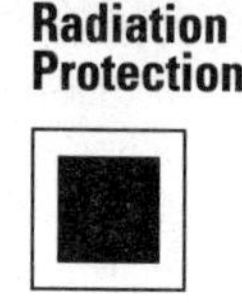

Patient Position Seated at the end of the radiographic table with all potential artifacts removed from the part.

Part Position The elbow is maintained in whatever degree of flexion comfortable for the patient.

- First AP: place the elbow so that the forearm is parallel to the cassette.
- Second AP: place the elbow so that the humerus is parallel to the cassette.

Central Ray Perpendicular to the elbow joint.

Breathing Instructions Normal respiration.

Example Exposure Techniques
Measure at CR and Use Chart (p.42)

Room	cm	kVp	mAs	mA	Sec	Beam	Film	Grid	1Ø3Ø
	4.0								
	5.0								
	6.0								
	7.0								
	8.0								

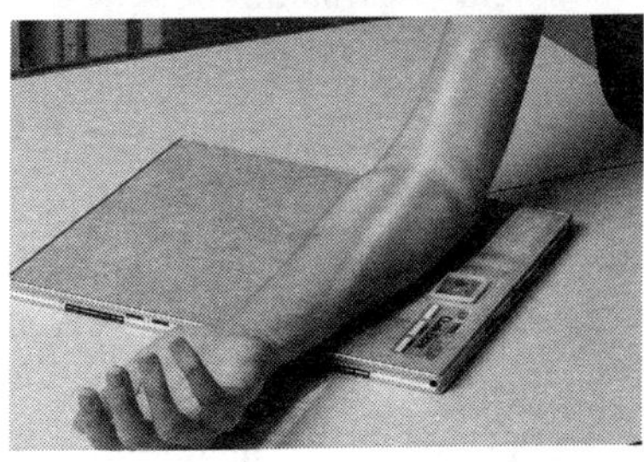

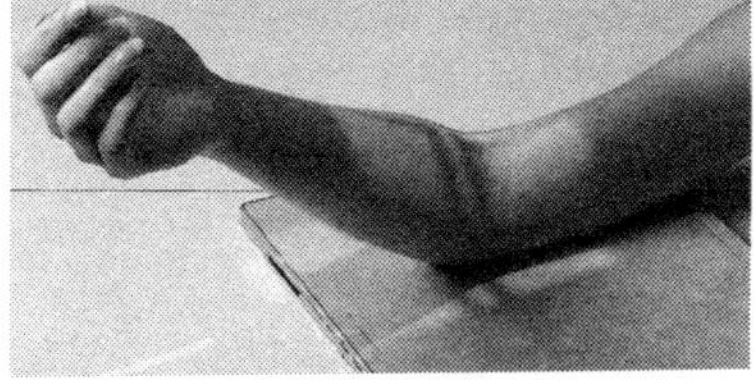

Evaluation Criteria

- Rotation of the epicondyles is minimal.
- Structures of the proximal radius/ulna should be best visualized on the AP with the forearm parallel to the film.
- Structures of the distal humerus should be best visualized on the AP with the humerus parallel to the film.

Exam Rationale These positions are used when injuries to the elbow do not allow the patient to fully extend the elbow joint for the routine AP. Structures demonstrated on the radiograph include the elbow joint space, proximal radius/ulna, and distal humerus.

Tip Trauma AP radiographs demonstrate similar structures as the routine AP; however, their radiographic appearance will be more distorted.

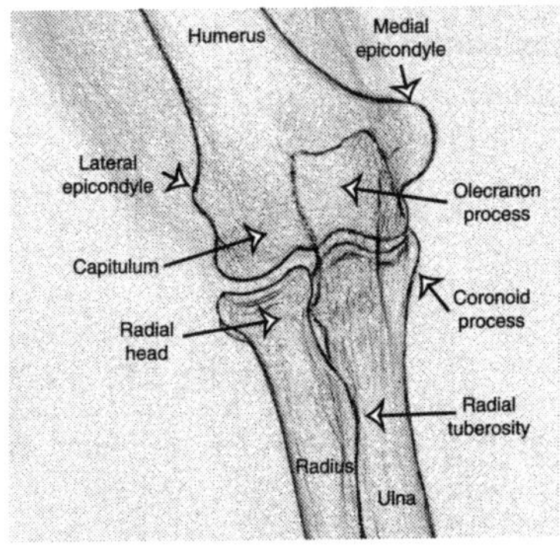

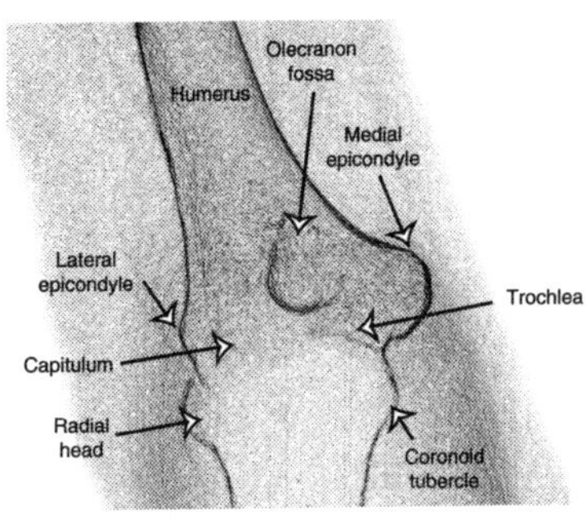

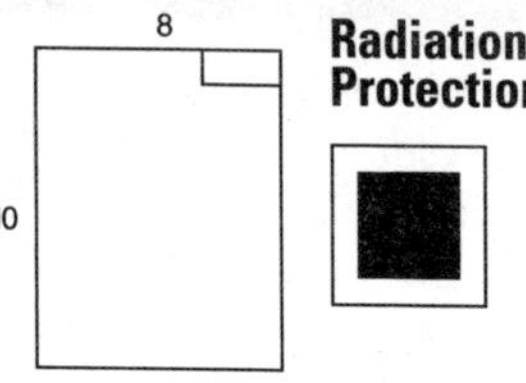

Technical Considerations

- Extremity screen/film
- Non-grid
- kVp range: 65–70
- SID: 40 inch (100 cm)

Patient Position Seated at the end of the radiographic table with all potential artifacts removed from the part.

Part Position Rest the posterior surface of the humerus on the cassette so that the humerus is parallel to the film; flex the elbow as much as possible; the epicondylar plane line should be parallel to the film.

Central Ray Perpendicular to the film and centered to the epicondyles.

Breathing Instructions Normal respiration.

Evaluation Criteria

- Distal humerus and proximal radius/ulna should be superimposed.
- Epicondyles and olecranon process should be visualized in profile.

Example Exposure Techniques **Measure at CR and Use Chart (p.42)**									
Room	cm	kVp	mAs	mA	Sec	Beam	Film	Grid	1Ø3Ø
	9.0								
	10.0								
	11.0								
	12.0								
	13.0								

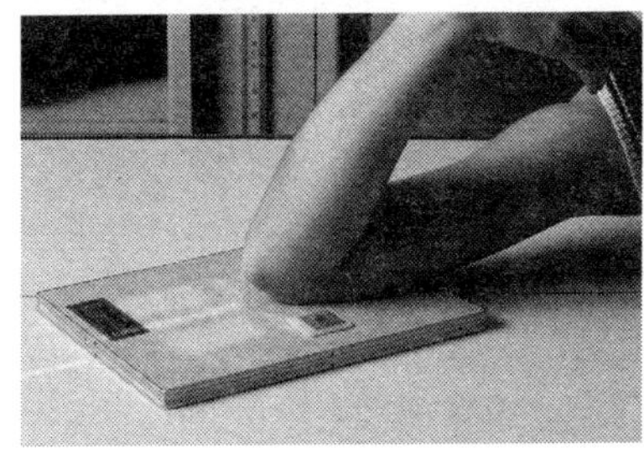

Exam Rationale This position is used primarily to demonstrate injuries to the olecranon process. Structures demonstrated on the radiograph include the olecranon process, proximal radius/ulna, and humeral epicondyles.

Tip Some department protocols call for 15° to 25° tube angulation toward the shoulder.

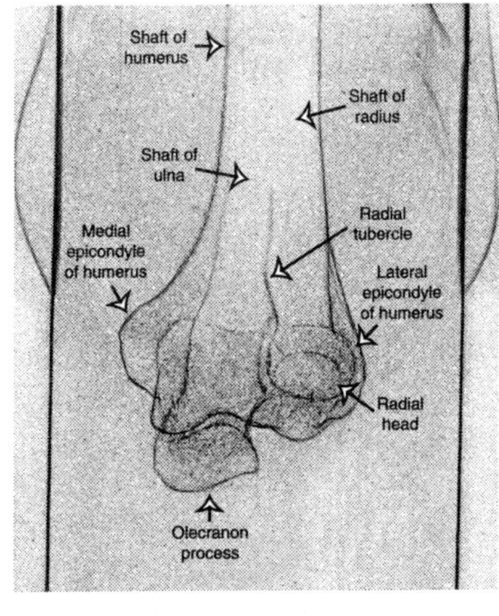

Technical Considerations
- Screen/film
- Grid
- kVp range: 70–80
- SID: 40 inch (100 cm)

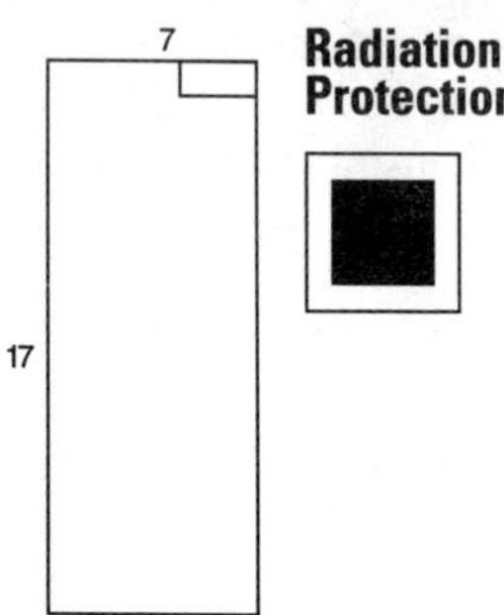

Patient Position Supine or upright, depending on patient condition, with the posterior surface of the body against the cassette; all potential artifacts removed from the part.

Part Position Fully extend the elbow and place the epicondylar line parallel to the film; align the long axis of the humerus to the long axis of the film, being certain to include 1/2 to 1 inch (1–3 cm) of both joints; the patient may be turned slightly toward the affected side to reduce object-film distance.

Central Ray Perpendicular to the midshaft.

Breathing Instructions Normal respiration.

Evaluation Criteria
- Both elbow and shoulder joints should be included.

Example Exposure Techniques
Measure at CR and Use Chart (p.42)

Room	cm	kVp	mAs	mA	Sec	Beam	Film	Grid	1Ø3Ø
	5								
	6								
	7								
	8								
	9								
	10								
	11								
	12								
	13								
	14								

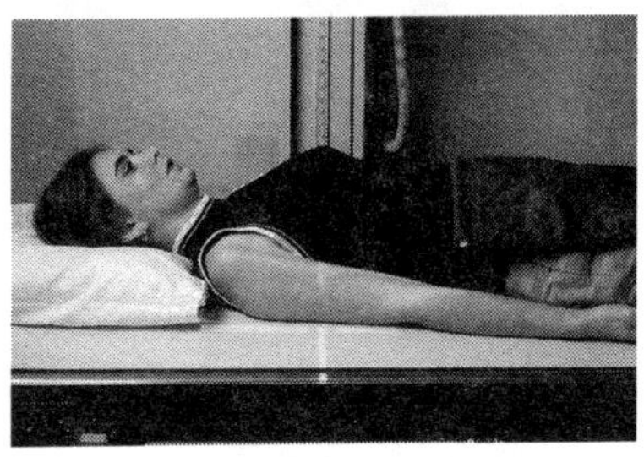

- Greater tubercle should be demonstrated in profile on the lateral aspect of the humerus.

Exam Rationale The most common indication for humerus examinations is trauma. Bony tumors and cysts are occasionally visualized on long bones such as the humerus. Structures demonstrated on the radiograph include the entire humerus and a portion of the elbow and shoulder joints.

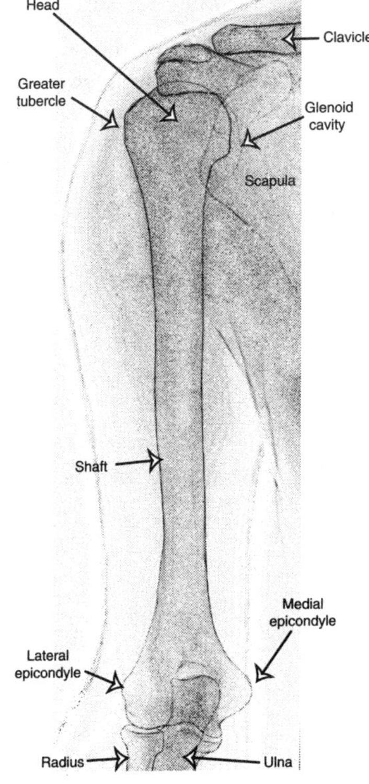

Tips

1. For parts measuring less than 12 cm, this projection can be done without a grid.
2. If acute trauma is evident or suspected, the AP is taken in whatever position the arm is presented. Do not attempt to rotate the arm of a patient with injuries to the humerus.
3. If both elbow and shoulder joints cannot be demonstrated on a single film, a separate AP of one joint should be done.
4. Some department protocols allow follow-up radiographs to include only the joint closest to the site of injury.

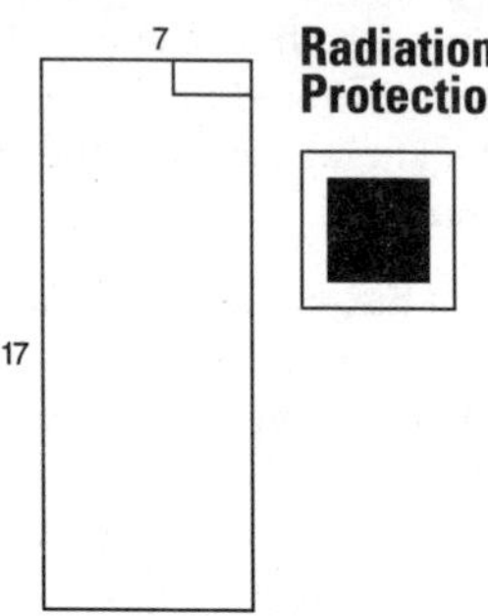

Technical Considerations

- Screen/film
- Grid
- kVp range: 70–80
- SID: 40 inch (100 cm)

Patient Position Supine or upright, depending on patient condition, with the posterior surface of the body against the cassette; all potential artifacts removed from the part.

Part Position Flex the elbow and rotate the arm medially to place the epicondylar line perpendicular to the film; align the long axis of the humerus to the long axis of the film, being certain to include 1/2 to 1 inch of both joints; the patient may be turned slightly toward the affected side to reduce object-film distance.

Central Ray Perpendicular to the midshaft.

Breathing Instructions Normal respiration.

Example Exposure Techniques **Measure at CR and Use Chart (p.42)**									
Room	**cm**	**kVp**	**mAs**	**mA**	**Sec**	**Beam**	**Film**	**Grid**	**1Ø3Ø**
	5								
	6								
	7								
	8								
	9								
	10								
	11								
	12								
	13								
	14								

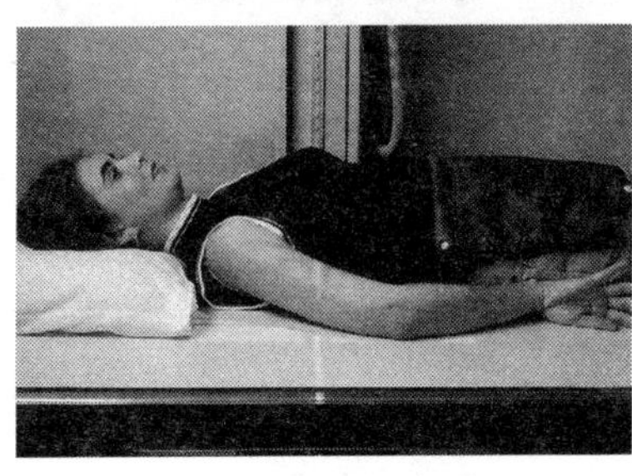

Evaluation Criteria

- Both elbow and shoulder joints should be included.
- Epicondyles should be superimposed.
- Lesser tubercle should be demonstrated in profile on the medial aspect of the humerus.

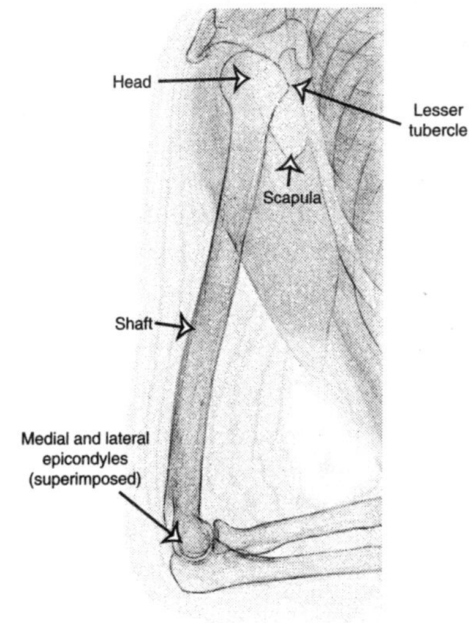

Exam Rationale The lateral is one of two routine positions of the humerus. Structures demonstrated on the radiograph include the entire humerus and a portion of the elbow and shoulder joints.

Tips

1. For parts measuring less than 12 cm, this projection can be done without a grid.
2. If acute trauma is evident or suspected, the trauma lateral or transthoracic lateral should be substituted. Do not attempt to rotate the arm of a patient with injuries to the humerus.
3. If both elbow and shoulder joints cannot be demonstrated on a single film, a separate lateral of one joint should be done.
4. Some department protocols allow follow-up radiographs to include only the joint closest to the site of injury.

Technical Considerations
- Screen/film
- Grid
- kVp range: 70–80
- SID: 40 inch (100 cm)
- Long exposure time (see Breathing Instructions below)

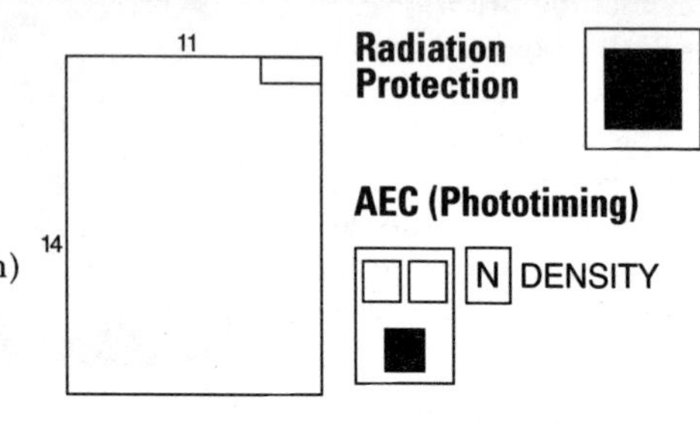

Patient Position Upright with affected arm against film holder; all potential artifacts removed from the part.

Part Position The affected arm is maintained in a neutral position; the top of the film should be placed 1 inch (3 cm) above the top of the affected shoulder; the opposite arm is raised over the head, elevating the unaffected shoulder as much as possible.

Central Ray Horizontal and perpendicular to the film, directed to exit at the midshaft of the affected humerus.

Breathing Instructions Normal respiration. The patient is allowed to continue normal breathing during the exposure because this will blur thorax shadows, which frequently obscure bony detail.

Example Exposure Techniques
Measure at CR and Use Chart (p.42)

Room	cm	kVp	mAs	mA	Sec	Beam	Film	Grid	1Ø3Ø
	22								
	24								
	26								
	28								
	30								
	32								
	34								
	36								
	38								
	40								

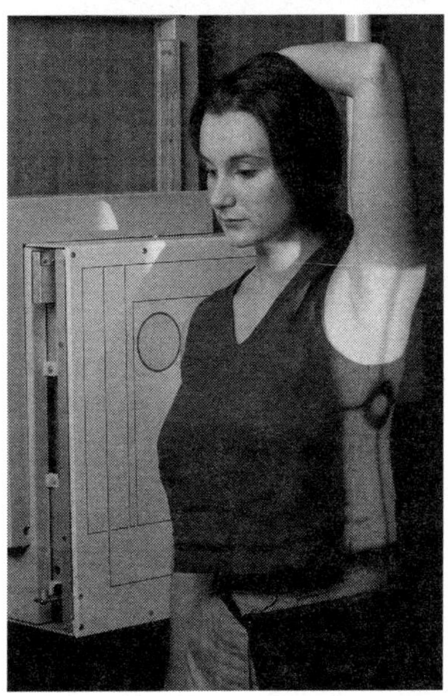

Evaluation Criteria

- Proximal two-thirds of the humerus and the relationship of the humeral head to the glenohumeral joint should be demonstrated.

Exam Rationale The transthoracic lateral is an alternate position taken primarily in cases of acute trauma to the upper arm or shoulder or when the patient is otherwise unable to rotate the arm. Structures demonstrated on the radiograph include the head and shaft of the humerus in a lateral perspective, superimposed on rib and lung anatomy.

Tips

1. For parts measuring less than 12 cm, this projection can be done without a grid.
2. A 15° cephalad angle can be used to prevent superimposition of the shoulders if the patient is unable to raise the unaffected arm high over the head.
3. An exposure time of at least 2 seconds is needed to accommodate the breathing technique.
4. This projection may be done in the supine position or with the patient seated in a wheelchair.

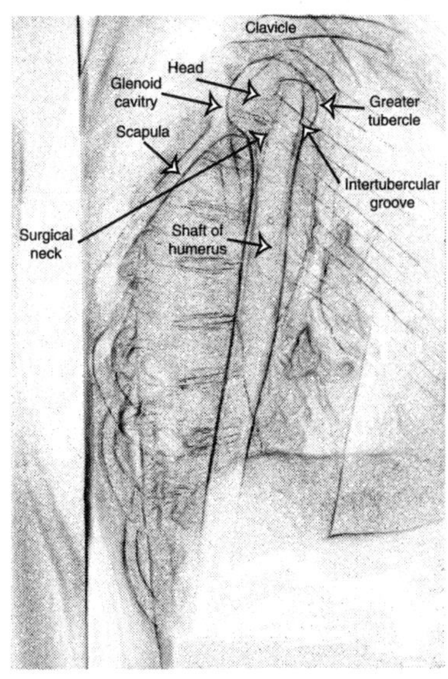

Technical Considerations
- Regular screen/film
- Grid:
- kVp range: 70–80
- SID: 40 inch (100 cm)

12

10

Radiation Protection

AEC (Phototiming)

N DENSITY

Patient Position Supine or upright, depending on patient condition, with the posterior surface of the body against the cassette; all potential artifacts removed from the part.

Part Position Place the affected arm by the patient's side with the back of the hand resting on the thigh to place the intercondylar line perpendicular to the film.

Central Ray Perpendicular to the coracoid process.

Breathing Instructions Suspend on inspiration.

Example Exposure Techniques
Measure at CR and Use Chart (p.42)

Room	cm	kVp	mAs	mA	Sec	Beam	Film	Grid	1Ø3Ø
	8								
	9								
	10								
	11								
	12								
	13								
	14								
	15								
	16								
	17								

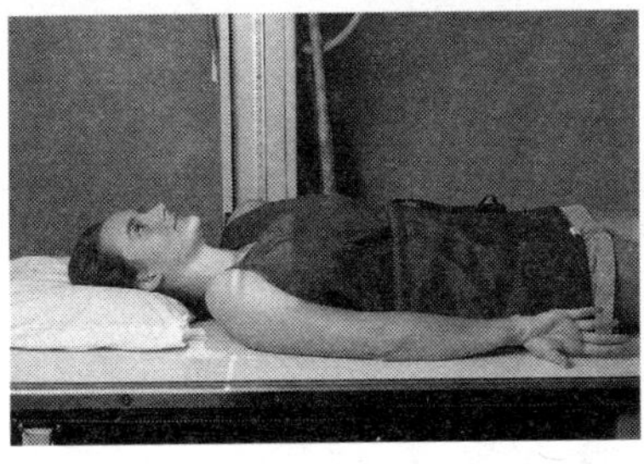

Evaluation Criteria

- Proximal humerus, at least the distal two-thirds of the clavicle, and most of the scapula should be included.
- Lesser tubercle should be demonstrated in profile on the medial aspect of the humerus.
- Humeral head should be slightly more superimposed on the glenoid fossa as compared to the neutral position.

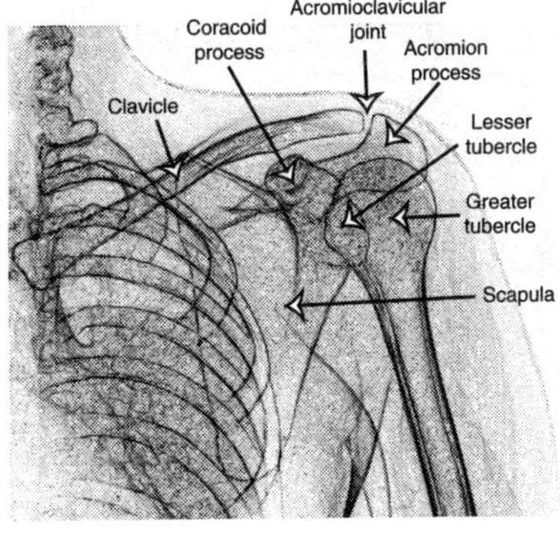

Exam Rationale Indications for shoulder examinations are numerous and include fracture, dislocation, bursitis, tendon or ligament damage, bony tumors, and cysts. Structures demonstrated on the radiograph include the proximal humerus and most of the clavicle and scapula.

Tip The internal rotation should never be done if acute trauma is evident or suspected.

Technical Considerations

- Regular screen/film
- Grid:
- kVp range: 70–80
- SID: 40 inch (100 cm)

12

10

Radiation Protection

AEC (Phototiming)

N DENSITY

Patient Position Supine or upright, depending on patient condition, with the posterior surface of the body against the cassette; all potential artifacts removed from the part.

Part Position Place the affected arm by the patient's side with the hand supinated to place the intercondylar line parallel to the film.

Central Ray Perpendicular to the coracoid process.

Breathing Instructions Suspend on inspiration.

Example Exposure Techniques
Measure at CR and Use Chart (p.42)

Room	cm	kVp	mAs	mA	Sec	Beam	Film	Grid	1Ø3Ø
	8								
	9								
	10								
	11								
	12								
	13								
	14								
	15								
	16								
	17								

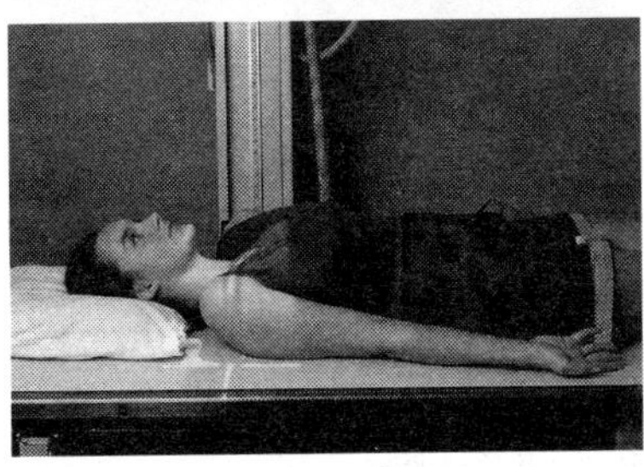

Evaluation Criteria

- Proximal humerus, at least the distal two-thirds of the clavicle, and most of the scapula should be demonstrated.
- Greater tubercle should be demonstrated in profile on the lateral aspect of the humerus.
- Humeral head should be slightly superimposed on the glenoid fossa.

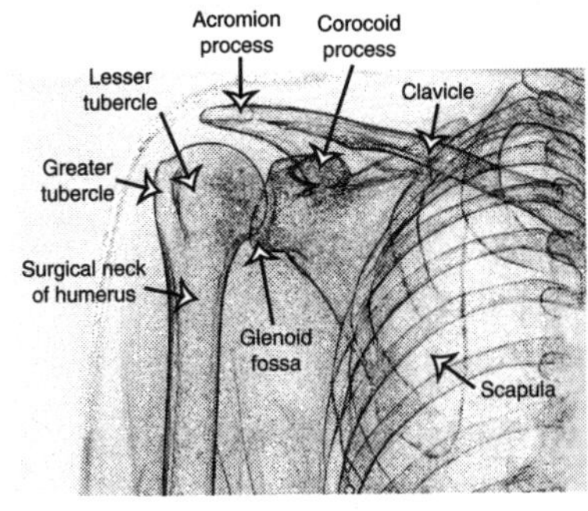

Exam Rationale

Indications for shoulder examinations are numerous and include fracture, dislocation, bursitis, tendon or ligament damage, bony tumors, and cysts. Structures demonstrated on the radiograph include the proximal humerus and most of the clavicle and scapula.

Tip The external rotation should never be done if acute trauma is evident or suspected.

Technical Considerations
- Regular screen/film
- Grid:
- kVp range: 70–80
- SID: 40 inch (100 cm)

12

10

Radiation Protection

AEC (Phototiming)

N DENSITY

Patient Position Supine or upright, depending on patient condition, with the posterior surface of the body against the cassette; all potential artifacts removed from the part.

Part Position Place the affected arm by the patient's side with the palm resting on the thigh.

Central Ray Perpendicular to the coracoid process.

Breathing Instructions Suspend on inspiration.

Example Exposure Techniques
Measure at CR and Use Chart (p.42)

Room	cm	kVp	mAs	mA	Sec	Beam	Film	Grid	1Ø3Ø
	8								
	9								
	10								
	11								
	12								
	13								
	14								
	15								
	16								
	17								

Evaluation Criteria

- Proximal humerus, at least the distal two-thirds of the clavicle, and most of the scapula should be demonstrated.
- Humeral head should be slightly superimposed on the glenoid fossa.
- Neither the greater nor lesser tubercle should appear in profile.

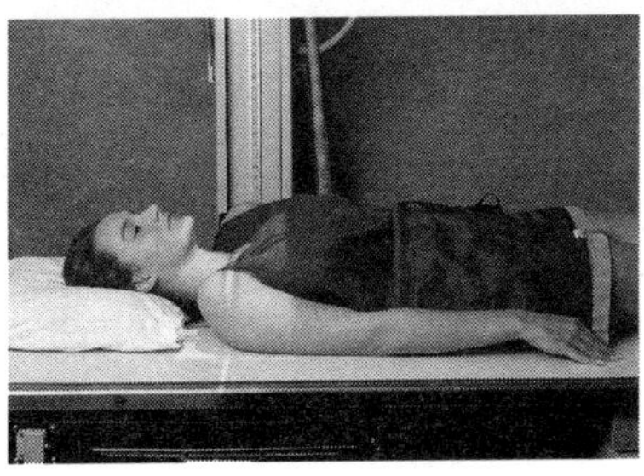

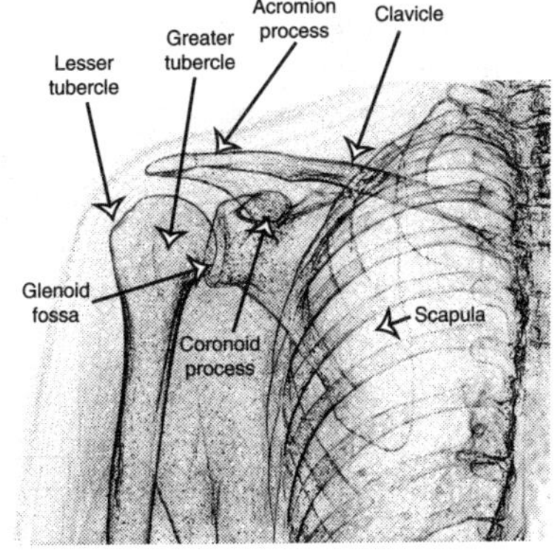

Exam Rationale

Indications for shoulder examinations are numerous and include fracture, dislocation, bursitis, tendon or ligament damage, bony tumors, and cysts. Structures demonstrated on the radiograph include the proximal humerus and most of the clavicle and scapula.

Tip The neutral position is generally used with trauma patients because the arm should not be rotated in cases of acute injury.

Technical Considerations

- Regular screen/film
- Grid or non-grid
- kVp range: 70–80
- SID: 40 inch (100 cm)

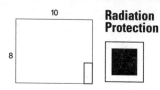

10

8

Radiation Protection

Patient Position Supine with all potential artifacts removed from the part .

Part Position Place the cassette perpendicular to the table, as close to neck as possible; adduct the affected arm 90° from the body; turn the patient's head away from the affected shoulder; a nonopaque sponge may be placed under the affected shoulder to center the part to the film.

Central Ray Horizontal, directed through the axilla to exit at the acromioclavicular joint at the midpoint of film.

Breathing Instructions Suspend on inspiration.

Example Exposure Techniques
Measure at CR and Use Chart (p.42)

Room	cm	kVp	mAs	mA	Sec	Beam	Film	Grid	1Ø3Ø
	7								
	8								
	9								
	10								
	11								
	12								
	13								
	14								
	15								
	16								

Evaluation Criteria

- Lesser tubercle should be visualized in profile superiorly.
- Glenohumeral joint should be clearly demonstrated.

Exam Rationale The inferosuperior axial projection is used primarily to obtain a lateral view of the proximal humerus and its relationship to the glenoid fossa. Structures demonstrated on the radiograph include the glenoid fossa and the proximal humerus.

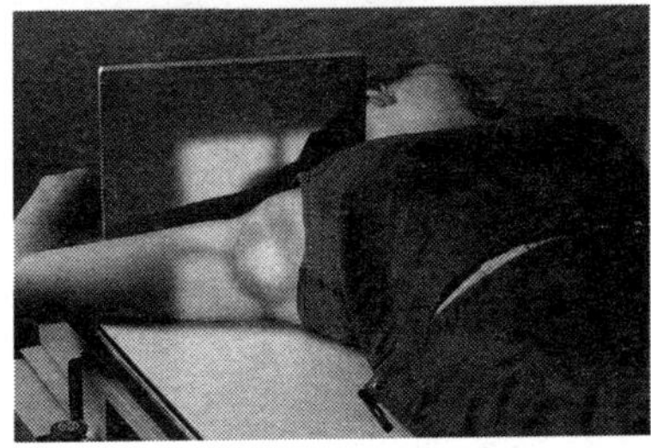

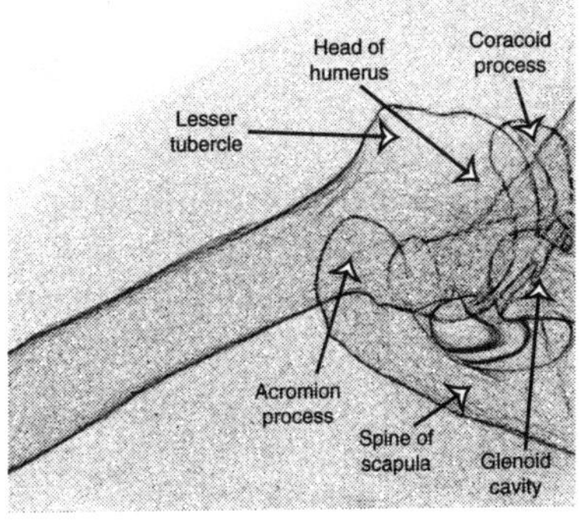

Tips

1. A similar radiograph may be obtained with a superoinferior axial projection.
2. It is desirable to keep the beam as close to perpendicular to the film as possible; however, a 15° to 20° medial angulation may be necessary to align the tube, part, and film accurately.

Technical Considerations
- Regular screen/film
- Grid:
- kVp range: 70–80
- SID: 40 inch (100 cm)

12

10

Radiation Protection

AEC (Phototiming)

N DENSITY

Patient Position Supine or upright, depending on patient condition, with the posterior surface of the body against the cassette; all potential artifacts removed from the part.

Part Position Place the affected arm by the patient's side in a neutral position or rest the forearm on the chest; turn patient 35° to 45° toward the affected side to place the scapula parallel to the film (LPO for injuries to the left side and RPO for injuries to the right side).

Central Ray Perpendicular to the glenohumeral joint space, 1 to 2 inches lateral to the coracoid process.

Example Exposure Techniques
Measure at CR and Use Chart (p.42)

Room	cm	kVp	mAs	mA	Sec	Beam	Film	Grid	1Ø3Ø
	8								
	9								
	10								
	11								
	12								
	13								
	14								
	15								
	16								
	17								

Breathing Instructions
Suspend on inspiration.

Evaluation Criteria

- Glenoid fossa should be visualized free from superimposition of the humeral head.

Exam Rationale The Grashey position is an alternate view of the shoulder that is taken primarily to demonstrate possible dislocations of the head of the humerus. Structures demonstrated on the radiograph include the proximal humerus, a portion of the clavicle and scapula, and the glenoid fossa free from superimposition from the humeral head.

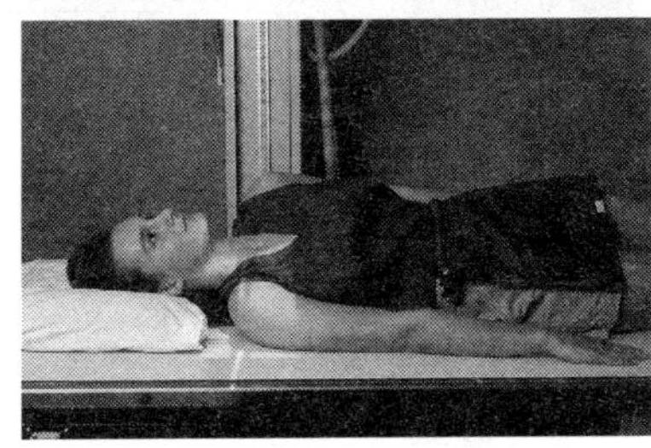

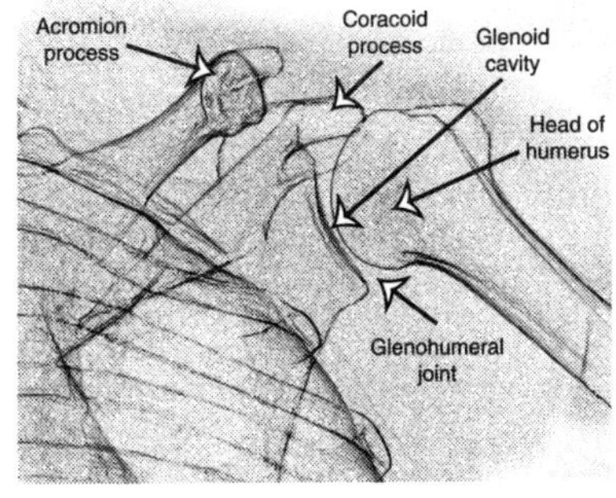

Technical Considerations
- Regular screen/film
- Grid:
- kVp range: 70–80
- SID: 40 inch (100 cm)

10

12

Radiation Protection

AEC (Phototiming)

N DENSITY

Patient Position
Supine or upright, depending on patient condition, with the posterior surface of the body against the cassette; all potential artifacts removed from the part.

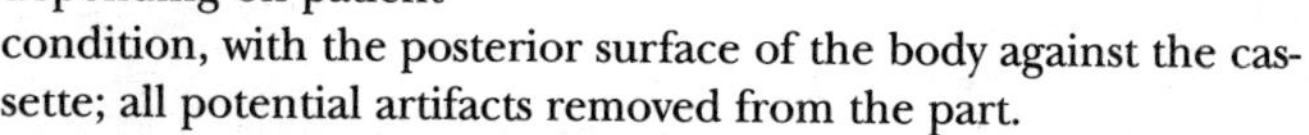

Part Position Place the affected arm by the patient's side in a neutral position; turn the patient 30° away from the affected side (LPO for injuries to the right side and RPO for injuries to the left side).

Central Ray Perpendicular to the glenohumeral joint, 2 to 3 inches below the acromion process.

Breathing Instructions Suspend on inspiration.

Example Exposure Techniques
Measure at CR and Use Chart (p.42)

Room	cm	kVp	mAs	mA	Sec	Beam	Film	Grid	1Ø3Ø
	10								
	11								
	12								
	13								
	14								
	15								
	16								
	17								
	18								
	19								

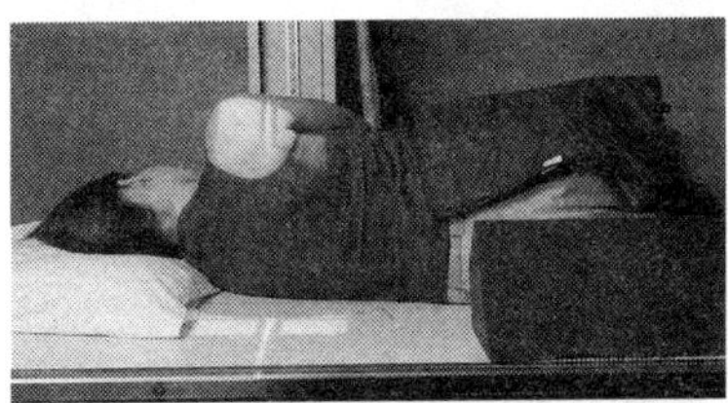

Evaluation Criteria

- Scapula should be in truly lateral position, free from rib superimposition.
- Shaft of the humerus should be superimposed on the body of the scapula.

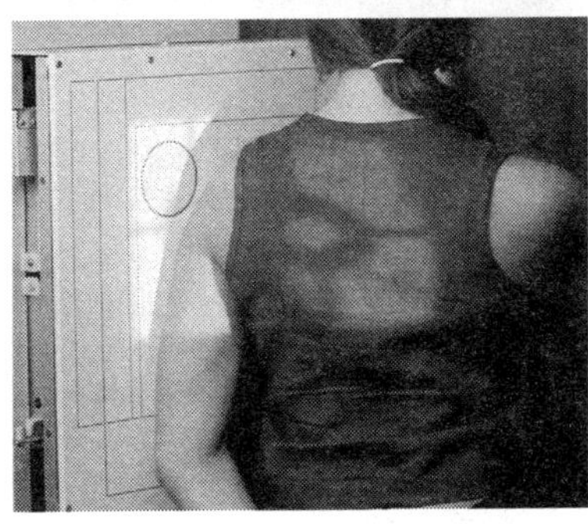

Exam Rationale The scapular Y is an alternate view of the shoulder used primarily with trauma patients to demonstrate possible dislocations of the head of the humerus. Structures demonstrated on the radiograph include the glenoid cavity, humeral head, and most of the scapula.

Tip If patient condition allows, anterior obliques may be done upright to achieve less object-film distance. With the patient facing the film, rotate the patient into a 60° anterior oblique (30° from lateral). The RAO is used for injuries to the right side, and the LAO for injuries to the left side.

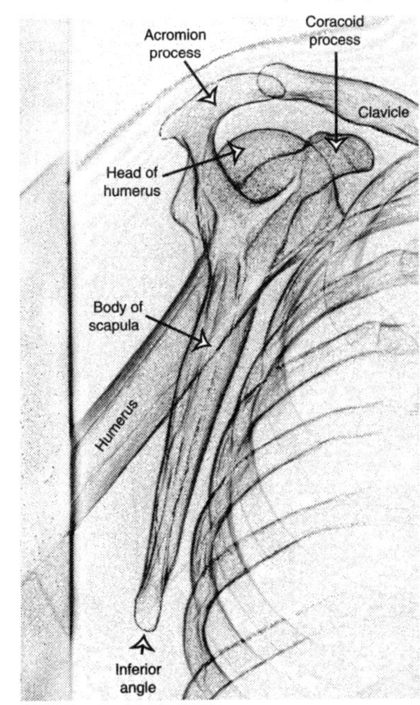

Technical Considerations

- Regular screen/film
- Grid:
- kVp range: 70–80
- SID: 40 inch (100 cm)

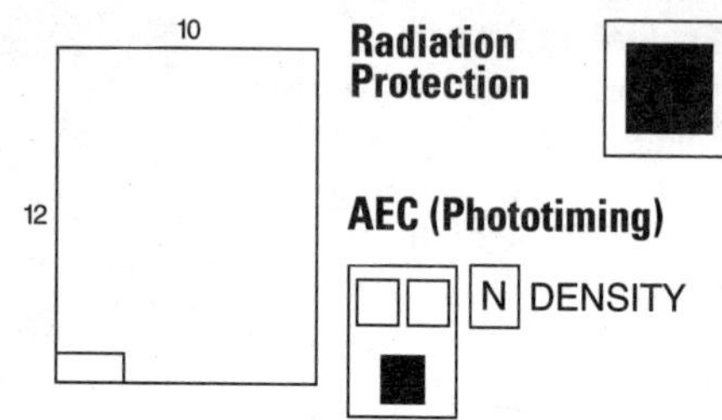

Patient Position

Supine or upright, depending on patient condition, with the posterior surface of the body against the cassette; all potential artifacts removed from the part.

Part Position With the elbow flexed, adduct the arm 90° from the body to place the scapula in better contact with the table; the top of the film is placed 1 to 2 inches above the acromion process.

Central Ray Perpendicular to the midscapula, 1 to 2 inches inferior to the coracoid process.

Breathing Instructions Normal respiration. The patient is allowed to continue normal breathing during the exposure because this will blur thorax shadows, which frequently obscure bony detail.

Example Exposure Techniques
Measure at CR and Use Chart (p.42)

Room	cm	kVp	mAs	mA	Sec	Beam	Film	Grid	1Ø3Ø
	9								
	10								
	11								
	12								
	13								
	14								
	15								
	16								
	17								
	18								

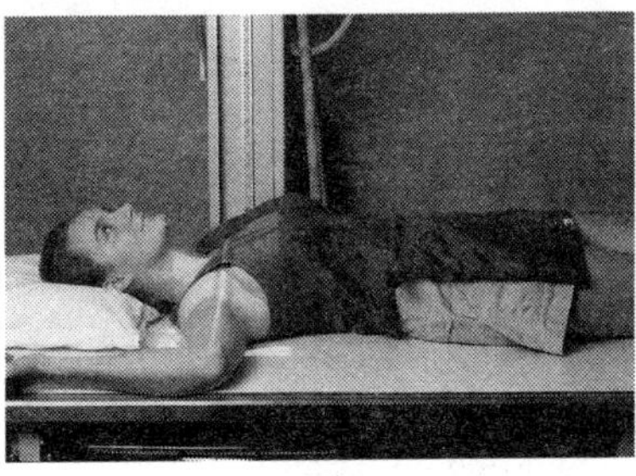

Evaluation Criteria

- Entire scapula must be included.
- Most of the scapula should be superimposed over the lung and ribs.
- Lateral border of the scapula should be mostly free from superimposing rib and lung anatomy.

Exam Rationale The most common indication for scapula examinations is trauma. Structures demonstrated on the radiograph include the scapular body, acromion process, glenoid fossa, and the scapular spine, mostly superimposed on the ribs and lungs.

Tip In cases of acute trauma, the arm is kept in a neutral position and the patient may be turned slightly toward the affected side to place the scapula flat on the table.

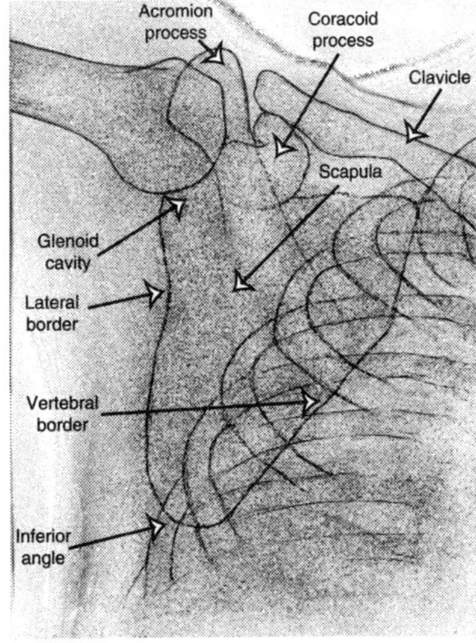

Technical Considerations

- Regular screen/film
- Grid:
- kVp range: 70–80
- SID: 40 inch (100 cm)

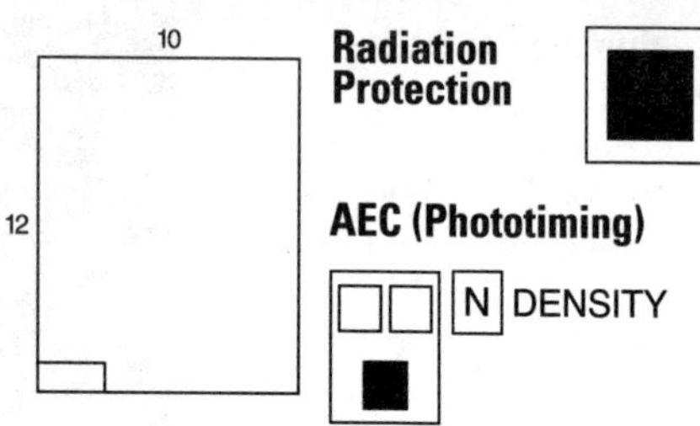

Patient Position Recumbent or upright, depending on patient condition; all potential artifacts removed from the part.

Part Position Start from the supine position and have the patient reach across the chest and grasp the unaffected shoulder; rotate the patient 30° away from the affected side (LPO for injuries to the right side and RPO for injuries to the left side); adjust the patient's obliquity to place the scapula perpendicular to the film; the top of the film is placed 1 to 2 inches above the acromion process.

Central Ray Perpendicular to the midscapula, 1 to 2 inches inferior to the coracoid process.

Breathing Instructions Suspend on inspiration.

Example Exposure Techniques
Measure at CR and Use Chart (p.42)

Room	cm	kVp	mAs	mA	Sec	Beam	Film	Grid	1Ø3Ø
	10								
	11								
	12								
	13								
	14								
	15								
	16								
	17								
	18								
	19								

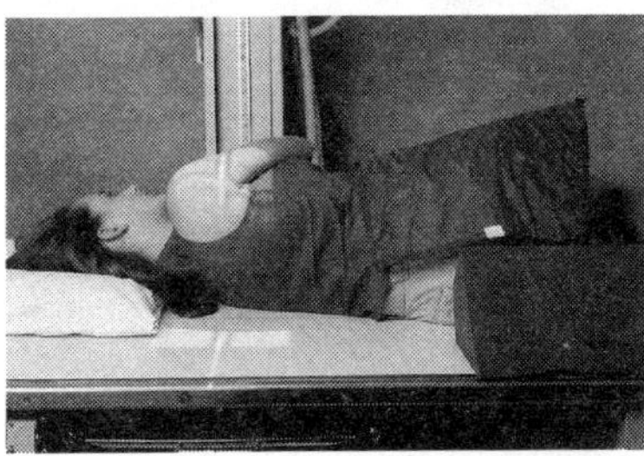

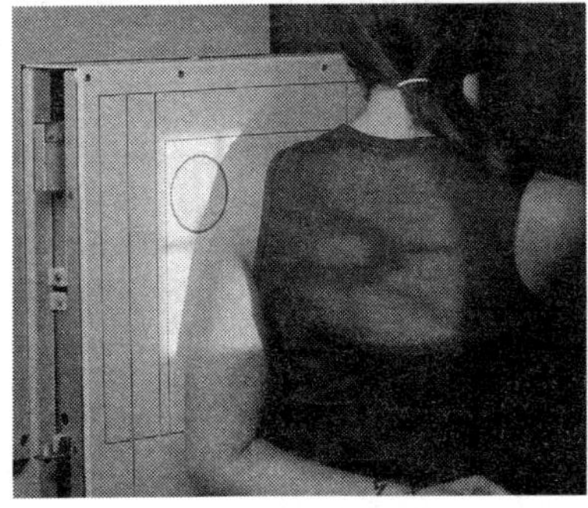

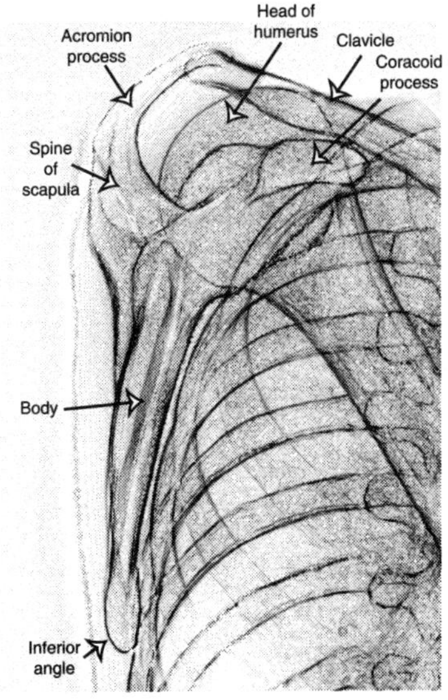

Evaluation Criteria

- Entire scapula should be demonstrated free of superimposition from ribs.
- Coracoid process should be projected anteriorly.
- Acromion process should be projected posteriorly.
- Unlike the scapular Y projection, which has similar positioning, the shaft of the humerus should not be superimposed on the body of the scapula on the lateral scapula radiograph.

Exam Rationale The lateral is one of two routine positions of the scapula. Structures demonstrated on the radiograph include the coracoid process, acromion process, and the body of the scapula in a lateral perspective, free from superimposing rib and lung anatomy.

Tip If patient condition allows, anterior obliques may be done on the upright to achieve less object-film distance. With the patient facing the film, rotate the patient into a 60° oblique (30° from lateral). The RAO is used for injuries to the right side, and the LAO for injuries to the left side.

Technical Considerations

- Regular screen/film
- Grid:
- kVp range: 70–80
- SID: 40 inch (100 cm)

12

10

Radiation Protection

AEC (Phototiming)

N DENSITY

Patient Position

Prone or upright, depending on patient condition, with the anterior surface of the body facing the cassette; all potential artifacts, including radiopaque pillows, removed from the part.

Part Position Place the affected arm by the patient's side in a neutral position.

Central Ray Perpendicular to the midclavicle.

Breathing Instructions Suspend on inspiration.

Example Exposure Techniques

Measure at CR and Use Chart (p.42)

Room	cm	kVp	mAs	mA	Sec	Beam	Film	Grid	1Ø3Ø
	10								
	11								
	12								
	13								
	14								
	15								
	16								
	17								
	18								
	19								

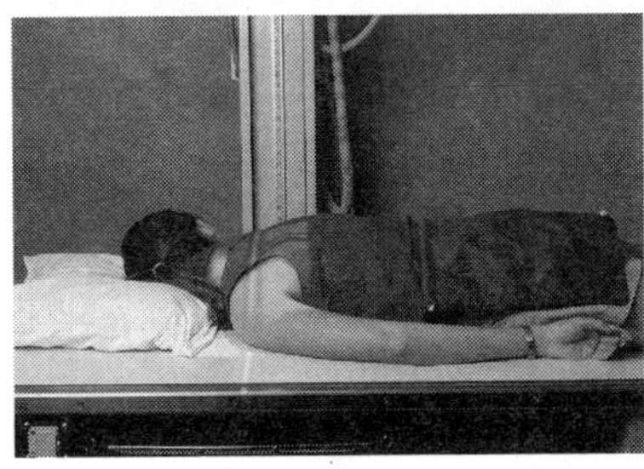

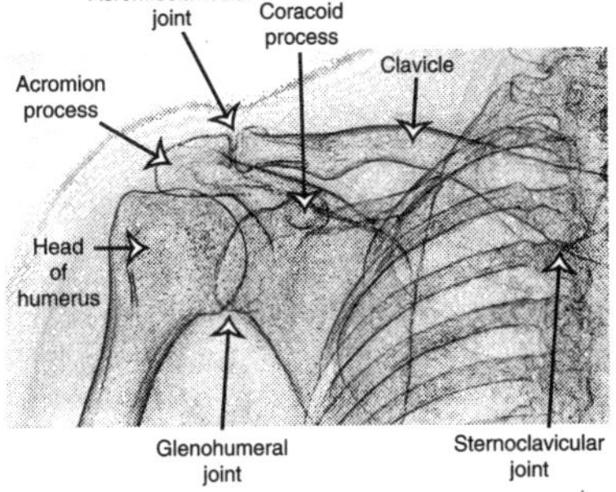

Evaluation Criteria

- Both acromioclavicular and sternoclavicular joints should be demonstrated.
- Proximal one-third of clavicle will be superimposed on thorax shadows.

Exam Rationale The most common indication for clavicle examinations is trauma. Structures demonstrated on the radiograph include the entire clavicle, including the acromioclavicular and sternoclavicular joints.

Tip The PA axial projection is sometimes used to project more of the clavicle off the thorax shadows. The tube angle for a PA axial varies from 10° to 30° caudal, depending on department protocol and the size of the patient. Thinner patients require a larger tube angle.

Technical Considerations
- Regular screen/film
- Grid:
- kVp range: 70–80
- SID: 40 inch (100 cm)

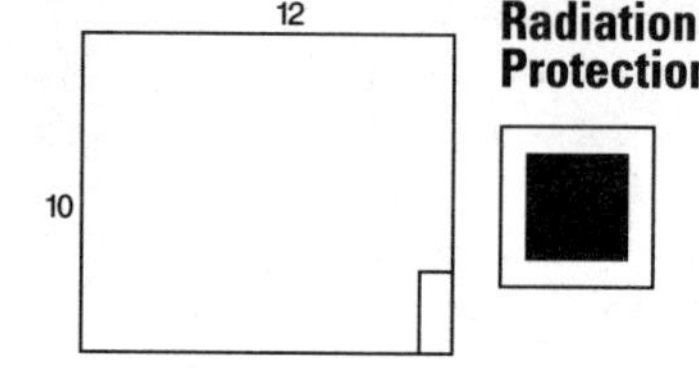

Patient Position Supine or upright, depending on patient condition, with the posterior surface of the body against the cassette; all potential artifacts, including radiopaque pillows, removed from the part.

Part Position Place the affected arm by the patient's side in a neutral position.

Central Ray Directed to the midclavicle at a 15° to 25° cephalad angle.

Breathing Instructions Suspend on inspiration.

Example Exposure Techniques **Measure at CR and Use Chart (p.42)**									
Room	**cm**	**kVp**	**mAs**	**mA**	**Sec**	**Beam**	**Film**	**Grid**	**1Ø3Ø**
	10								
	11								
	12								
	13								
	14								
	15								
	16								
	17								
	18								
	19								

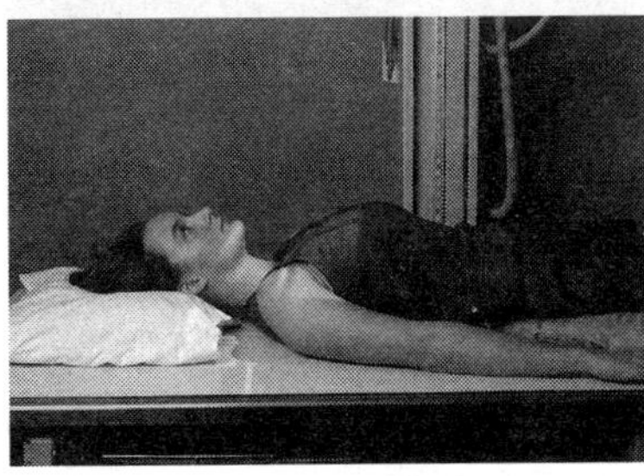

Evaluation Criteria

- Acromioclavicular and sternoclavicular joints should both be demonstrated.
- Clavicle may be superimposed on thorax shadows, depending on degree of tube angle.

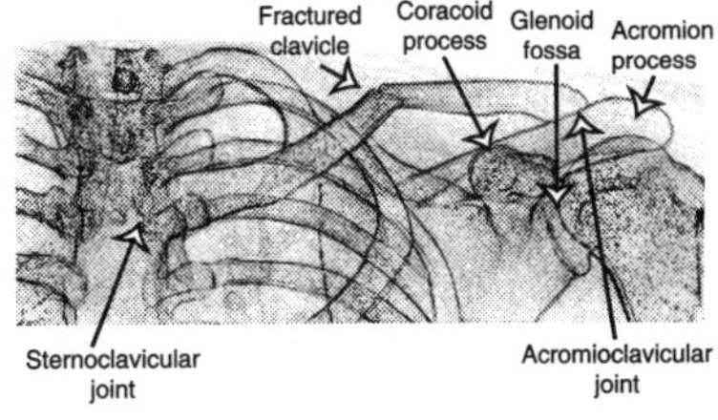

Exam Rationale The most common indication for clavicle examinations is trauma. The AP clavicle is performed when the patient cannot be placed into a prone position. Although the AP clavicle demonstrates the same structures as the PA, the AP results in more magnification of the structures of interest.

Tips

1. Tube angle varies from 10° to 30° depending on department protocol and the size of the patient. Thinner patients require a larger tube angle.
2. Greater tube angles project the clavicle away from rib and thorax superimposition, although these angles also create more image distortion.

Technical Considerations

- Regular screen/film
- Grid
- kVp range: 70–80
- SID: 40 or 72 inch (100 or 180 cm)

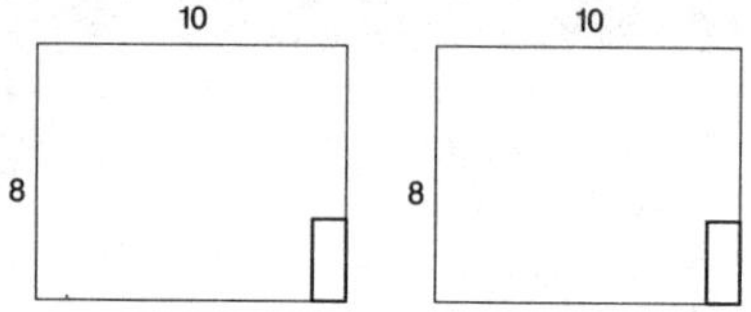

10
8

10
8

Radiation Protection

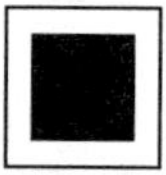

AEC (Phototiming)

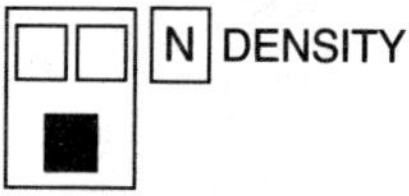

N DENSITY

Patient Position Upright with arms placed by the patient's sides.

Part Position

- Bilateral film without stress or weights.
- Bilateral film with the patient holding a 10- to 15-lb weight in each hand; weights must be equal and the arms relaxed for the weight to stress the joint.

Central Ray Perpendicular to the midpoint between the acromioclavicular joints, centered 1 to 2 inches above the jugular notch.

Breathing Instructions Suspend on inspiration.

Example Exposure Techniques
Measure at CR and Use Chart (p.6)

Room	cm	kVp	mAs	mA	Sec	Beam	Film	Grid	1Ø3Ø
	10								
	11								
	12								
	13								
	14								
	15								
	16								
	17								
	18								
	19								

Evaluation Criteria

- Acromioclavicular joint space should be well demonstrated.
- Rotation, as observed by symmetry of the sternoclavicular joints, should not be evident.

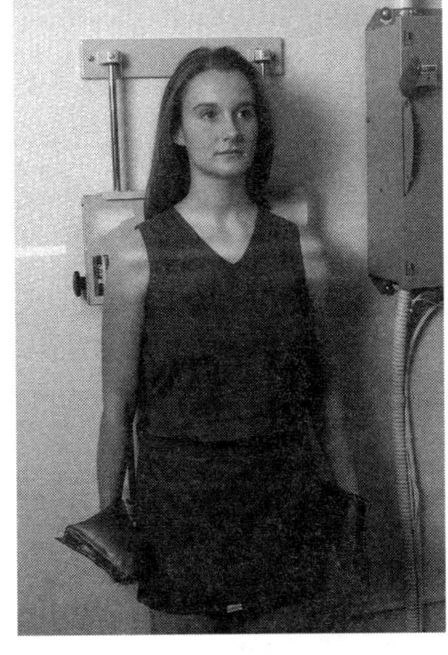

Exam Rationale The AP acromioclavicular joint projection is taken to demonstrate dislocations. Because dislocations are often subtle, a complete series includes both right and left acromioclavicular joints for comparison. To demonstrate small dislocations, the joint must be stressed by the use of weights.

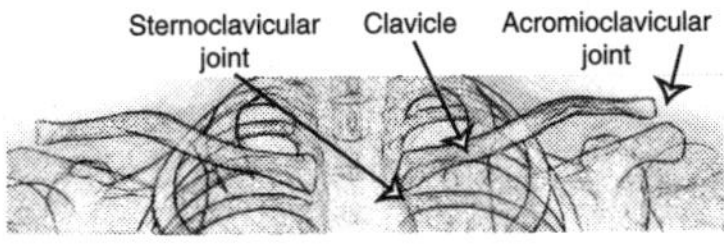

Tips

1. Technical factors require some reduction in mAs from an AP shoulder to demonstrate the soft tissue of the acromioclavicular joint.
2. Breathing is suspended after expiration because this usually depresses the shoulders.
3. Whenever possible, these films should be done with the patient in an upright position. If the patient cannot stand, the films may be taken with the patient supine. To stress the joints, the arms must be gently pulled down.

Pediatric Considerations Pediatric patients require special handling in the radiography department. Good images of the extremities nearly always require some form of immobilization for infants and young children. Sandbags are usually effective in immobilizing extremities.

LOWER LIMB AND PELVIS

ROUTINE AND ALTERNATIVE POSITIONS/PROJECTIONS

Part	Routine	Page	Alternative	Page
Toes	AP	108		
	Oblique	110		
	Lateral	112		
			Tangential sesamoids (Lewis)	114
Foot	AP (dorsoplantar)	116	AP weight-bearing	122
	Oblique	118		
	Lateral	120	Lateral weight-bearing	124
Calcaneus	Axial (plantodorsal)	126		
	Lateral	128		
			Lateral subtalar joint (Broden)	130
Ankle	AP	132	AP mortise	138
			AP stress	140
	Oblique	134		
	Lateral	136		
Lower leg	AP	142		
	Lateral	144		
			Oblique	146
Knee	AP	148	AP weight-bearing	154
	Internal oblique	150	External oblique	156
	Lateral	152		
Patella	PA	158		
	Lateral	160		
			Tangential (Settegast)	162
			Tangential (Hughston)	164
			Tangential (Merchant)	166
Intercondyloid fossa	Axial (Holmblad)	168	Axial (Camp-Coventry)	170
			Axial (Beclere)	172
Femur	AP	174		
	Lateral	176	Translateral	178
Pelvis	AP	180	Axial AP (Taylor)	182
Hip	AP	184		
	Lateral (frog)	186	Bilateral (Modified Cleaves)	188
			Superoinferior (Danelius-Miller)	190
			Superoinferior (Clements-Nakayama)	192
Sacroiliac joints	Axial AP	194		
	Oblique	196		

Technical Considerations

- Extremity screen/film
- Non-grid
- kVp range: 55–60
- SID: 40 inch (100 cm)

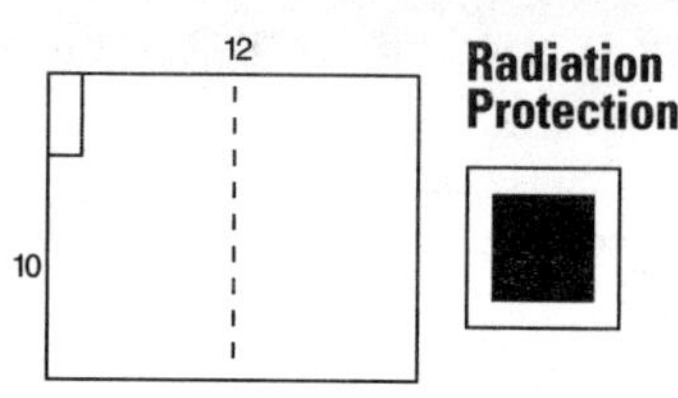

Patient Position Seated on the table with the knee flexed; all potential artifacts, including shoe and sock, removed from the part.

Part Position Place the foot flat on the cassette with the toes centered to the unexposed portion of the cassette.

Central Ray Perpendicular to the second metatarsophalangeal joint.

Breathing Instructions Normal respiration.

Evaluation Criteria

- Phalanges should not be rotated; toes should be slightly separated from each other; and distal ends of the metatarsals should be included.

Example Exposure Techniques
Measure at CR and Use Chart (p.42)

Room	cm	kVp	mAs	mA	Sec	Beam	Film	Grid	1Ø3Ø
	2.0								
	3.0								
	4.0								
	5.0								
	6.0								

Exam Rationale The most common indication for examination of the toe(s) is trauma. Structures demonstrated on the AP projection include the phalanges, the interphalangeal joints, and the distal ends of the metatarsals; the metatarsophalangeal joints are not well visualized.

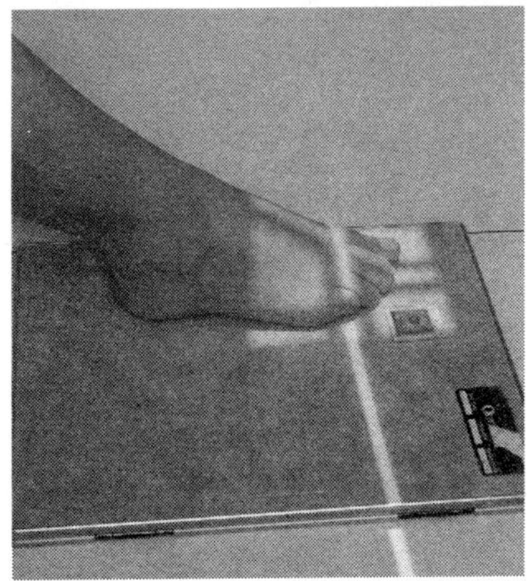

Tips

1. To open joint spaces, angle central ray 15° posteriorly.
2. Many department protocols require that, on initial examination, the entire foot be demonstrated on the AP projection; this can be done on half a 10 × 12 (25 × 30 cm) with the oblique and lateral of only the toe on the other half of the cassette.

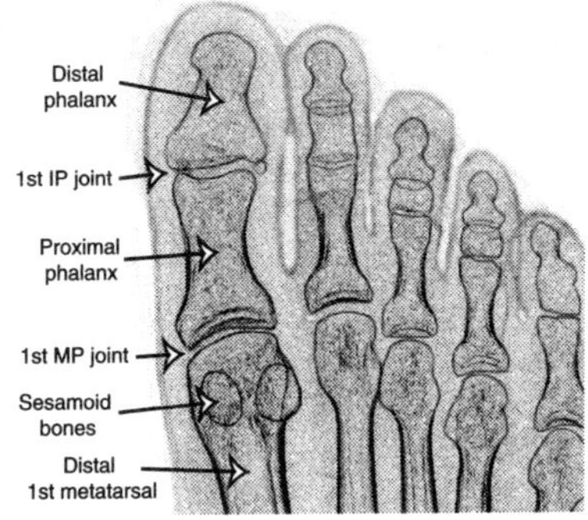

Technical Considerations

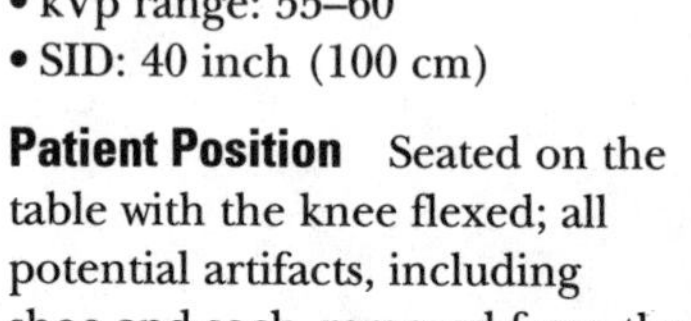

- Extremity screen/film
- Non-grid
- kVp range: 55–60
- SID: 40 inch (100 cm)

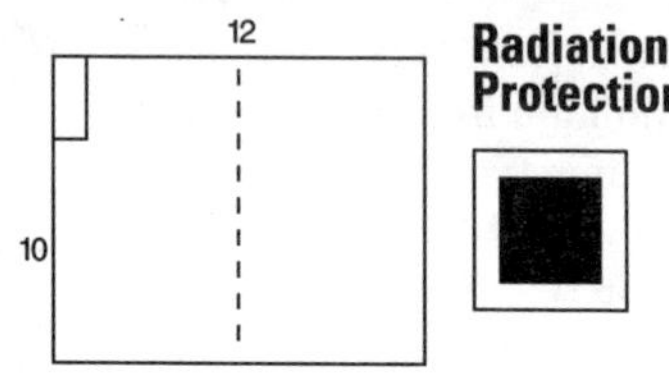

Patient Position Seated on the table with the knee flexed; all potential artifacts, including shoe and sock, removed from the part.

Part Position Place the foot flat on the cassette with the toes centered to the unexposed portion of the cassette; rotate the foot internally 30°.

Central Ray Perpendicular to the third metatarso-phalangeal joint.

Breathing Instructions Normal respiration.

Evaluation Criteria

- All phalanges of the digit should be seen; toes should be slightly separated from each other.

Example Exposure Techniques **Measure at CR and Use Chart (p.42)**									
Room	**cm**	**kVp**	**mAs**	**mA**	**Sec**	**Beam**	**Film**	**Grid**	**1Ø3Ø**
	3.0								
	4.0								
	5.0								
	6.0								
	7.0								

- Obliquity of the toes should be evident; interphalangeal and second through fifth metatarsophalangeal joint spaces should be open; first meta-tarsophalangeal joint space is not always open.
- Distal ends of the metatarsals should be included.

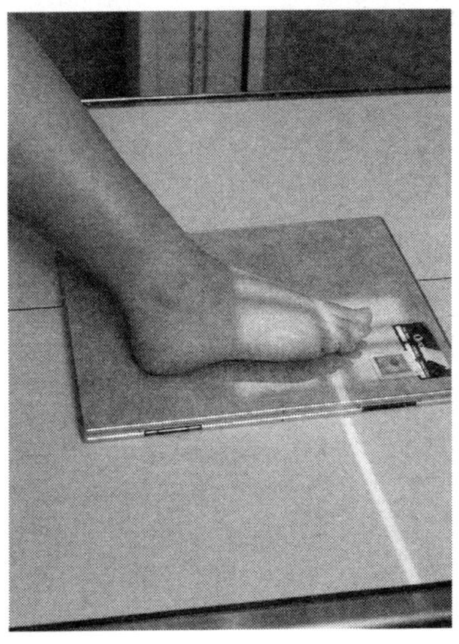

Exam Rationale The oblique is a routine position of the toes that gives a different perspective than that of the AP. Structures demonstrated on the radiograph include the phalanges, the interphalangeal joints, and the distal ends of the metatarsals.

Tip Some department protocols call for a 45° rotation of the foot.

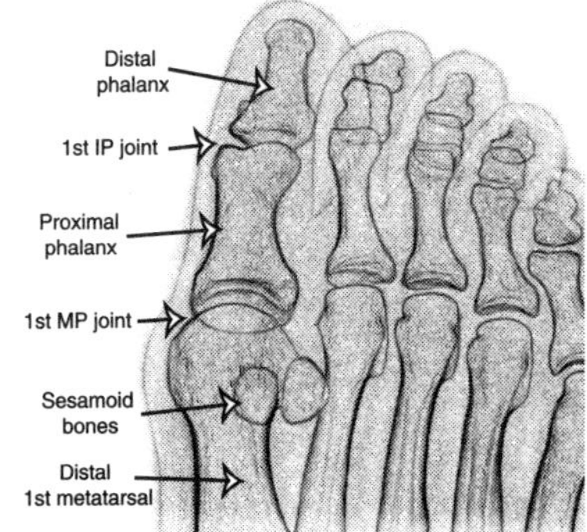

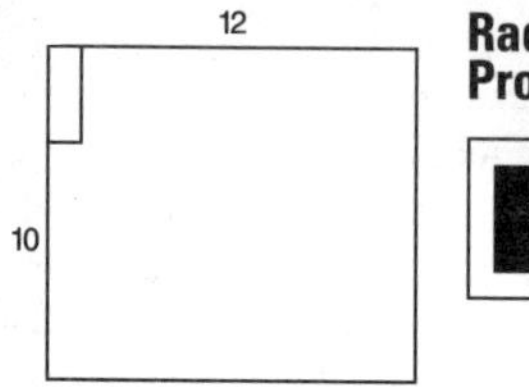

Radiation Protection

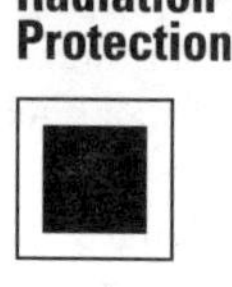

Technical Considerations
- Extremity screen/film
- Non-grid
- kVp range: 55–60
- SID: 40 inch (100 cm)

Patient Position Lateral recumbent position; potential artifacts, including shoe and sock, removed from the part.

Part Position Center the toes to the unexposed portion of the cassette; rest the foot on its medial surface for toes one, two, and three; on the lateral surface for toes four and five; use a strip of gauze to gently pull the affected toe forward or backward from the other toes to prevent superimposition.

Central Ray For toe one, perpendicular to the interphalangeal joint; for toes two through five, perpendicular to the proximal interphalangeal joint of the affected toe.

Breathing Instructions Normal respiration.

Example Exposure Techniques
Measure at CR and Use Chart (p.42)

Room	cm	kVp	mAs	mA	Sec	Beam	Film	Grid	1Ø3Ø
	2.0								
	3.0								
	4.0								
	5.0								
	6.0								

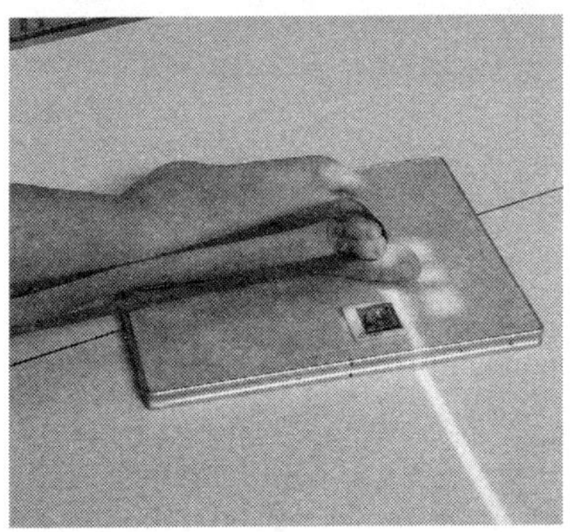

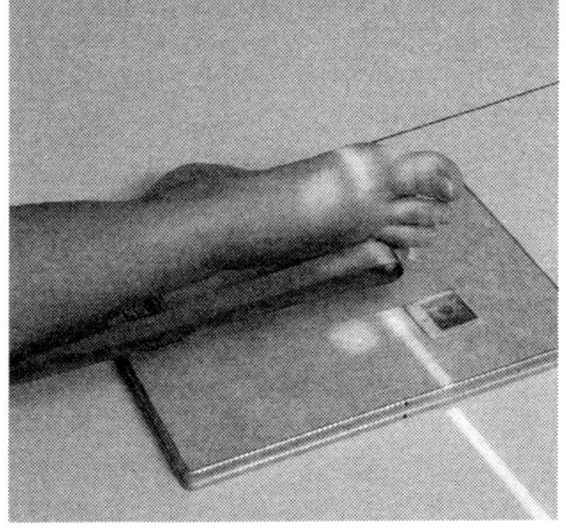

Evaluation Criteria

- Phalanx of interest should be seen in profile.
- Phalanx of interest should be seen without superimposition of the other toes; when complete separation is not possible, the proximal phalanx should be visualized through the superimposed structures.
- Interphalangeal and metatarsophalangeal joint spaces should be open.

Exam Rationale This projection provides a lateral view of the affected toe free of superimposition from other phalanges. Structures demonstrated on the radiograph include the phalanges and interphalangeal joints of the affected toe.

Technical Considerations

- Extremity screen/film
- Non-grid
- kVp range: 55–60
- SID: 40 inch (100 cm)

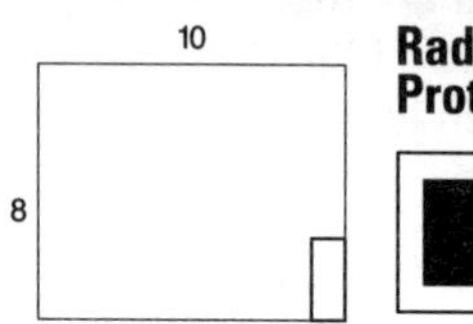

Radiation Protection

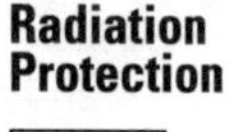

Patient Position Prone on the table; all potential artifacts, including shoe and sock, removed from the part.

Part Position With the toes centered to the cassette, rest the foot on the plantar surface of the great toe; dorsiflex the foot until the ball of the foot is perpendicular to the cassette.

Central Ray Perpendicular and tangential to the second metatarsophalangeal joint.

Breathing Instructions Normal respiration.

Evaluation Criteria

- Sesamoids should be projected free of superimposition by the metatarsal heads.
- Metatarsal heads should be visualized.

Example Exposure Techniques **Measure at CR and Use Chart (p.42)**									
Room	cm	kVp	mAs	mA	Sec	Beam	Film	Grid	1Ø3Ø
	4								
	5								
	6								
	7								
	8								
	9								
	10								

Exam Rationale The most common indication for an examination of the sesamoids is possible fracture. Structures demonstrated on the radiograph include a profile view of the sesamoids and the metatarsal heads.

Tip If the patient is unable to assume the prone position, Holly described an alternative with the patient in the supine position; with the patient seated and the knee extended, center the heel to the cassette and adjust the foot so its medial border is perpendicular to the cassette and the plantar surface is at an angle of 75°; the patient uses gauze to place/maintain the toes in flexed position; the central ray is directed perpendicular to the head of the first metatarsal.

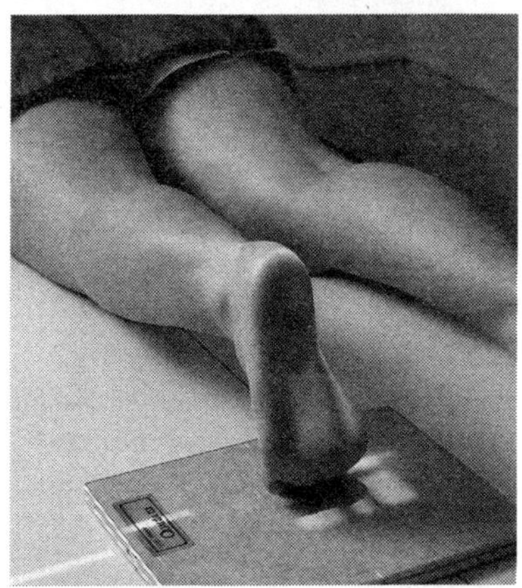

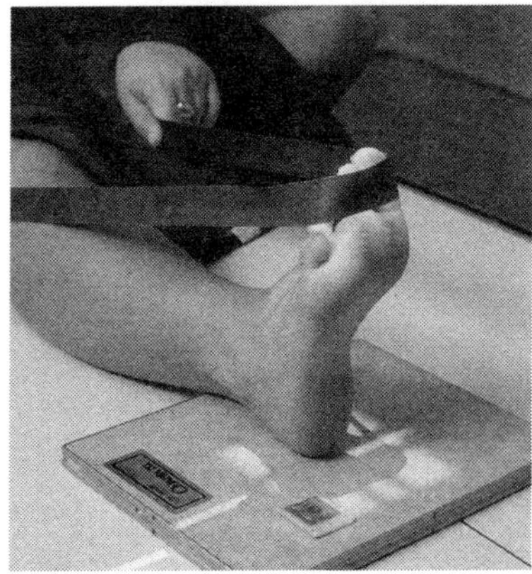

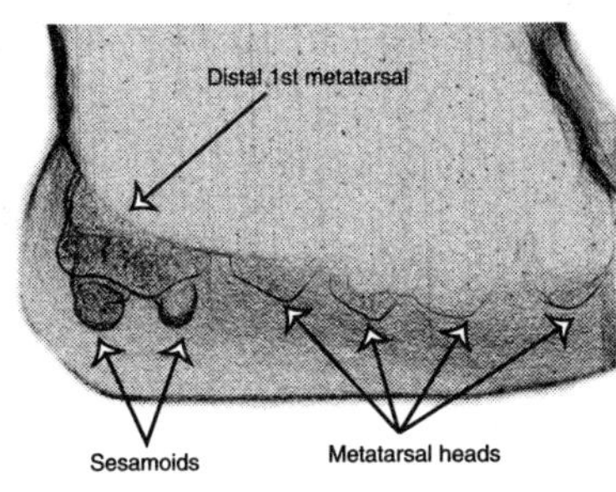

Technical Considerations

- Extremity screen/film
- Non-grid
- kVp range: 55–60
- SID: 40 inch (100 cm)

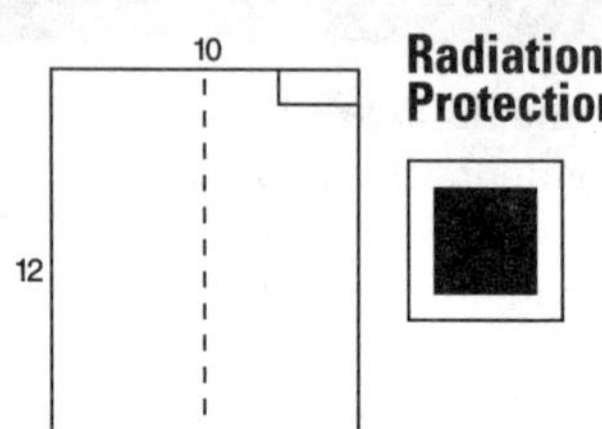

Patient Position Seated on the table with knee flexed; all potential artifacts, including shoe and sock, removed from the part.

Part Position Place the plantar surface of the foot flat on the cassette with the foot centered to the unexposed portion of the cassette.

Central Ray Perpendicular to the base of the third metatarsal, or 10° cephalic angle to the base of the third metatarsal.

Breathing Instructions Normal respiration.

Evaluation Criteria

- Foot should not be rotated as evidenced by equal space between midshafts of adjacent metatarsals (2–4) and overlap of bases of second, third, and fourth metatarsals.

Example Exposure Techniques
Measure at CR and Use Chart (p.42)

Room	cm	kVp	mAs	mA	Sec	Beam	Film	Grid	1Ø3Ø
	4.0								
	5.0								
	6.0								
	7.0								
	8.0								

Exam Rationale The most common indication for an examination of the foot is trauma. The AP projection provides a general survey of the bones of the foot, including demonstration of the phalanges, the metatarsals, and the tarsals anterior to the talus.

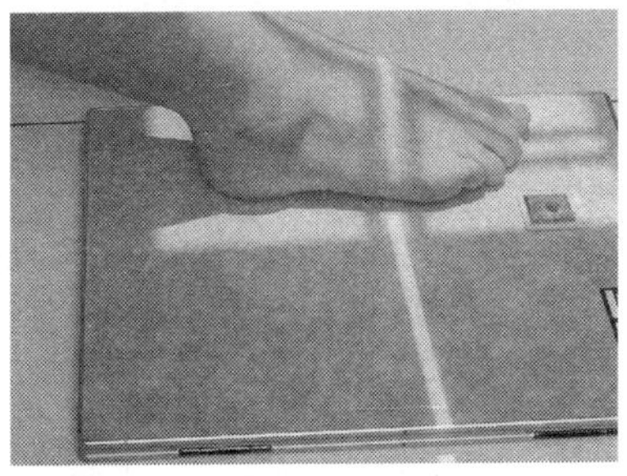

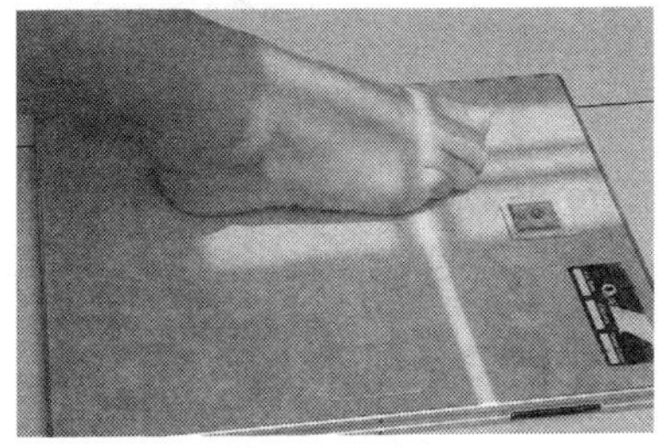

Tips

1. Use of central ray angulation demonstrates more open metatarsophalangeal joints.
2. Use of a compensating filter is helpful in achieving consistent density throughout the foot.

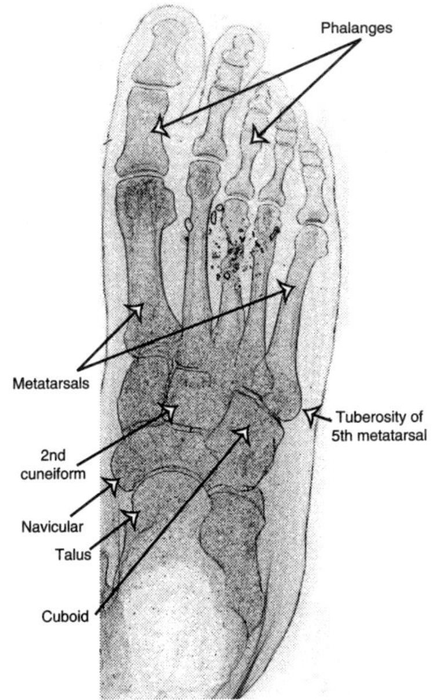

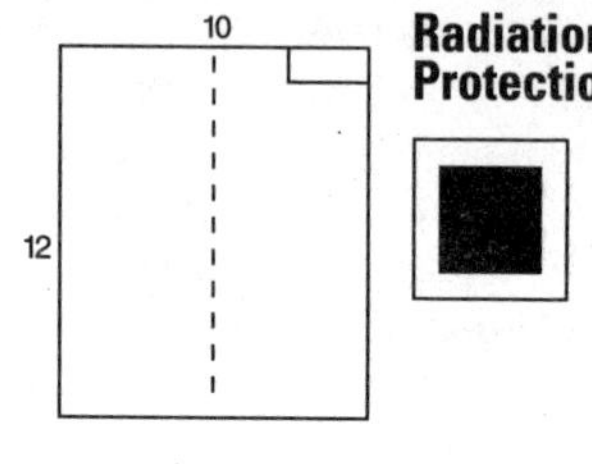

Technical Considerations

- Extremity screen/film
- Non-grid
- kVp range: 55–60
- SID: 40 inch (100 cm)

Patient Position Seated on the table with the knee flexed; all potential artifacts, including shoe and sock, removed from the part.

Part Position Place the plantar surface of the foot on the cassette with the foot centered to the unexposed portion of the cassette; rotate the foot medially 30°.

Central Ray Perpendicular to the base of the third metatarsal.

Breathing Instructions Normal respiration.

Evaluation Criteria

- Third to fifth metatarsal bases should be free of superimposition; bases of the first and second metatarsals should be superimposed.
- Sinus tarsi should be visualized.

Example Exposure Techniques **Measure at CR and Use Chart (p.42)**									
Room	**cm**	**kVp**	**mAs**	**mA**	**Sec**	**Beam**	**Film**	**Grid**	**1Ø3Ø**
	5.0								
	6.0								
	7.0								
	8.0								
	9.0								

- Tuberosity of the fifth metatarsal should be visualized
- Equal amount of space should exist between shafts of the second through fifth metatarsals.

Exam Rationale The oblique is a routine position of the foot that gives a different perspective than that of the AP. Structures demonstrated on the radiograph include the phalanges; metatarsals; sinus tarsi; and the following interspaces: between the cuboid and the calcaneus, between the cuboid and the fourth and fifth metatarsals, between the cuboid and the lateral cuneiform, and between the talus and the scaphoid.

Tip The foot can be rotated laterally 30° to better demonstrate the interspace between the first and second metatarsals and between the medial and intermediate cuneiform.

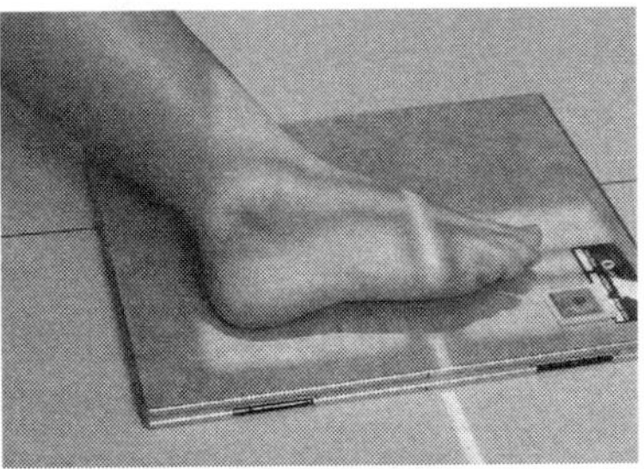

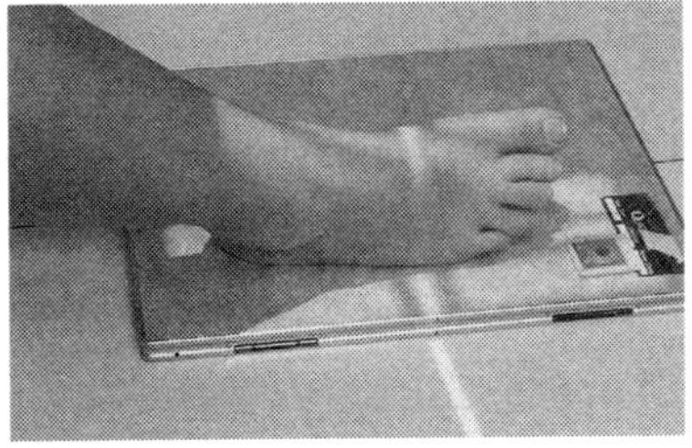

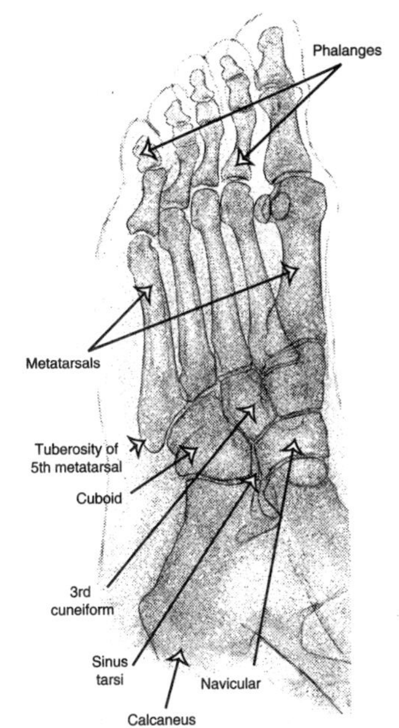

Technical Considerations

- Extremity screen/film
- Non-grid
- kVp range: 55–60
- SID: 40 inch (100 cm)

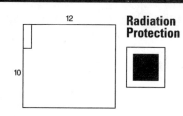

Radiation Protection

Patient Position Lateral recumbent on the affected side with the unaffected leg behind the affected leg; all potential artifacts, including shoe and sock, removed from the part.

Part Position Rest the lateral surface on the cassette with the foot centered to the cassette; dorsiflex the foot and adjust it so the plantar surface is perpendicular to the cassette.

Central Ray Perpendicular to the middle of the foot.

Breathing Instructions Normal respiration.

Evaluation Criteria

- Metatarsals should be nearly superimposed on each other.
- Should include the distal tibia and fibula with the fibula slightly overlapping the posterior tibia.
- Tibiotalar joint should be visualized.

Example Exposure Techniques
Measure at CR and Use Chart (p.42)

Room	cm	kVp	mAs	mA	Sec	Beam	Film	Grid	1Ø3Ø
	5.0								
	6.0								
	7.0								
	8.0								
	9.0								

Exam Rationale The lateral, taken at 90° from the AP, is used to demonstrate anterior/posterior displacements of bony structures and to localize foreign bodies. Structures demonstrated on the radiograph include the foot in profile, the ankle joint, and the distal ends of the tibia and fibula.

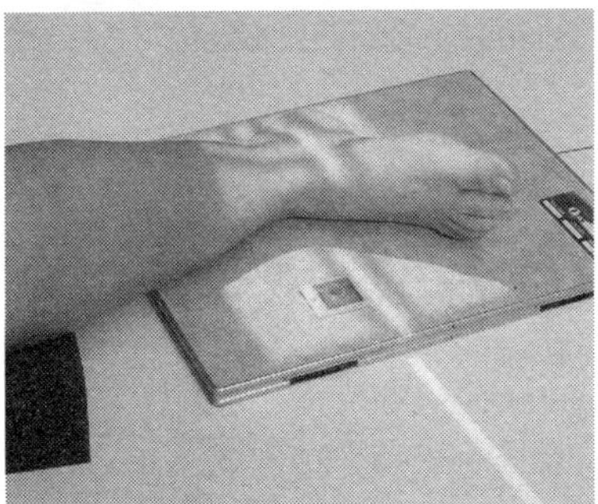

Tips

1. Placing a support under the knee may be helpful in maintaining the foot in a true lateral position.
2. If patient condition permits, the patient can be placed in the lateral recumbent position on the unaffected side; the foot should rest on its medial surface (lateromedial) and should be adjusted so the plantar surface is perpendicular to the cassette. This provides a truer lateral view of the foot, ankle joint, and distal tibia and fibula.

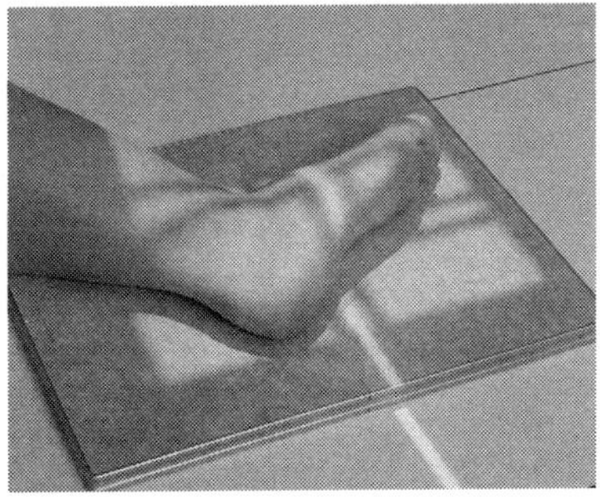

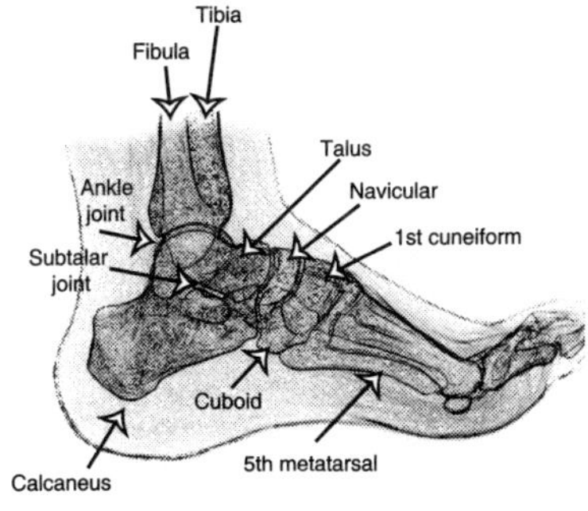

Technical Considerations

- Extremity screen/film
- Non-grid
- kVp range: 55–60
- SID: 40 inch (100 cm)

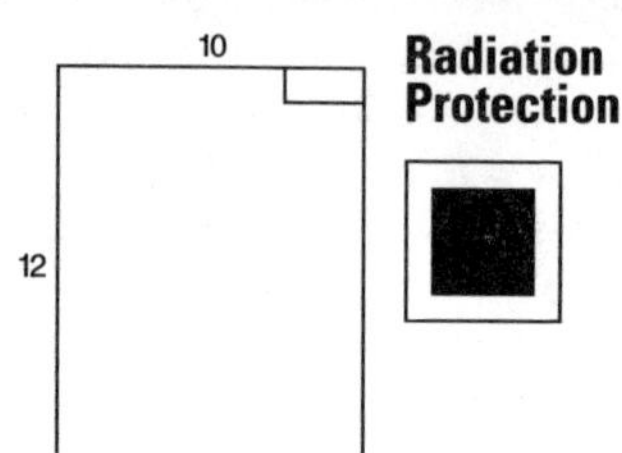

Patient Position Standing, all potential artifacts, including shoe and sock, removed from the part.

Part Position Place the plantar surface of the foot flat, centering the foot to the cassette:

- Exposure 1: unaffected foot should be approximately 12 inches (30 cm) behind the affected foot.
- Exposure 2: unaffected foot should be approximately 12 inches (30 cm) ahead of the affected foot.

Both exposures are made using a single cassette, superimposing the two images of the foot.

Central Ray

- Exposure 1: 15° posterior angulation to the scaphoid.
- Exposure 2: 25° anterior angulation to the posterior ankle so that it exits at the level of the lateral malleolus.

Example Exposure Techniques
Measure at CR and Use Chart (p.42)

Room	cm	kVp	mAs	mA	Sec	Beam	Film	Grid	1Ø3Ø
	4.0								
	5.0								
	6.0								
	7.0								
	8.0								

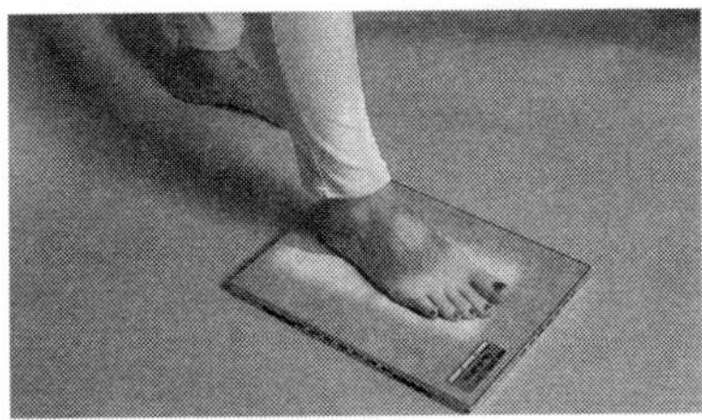

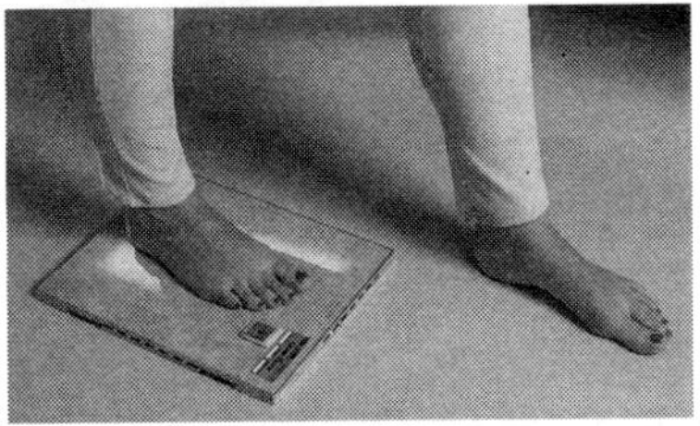

Breathing Instructions

Normal respiration.

Evaluation Criteria

- Foot should not be rotated, as evidenced by an equal amount of space between the midshafts of the adjacent metatarsals (2–4) and overlap of the bases of the second, third, and fourth metatarsals.
- All tarsals should be seen.

Exam Rationale This position is used to demonstrate a weight-bearing, axial projection of all the bones of the foot, projected free from the distal lower leg.

Tip Care must be taken that the patient carefully maintains the position of the affected foot while moving the unaffected leg between the first and second exposures.

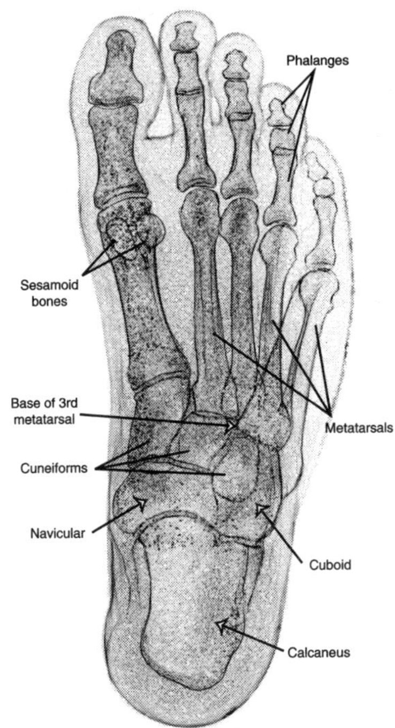

Technical Considerations

- Extremity screen/film
- Non-grid
- kVp range: 55–60
- SID: 40 inch (100 cm)

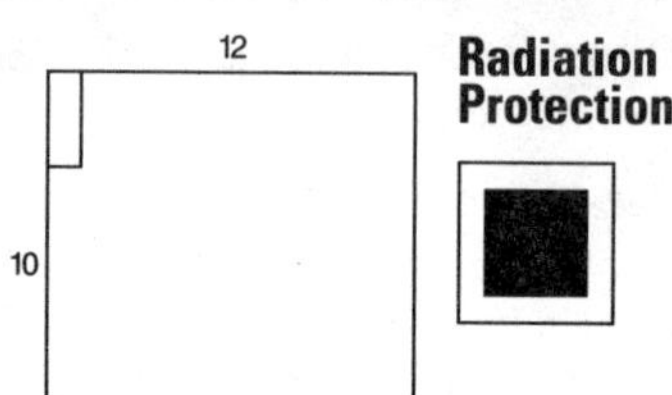

Patient Position Standing; all potential artifacts, including shoes and socks, removed.

Part Position The feet should be flat in a natural position with the weight equally distributed on the feet, one on each side of the cassette.

Central Ray Perpendicular (horizontal) to a point just above the base of the fifth metatarsal.

Breathing Instructions Normal respiration.

Evaluation Criteria

- Plantar surfaces of the metatarsal heads should be superimposed.
- Should include the entire foot and the distal tibia and fibula, with the fibula overlapping the posterior tibia.

Example Exposure Techniques **Measure at CR and Use Chart (p.42)**									
Room	**cm**	**kVp**	**mAs**	**mA**	**Sec**	**Beam**	**Film**	**Grid**	**1Ø3Ø**
	5.0								
	6.0								
	7.0								
	8.0								
	9.0								

Exam Rationale This projection is used to demonstrate the structural status of the longitudinal arch. Both sides are examined for comparison.

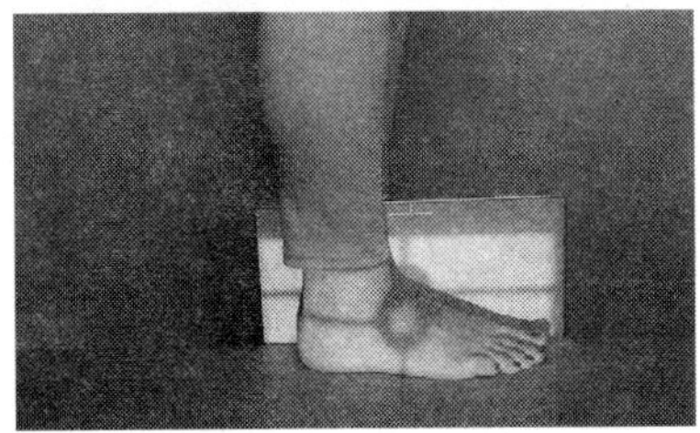

Tip

It may be necessary to have the patient stand on a step stool or other low bench to raise the feet to tube level.

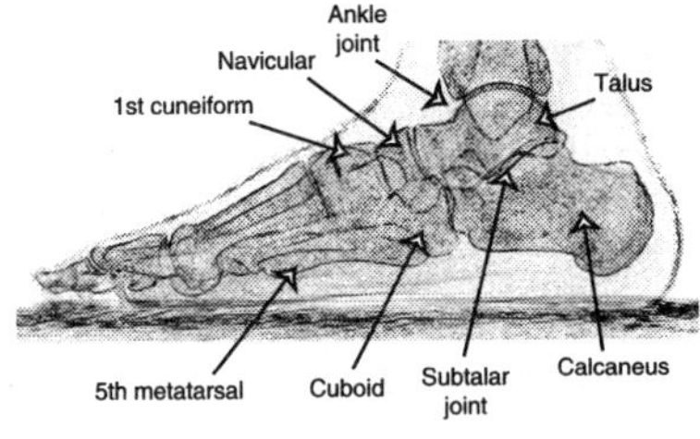

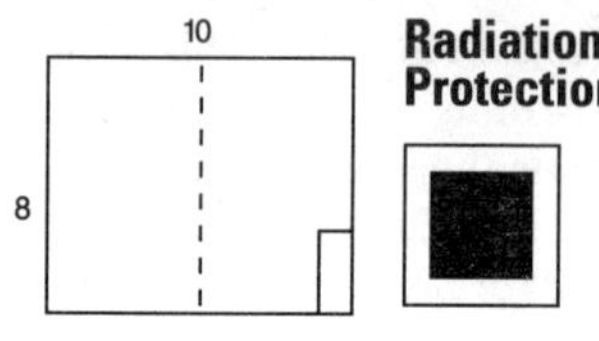

Technical Considerations
- Extremity screen/film
- Non-grid
- kVp range: 55–60
- SID: 40 inch (100 cm)

Patient Position Seated on the table with the knee extended; all potential artifacts, including shoe and sock, removed from the part.

Part Position With the heel centered to the unexposed portion of the cassette, adjust the foot so it is not rotated and dorsiflex the foot until the plantar surface is perpendicular to the cassette.

Central Ray 40° cephalic angle to the midpoint of the plantar surface of the foot at the level of the base of the third metatarsal.

Breathing Instructions Normal respiration.

Evaluation Criteria
- All of the calcaneus and the talocalcaneal joint should be visualized.
- Calcaneus should not be rotated as evidenced by the first and fifth metatarsals not being visible on either side of the foot.

Example Exposure Techniques **Measure at CR and Use Chart (p.42)**									
Room	**cm**	**kVp**	**mAs**	**mA**	**Sec**	**Beam**	**Film**	**Grid**	**1Ø3Ø**
	4								
	5								
	6								
	7								
	8								
	9								
	10								
	11								
	12								

Exam Rationale The most common indication for an examination of the heel is trauma. Structures demonstrated on the radiograph include the entire calcaneus and the talocalcaneal joint.

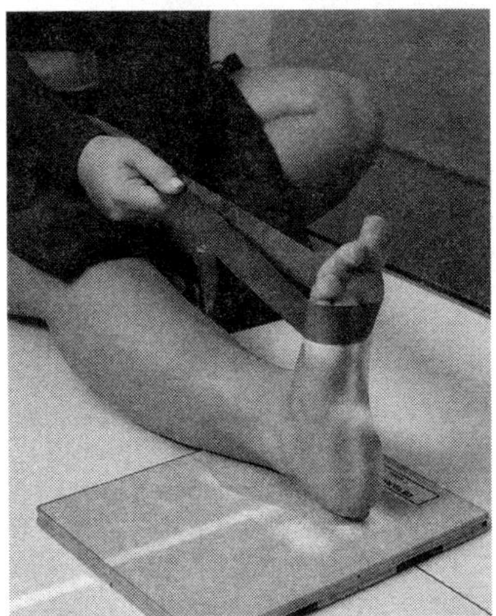

Tips

1. A gauze strip may be placed around the ball of the foot and held by the patient to assist in adjusting/maintaining the plantar surface perpendicular to the film.
2. The density should be appropriate to visualize the talocalcaneal joint without "burning out" the tuberosity of the calcaneus.

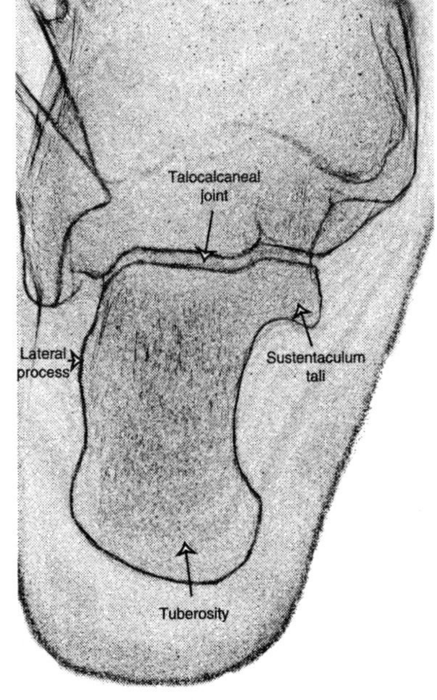

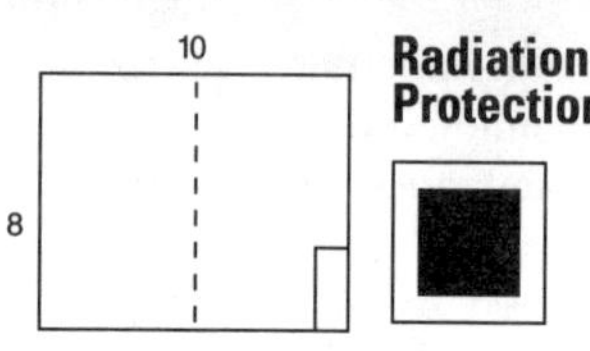

Technical Considerations
- Extremity screen/film
- Non-grid
- kVp range: 55–60
- SID: 40 inch (100 cm)

Patient Position Lateral recumbent on the affected side with the unaffected leg behind the affected leg; all potential artifacts, including shoe and sock, removed from the part.

Part Position With the heel centered to the unexposed portion of the cassette, dorsiflex the foot and rest its lateral surface on the cassette; adjust so the plantar surface is perpendicular to the cassette.

Central Ray Perpendicular to the midportion of the calcaneus (about 1 to 1 1/2 inches [3–4 cm] distal to the medial malleolus).

Breathing Instructions Normal respiration.

Evaluation Criteria
- Calcaneus should not be rotated.
- Sinus tarsi should be visualized.
- Ankle joint and adjacent tarsals should be included.

Example Exposure Techniques
Measure at CR and Use Chart (p.42)

Room	cm	kVp	mAs	mA	Sec	Beam	Film	Grid	1Ø3Ø
	5.0								
	6.0								
	7.0								
	8.0								
	9.0								

Exam Rationale The lateral shows the heel in profile and is used to demonstrate anterior/posterior displacements of bony pieces.

Tip Placing a support under the knee may be helpful in maintaining the foot in true lateral position.

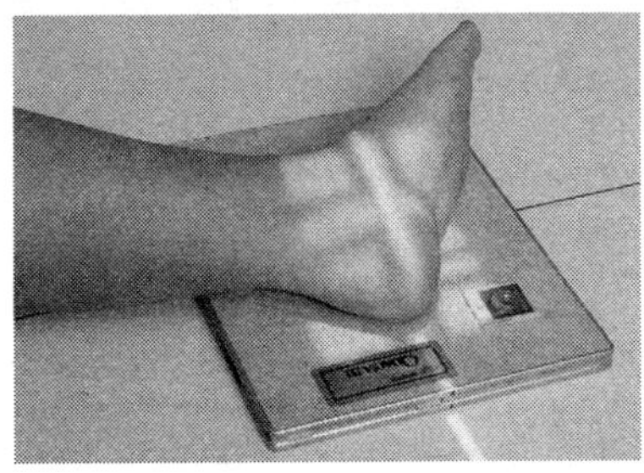

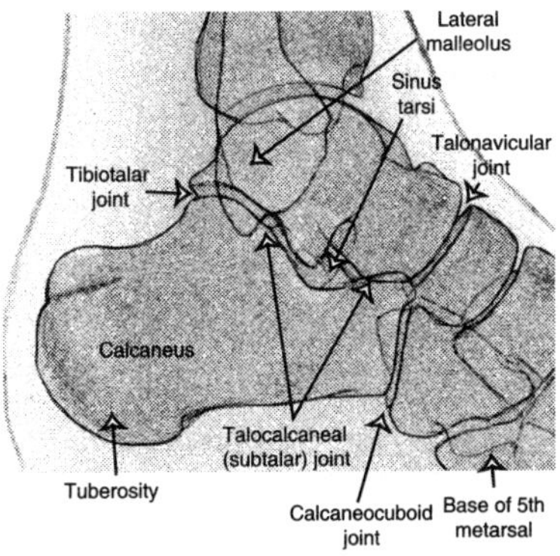

Technical Considerations

- Extremity screen/film
- Non-grid
- kVp range: 55–60
- SID: 40 inch (100 cm) 23

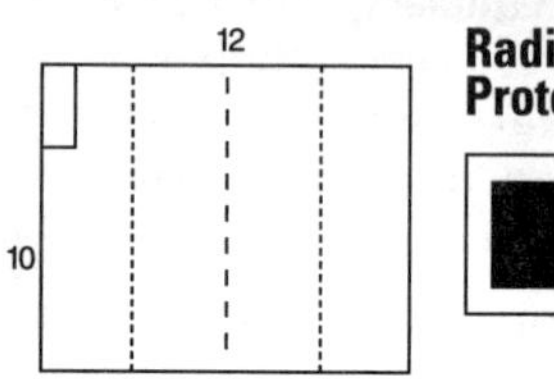

Patient Position Seated on the table with the knee extended; all potential artifacts, including shoe and sock, removed from the part.

Part Position With the heel positioned approximately 1 inch (3 cm) above the lower end of the cassette, dorsiflex the foot until its plantar surface is perpendicular to the cassette; with the ankle maintained at the right angle flexion, rotate the leg and foot medially approximately 45°.

Central Ray Directed to a point approximately 1 inch (3 cm) superoanteriorly to the lateral malleolus; four exposures are made with the central ray angled cephalad at 40°, 30°, 20° and 10°.

Breathing Instructions Normal respiration.

Example Exposure Techniques
Measure at CR and Use Chart (p.42)

Room	cm	kVp	mAs	mA	Sec	Beam	Film	Grid	1Ø3Ø
	6.0								
	7.0								
	8.0								
	9.0								
	10.0								

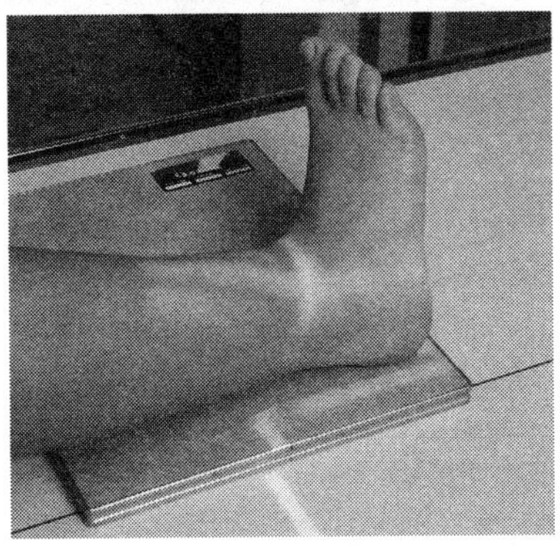

Evaluation Criteria

- All of the calcaneus and talocalcaneal joint should be visualized.

Exam Rationale An examination of the subtalar joint is indicated when joint involvement is suspected in cases of comminuted fractures. Structures demonstrated on the radiograph include the calcaneus and the talocalcaneus joint. The 40° angle best demonstrates the posterior articular facet of the calcaneus and the 10° angle the anterior articular facet; the articulation between the talus and sustentaculum is best demonstrated on one of the two intermediate angulations.

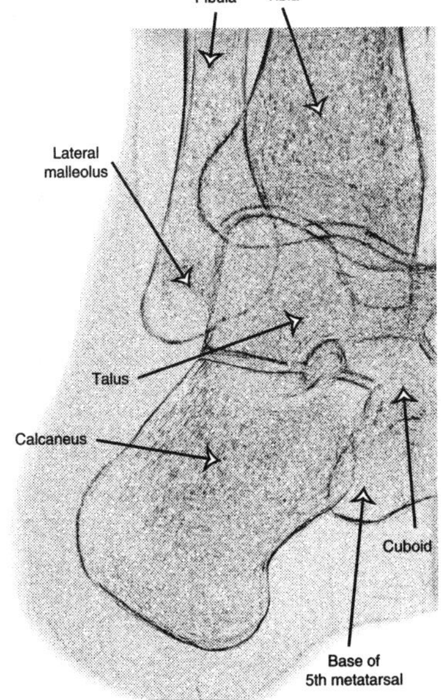

Tip A gauze strip may be placed around the ball of the foot to assist in adjusting/maintaining the plantar surface perpendicular to the film.

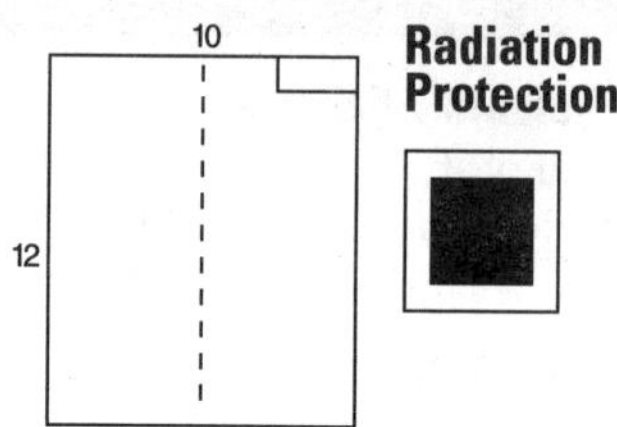

Technical Considerations

- Extremity screen/film
- Non-grid
- kVp range: 55–60
- SID: 40 inch (100 cm)

Patient Position Seated on the table with the knee extended; all potential artifacts, including shoe and sock, removed from the part.

Part Position Dorsiflex the foot so its plantar surface is perpendicular to the cassette; center the ankle to the unexposed portion of the cassette and adjust the foot so the ankle is in true AP position (intermalleolar plane will not be parallel with the film's surface).

Central Ray Perpendicular midway between the malleoli.

Breathing Instructions Normal respiration.

Evaluation Criteria

- Visualization of both the lateral and medial malleoli with moderate overlapping at the distal tibiofibular articulation.
- Visualization of the tibiotalar joint space with the medial tibiotalar articulation free of overlap.

Example Exposure Techniques **Measure at CR and Use Chart (p.42)**									
Room	**cm**	**kVp**	**mAs**	**mA**	**Sec**	**Beam**	**Film**	**Grid**	**1Ø3Ø**
	6.0								
	7.0								
	8.0								
	9.0								
	10.0								

Exam Rationale The most common indication for an examination of the ankle is trauma. Structures demonstrated on the AP projection include the distal tibia and fibula and the proximal portion of the talus.

Tip To visualize more of the tibia and fibula, position the ankle closer to the lower edge of the cassette; if the ankle joint is involved, the central ray should be directed through the ankle joint to prevent distortion of the joint space.

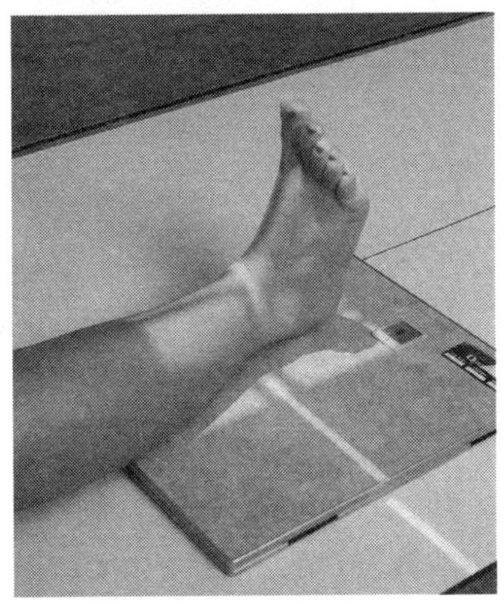

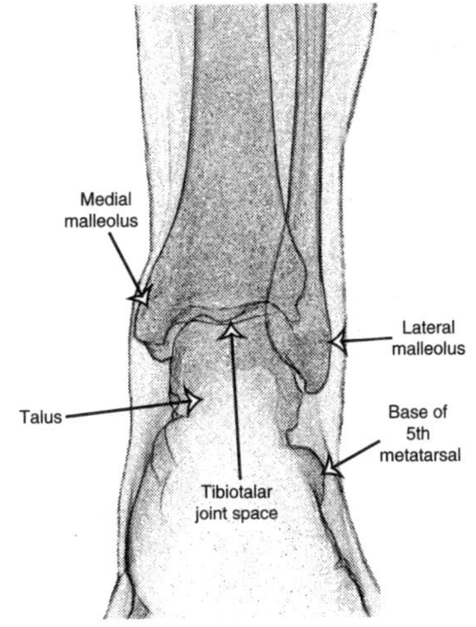

Technical Considerations

- Extremity screen/film
- Non-grid
- kVp range: 55–60
- SID: 40 inch (100 cm)

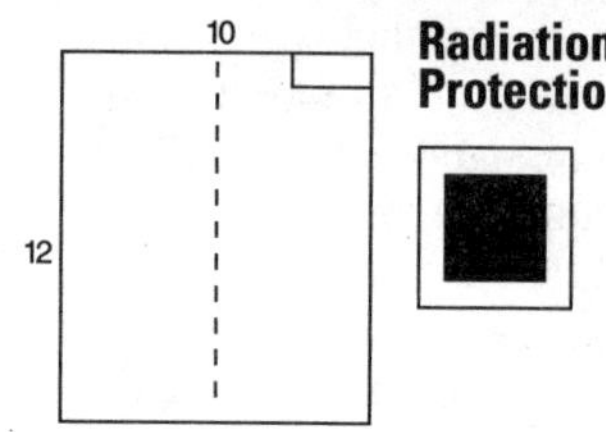

Patient Position Seated on the table with the knee extended; all potential artifacts, including shoe and sock, removed from the part.

Part Position Adjust the long axis of the ankle parallel with the long axis of the cassette and center the ankle to the unexposed portion of the cassette; rotate the entire leg and foot 45° and dorsiflex the foot to place its plantar surface perpendicular to the cassette.

Central Ray Perpendicular midway between the malleoli.

Breathing Instructions Normal respiration.

Evaluation Criteria

- Distal tibia and fibula should be somewhat overlapped.

Example Exposure Techniques **Measure at CR and Use Chart (p.42)**									
Room	**cm**	**kVp**	**mAs**	**mA**	**Sec**	**Beam**	**Film**	**Grid**	**1Ø3Ø**
	6.0								
	7.0								
	8.0								
	9.0								
	10.0								

Exam Rationale The oblique is a routine position of the ankle that gives a different perspective than that of the AP. Structures demonstrated on the radiograph include the distal tibia and fibula and the tibiotalar joint.

Tip To visualize more of the tibia and fibula, position the ankle closer to the lower edge of the cassette; if the ankle joint is involved, the central ray should be directed through the ankle joint to prevent distortion of the joint space.

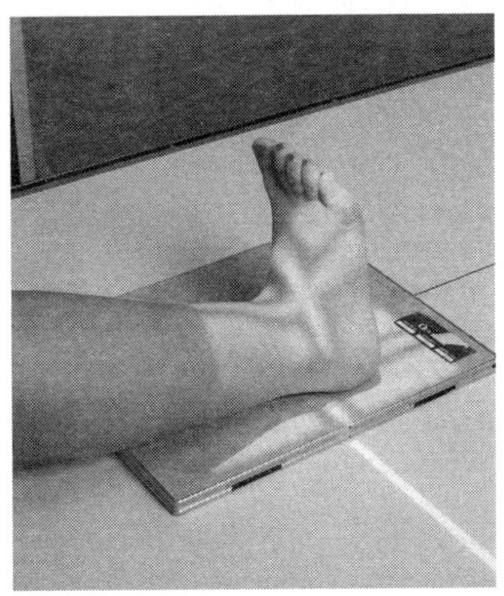

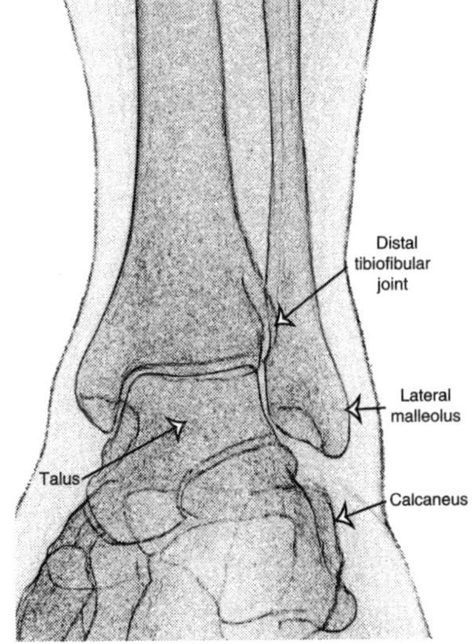

Technical Considerations

- Extremity screen/film
- Non-grid
- kVp range: 55–60
- SID: 40 inch (100 cm)

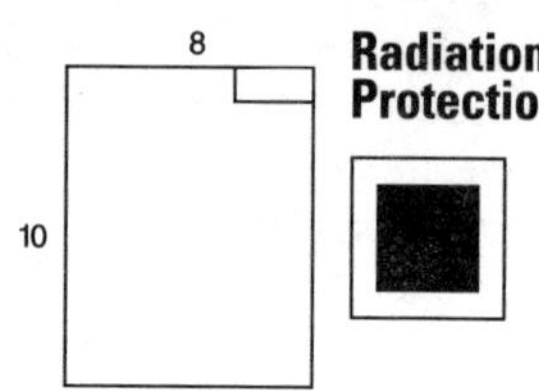

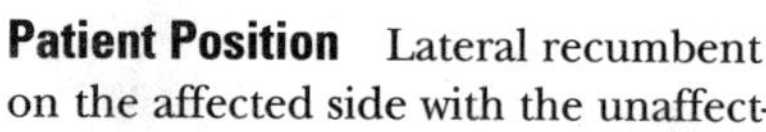

Patient Position Lateral recumbent on the affected side with the unaffected leg behind the affected leg; all potential artifacts, including shoe and sock, removed from the part.

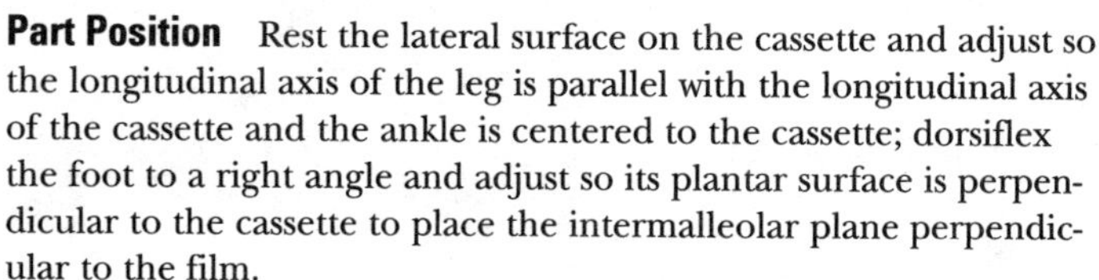

Part Position Rest the lateral surface on the cassette and adjust so the longitudinal axis of the leg is parallel with the longitudinal axis of the cassette and the ankle is centered to the cassette; dorsiflex the foot to a right angle and adjust so its plantar surface is perpendicular to the cassette to place the intermalleolar plane perpendicular to the film.

Central Ray Perpendicular to the medial malleolus.

Breathing Instructions Normal respiration.

Evaluation Criteria

- Fibula should be overlapped by the posterior tibia.

Example Exposure Techniques **Measure at CR and Use Chart (p.42)**									
Room	**cm**	**kVp**	**mAs**	**mA**	**Sec**	**Beam**	**Film**	**Grid**	**1030**
	5.0								
	6.0								
	7.0								
	8.0								
	9.0								

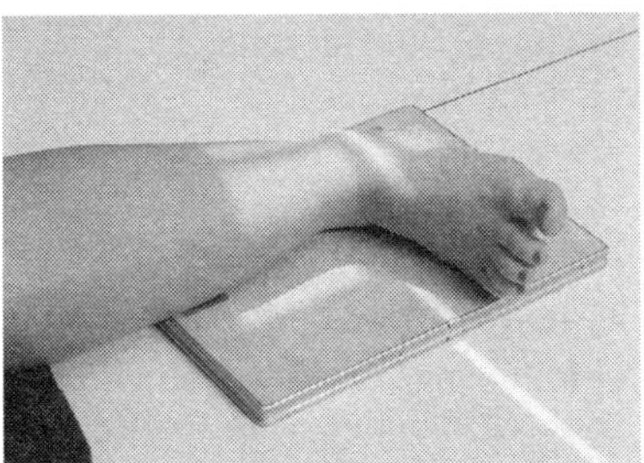

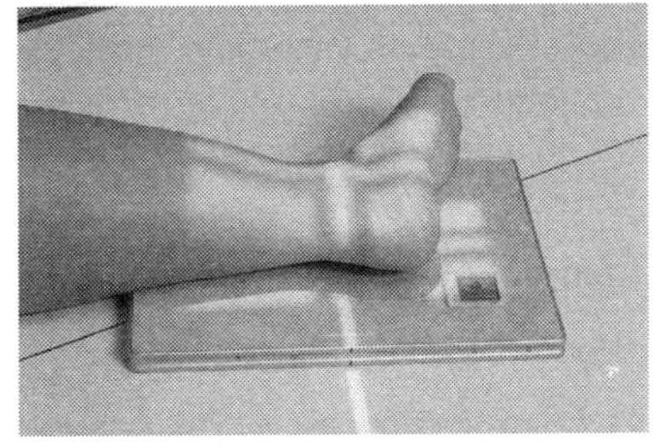

Exam Rationale The lateral, taken at 90° from the AP, is used to demonstrate anterior/posterior displacements of bony structures and to localize foreign bodies. Structures demonstrated on the radiograph include the distal tibia and fibula, the ankle joint, and the proximal tarsals.

Tips

1. Placing a support under the knee may be helpful in maintaining the foot in a true lateral position.
2. To visualize more of the tibia and fibula, position the ankle closer to the lower edge of the cassette; if the ankle joint is involved, the central ray should be directed through the ankle to prevent distortion of the joint space.
3. If patient condition permits, the patient can be placed in the lateral recumbent position on the unaffected side; the foot should rest on its medial surface (lateromedial) and should be adjusted so the plantar surface is perpendicular to the cassette. This provides a truer lateral view of the ankle joint and the distal tibia and fibula.

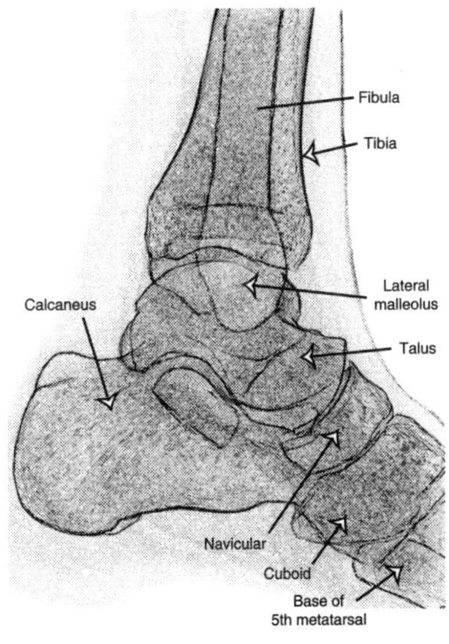

Technical Considerations

- Extremity screen/film
- Non-grid
- kVp range: 55–60
- SID: 40 inch (100 cm)

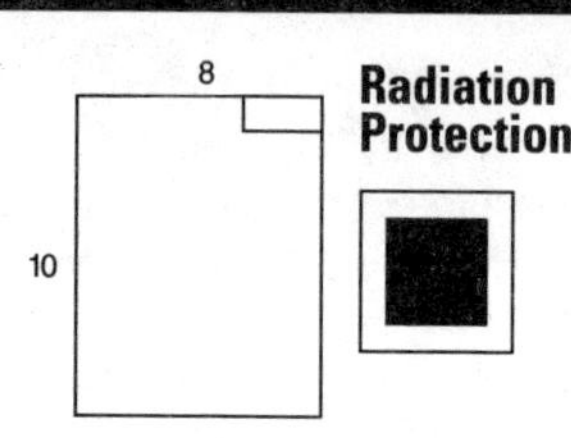

Patient Position Seated on the table with the knee extended; all potential artifacts, including shoe and sock, removed from the part.

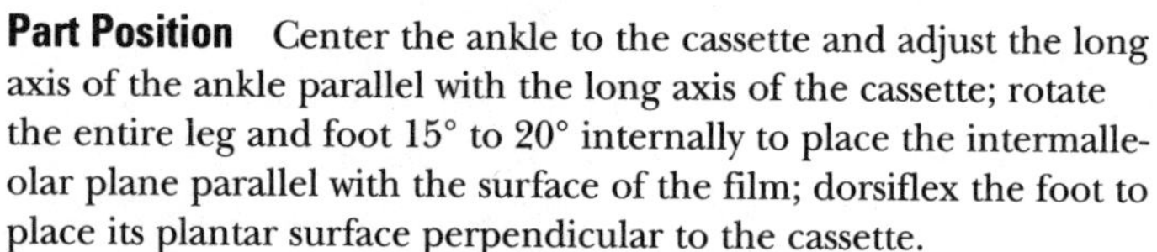

Part Position Center the ankle to the cassette and adjust the long axis of the ankle parallel with the long axis of the cassette; rotate the entire leg and foot 15° to 20° internally to place the intermalleolar plane parallel with the surface of the film; dorsiflex the foot to place its plantar surface perpendicular to the cassette.

Central Ray Perpendicular midway between the malleoli.

Breathing Instructions Normal respiration.

Evaluation Criteria

- Mortise joint should be projected free of both the tibia and fibula.

Example Exposure Techniques **Measure at CR and Use Chart (p.42)**									
Room	**cm**	**kVp**	**mAs**	**mA**	**Sec**	**Beam**	**Film**	**Grid**	**1Ø3Ø**
	6.0								
	7.0								
	8.0								
	9.0								
	10.0								

Exam Rationale This projection is an alternative view of the ankle that demonstrates the mortise joint free of superimposition of the talus or distal tibia and fibula.

Tip This view should supplement, not replace, a routine oblique projection of the ankle.

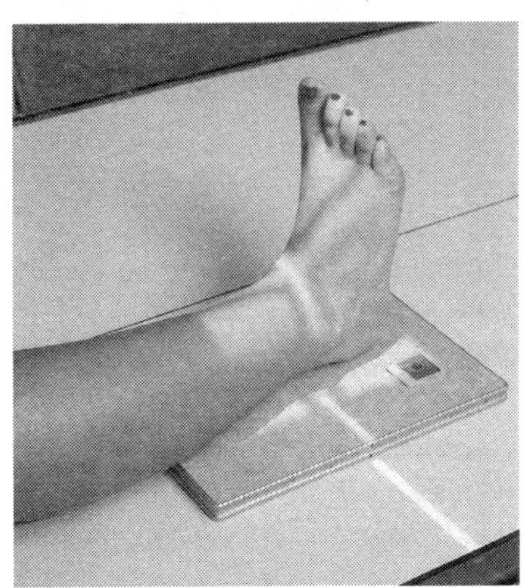

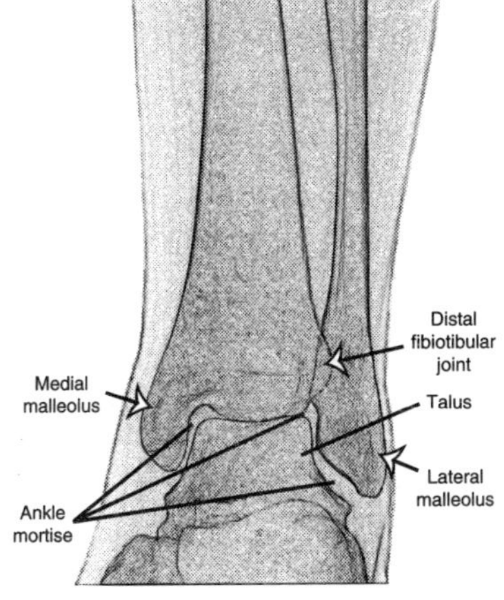

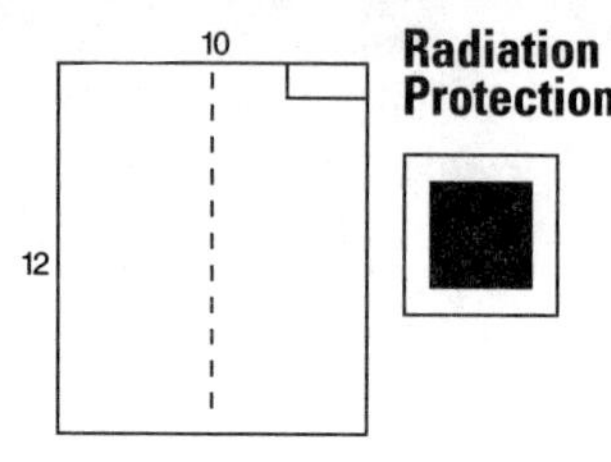

Technical Considerations

- Extremity screen/film
- Non-grid
- kVp range: 55–60
- SID: 40 inch (100 cm)

Patient Position Seated on the table with the knee extended; all potential artifacts, including shoe and sock, removed from the part.

Part Position With the ankle in the AP position, the foot is:

- Exposure 1: inverted as much as possible.
- Exposure 2: everted as much as possible.

Central Ray Perpendicular midway between the malleoli.

Breathing Instructions Normal respiration.

Evaluation Criteria

- Should include the distal tibia and fibula and talus.

Exam Rationale The most common indication for a stress study of the ankle is trauma resulting in a possible tear of ligaments.

Example Exposure Techniques
Measure at CR and Use Chart (p.42)

Room	cm	kVp	mAs	mA	Sec	Beam	Film	Grid	1Ø3Ø
	6.0								
	7.0								
	8.0								
	9.0								
	10.0								

Tips

1. If patient condition permits, a strip of gauze around the ball of the foot may be held by the patient and used to invert/evert the foot and maintain its position for the exposure.
2. For recent or very painful injuries, a local anesthetic may be required; placing and maintaining the foot in position is done by a physician or other health care personnel.

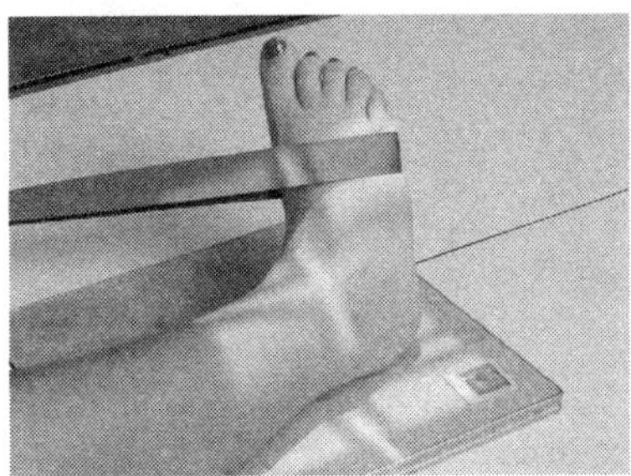

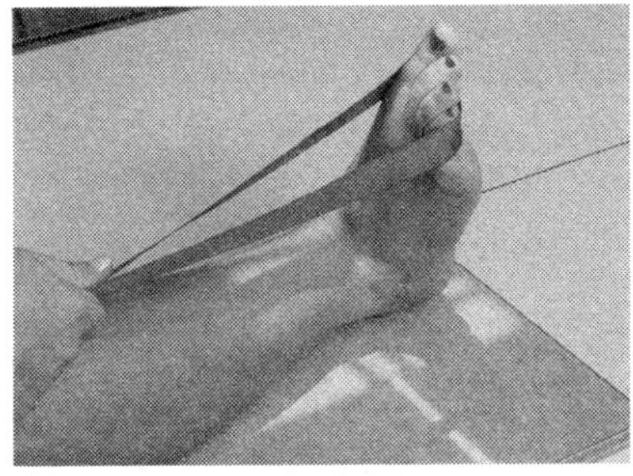

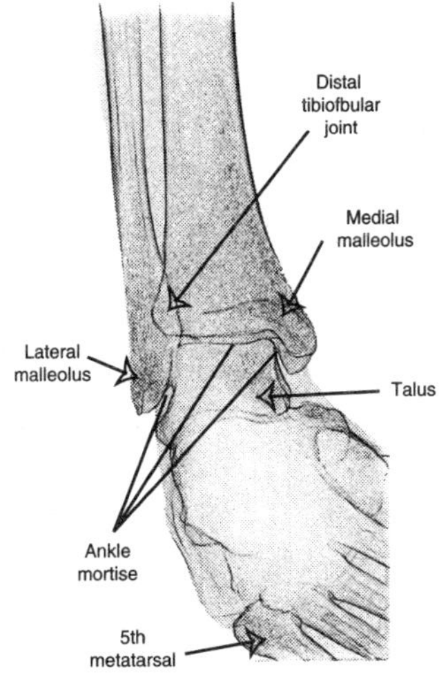

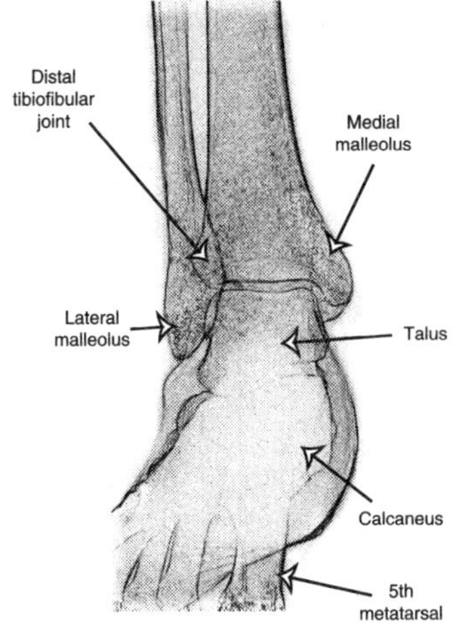

Technical Considerations

- Extremity screen/film
- Non-grid
- kVp range: 55–60
- SID: 40 inch (100 cm)

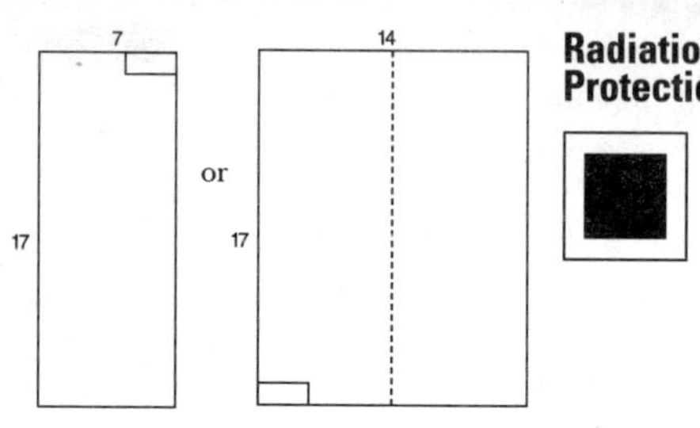

Patient Position

Seated on the table with the knee extended; all potential artifacts, including shoe and sock, removed from the knee down.

Part Position Center the leg to the cassette and adjust it into the AP position; dorsiflex the foot so it is perpendicular to the cassette.

Central Ray Perpendicular to the midpoint of the leg.

Breathing Instructions Normal respiration.

Evaluation Criteria

- Both the ankle and knee joints should be included; if necessary, a separate AP of one joint may be needed.
- Ankle and knee joints should be in true AP position.

Example Exposure Techniques **Measure at CR and Use Chart (p.42)**									
Room	**cm**	**kVp**	**mAs**	**mA**	**Sec**	**Beam**	**Film**	**Grid**	**1Ø3Ø**
	8								
	9								
	10								
	11								
	12								
	13								
	14								
	15								
	16								

- Tibia and fibula should be slightly overlapped at both the proximal and distal ends.

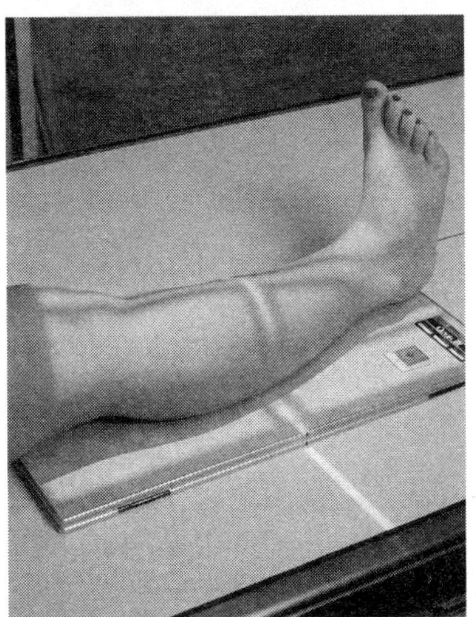

Exam Rationale The most common indication for an examination of the lower leg is trauma. Structures demonstrated on the radiograph include the tibia, fibula, and adjacent joints.

Tips

1. It may be necessary to invert the foot slightly to adjust the leg into the true AP position, but care must be taken to not rotate the entire leg.
2. It is important, on initial examination, to include both joints; some departmental protocols may permit follow-up examinations that include only the joint nearest the site of injury.
3. If the leg is too long to include both joints, the leg may be positioned diagonally on a 14 × 17 (36 × 43 cm) for each view.

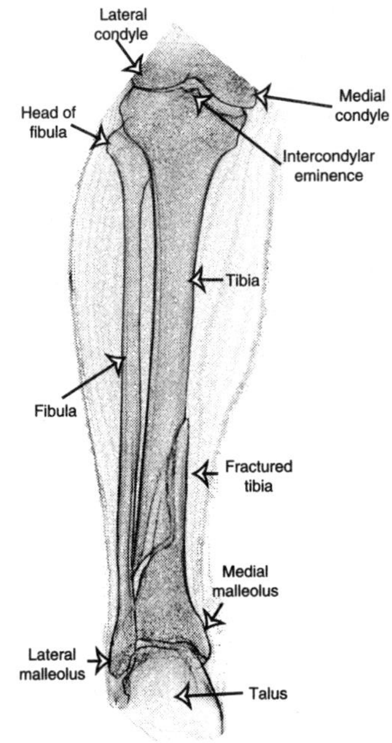

Technical Considerations

- Extremity screen/film
- Non-grid
- kVp range: 55–60
- SID: 40 inch (100 cm)

7

17

or

14

17

Radiation Protection

Patient Position

Lateral re-cumbent on the affected side with the unaffected leg behind the affected leg; all potential artifacts, including shoe and sock, removed from the knee down.

Part Position Dorsiflex the foot and rest the lateral surface of the leg on the cassette so the leg is centered to the cassette and the longitudinal axis of the leg is parallel with the longitudinal axis of the cassette; adjust the rotation of the leg so the patella is perpendicular to the cassette.

Central Ray Perpendicular to the midpoint of the leg.

Breathing Instructions Normal respiration.

Evaluation Criteria

- Both the ankle and knee joints should be included.
- There should be slight separation of the shafts of the tibia and fibula except at the proximal and distal ends.

Example Exposure Techniques
Measure at CR and Use Chart (p.42)

Room	cm	kVp	mAs	mA	Sec	Beam	Film	Grid	1Ø3Ø
	6								
	7								
	8								
	9								
	10								
	11								
	12								
	13								
	14								

- Proximally, there will be some overlap of the fibula and tibia.
- Distally, the fibula should overlap posterior tibia.

Exam Rationale The lateral, taken at 90° degrees from the AP, is used to demonstrate anterior/posterior displacements of bony structures. Structures demonstrated on the radiograph include the tibia, fibula, and adjacent joints.

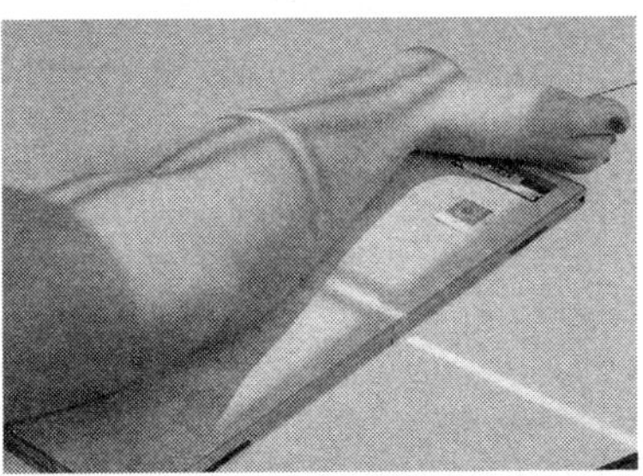

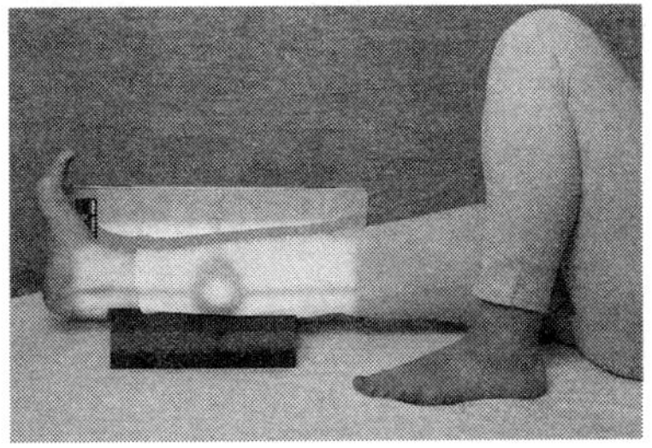

Tips

1. If patient condition does not permit turning the patient, a cross-table projection may be taken; the affected leg should be carefully lifted so that a firm support can be placed beneath it; the cassette is placed on the medial surface of the leg and the central ray directed from the lateral side.
2. It is important, on initial examination, to include both joints; some departmental protocols may permit follow-up examinations that include only the joint nearest the site of injury.
3. If the leg is too long to include both joints, it may be positioned diagonally on a 14 × 17 (36 × 43 cm) for each view.

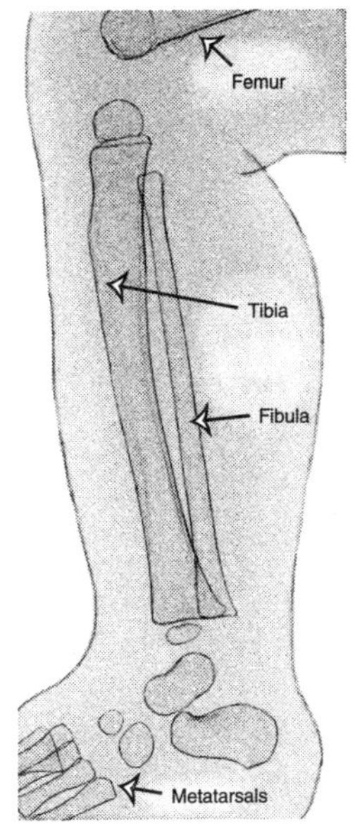

Technical Considerations

- Extremity screen/film
- Non-grid
- kVp range: 55–60
- SID: 40 inch (100 cm)

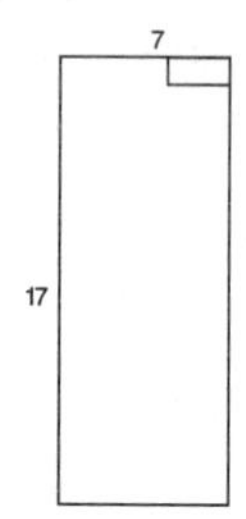

Radiation Protection

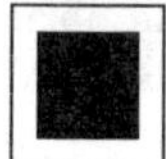

Patient Position Seated on the table with the knee extended; all potential artifacts, including shoe and sock, removed from the part.

Part Position Adjust the long axis of the leg so it is parallel with the long axis of the cassette; rotate the entire leg and foot 45° medially and dorsiflex the foot to place its plantar surface perpendicular to the cassette.

Central Ray Perpendicular to the midpoint of the leg.

Breathing Instructions Normal respiration.

Evaluation Criteria

- Both the ankle and knee joints should be included.
- Proximal and distal tibiofibular articulations should be visualized.
- Should demonstrate maximum space between the tibia and fibula.

Example Exposure Techniques **Measure at CR and Use Chart (p.42)**									
Room	cm	kVp	mAs	mA	Sec	Beam	Film	Grid	1Ø3Ø
	8								
	9								
	10								
	11								
	12								
	13								
	14								
	15								
	16								

Exam Rationale The oblique is an alternative position of the leg that is occasionally requested to demonstrate the tibiofibular articulations. Structures demonstrated on the radiograph include both the ankle and knee joints and the shafts of the tibia and fibula.

Tip Occasionally, a 45° external oblique may be requested; this will yield a radiograph that shows complete overlap of the tibia and fibula.

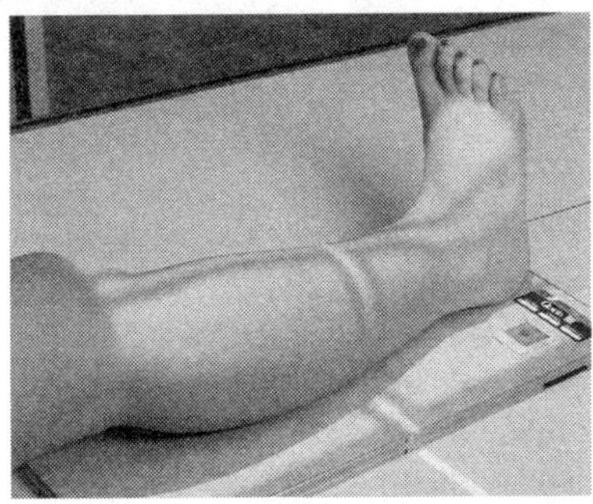

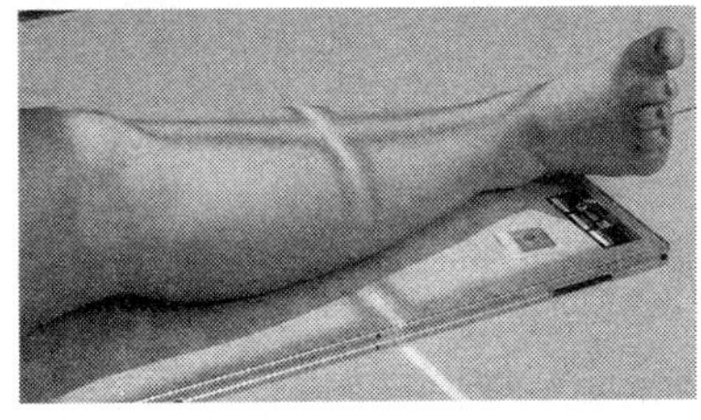

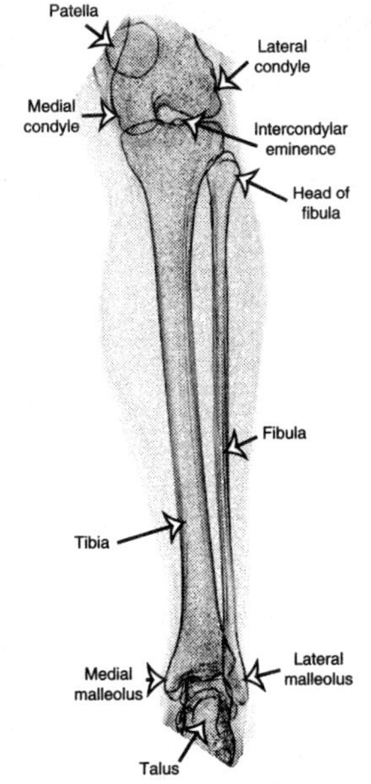

Technical Considerations

- Regular screen/film
- Grid
- kVp range: 60–70
- SID: 40 inch (100 cm)

10

12

Radiation Protection

AEC (Phototiming)

N DENSITY

Patient Position

Seated or supine on the table with the knee extended; all potential artifacts from the distal femur down removed.

Part Position Center the knee joint (1/2 inch distal to patellar apex) to the midline of the table and adjust the knee so the interepicondylar plane is parallel to the surface of the film; the patella will lie slightly to the medial side of the knee.

Central Ray One-half inch (1 cm) distal to the patellar apex at a 5° cephalic angle.

Breathing Instructions Normal respiration.

Evaluation Criteria

- Femur and tibia should be seen without rotation.
- Femorotibial joint space should be open.

Example Exposure Techniques **Measure at CR and Use Chart (p.42)**									
Room	**cm**	**kVp**	**mAs**	**mA**	**Sec**	**Beam**	**Film**	**Grid**	**1Ø3Ø**
	8								
	9								
	10								
	11								
	12								
	13								
	14								
	15								
	16								

- The head of the fibula will be slightly overlapped by the proximal tibia.
- Patella should be completely superimposed over the femur.
- In the normal knee, the femorotibial joint space should be equal on both sides.

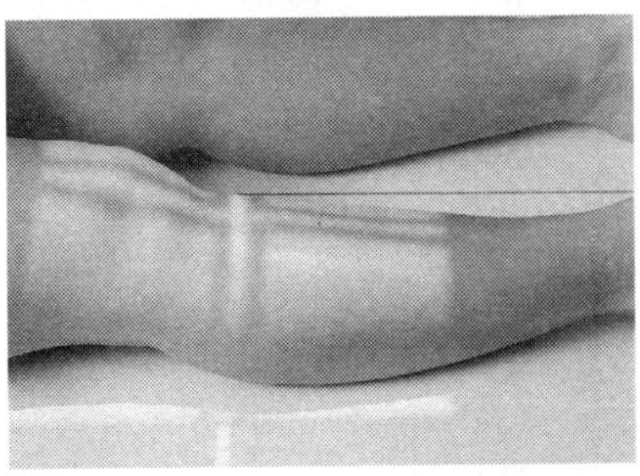

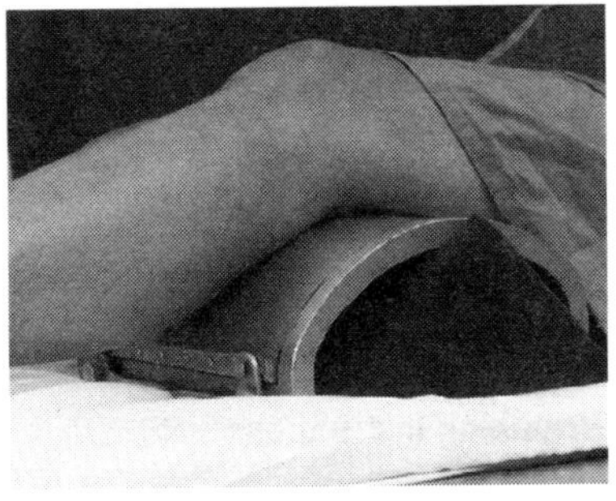

Exam Rationale

Radiographic examination of the knee is commonly indicated in cases of trauma or degenerative joint disease. Structures demonstrated include the knee joint, the proximal tibia and fibula, and the distal femur.

Tips

1. Non-grid method may be used for a knee that measures less than 11 cm.
2. When the primary interest is the distal femur or the proximal tibia and fibula, the central ray may be directed perpendicular through the knee joint.
3. In cases where the patient is unable to fully extend the knee, a curved cassette is recommended to reduce the part to image receptor distance.

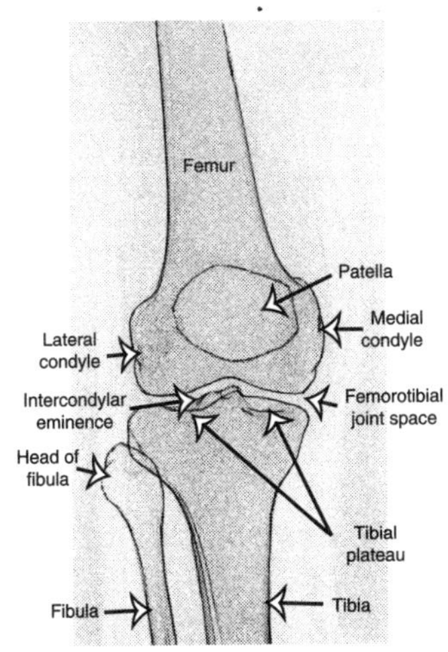

Technical Considerations

- Regular screen/film
- Grid
- kVp range: 60–70
- SID: 40 inch (100 cm)

10

12

Radiation Protection

AEC (Phototiming)

N DENSITY

Patient Position
Seated or supine on the table with the knee extended; all potential artifacts from the distal femur down removed.

Part Position With the knee centered to the midline of the table, rotate the affected leg 45° internally; this may require elevation of the hip on the affected side.

Central Ray 5° cephalic to the knee joint (1/2 inch/1 cm distal to patellar apex).

Breathing Instructions Normal respiration.

Example Exposure Techniques **Measure at CR and Use Chart (p.42)**									
Room	**cm**	**kVp**	**mAs**	**mA**	**Sec**	**Beam**	**Film**	**Grid**	**1Ø3Ø**
	8								
	9								
	10								
	11								
	12								
	13								
	14								
	15								
	16								

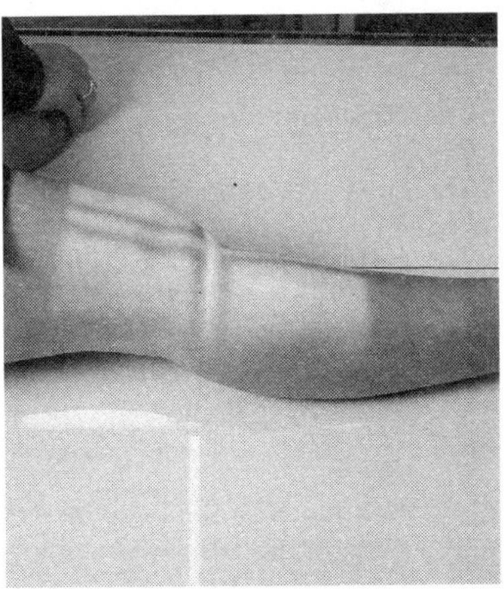

Evaluation Criteria

- Tibia and fibula should be separated at their proximal articulation.
- Lateral condyles of the femur and tibia should be visualized.
- Knee joint should be open.
- Both tibial plateaus should be visualized.
- Medial margin of the patella should be projected slightly beyond the medial margin of the femur.

Exam Rationale The oblique is an alternative position of the knee that is used to provide a different perspective from that of the AP and lateral. Structures demonstrated include the proximal tibia and fibula, the distal femur, and the knee joint. The internal oblique demonstrates particularly well the lateral femoral and tibial condyles, the lateral tibial plateau, and the head of the fibula.

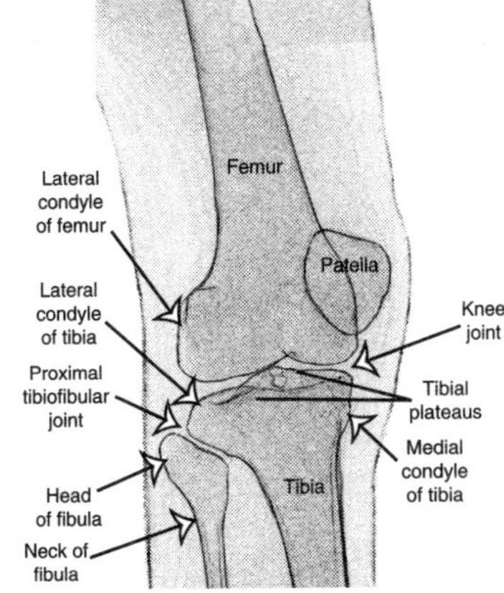

Tip Non-grid method may be used for a knee that measures less than 11 cm.

Technical Considerations

- Regular screen/film
- Grid
- kVp range: 60–70
- SID: 40 inch (100 cm)

10

12

Radiation Protection

AEC (Phototiming)

N DENSITY

Patient Position

Lateral recumbent on the affected side with the unaffected leg behind the affected leg; all potential artifacts from the distal femur down removed.

Part Position Rest the knee on its lateral surface and center it to the midline of the table; flex the knee 20° to 30° and adjust it so that the interepicondylar plane is perpendicular to the cassette.

Central Ray 5° cephalic to the knee joint (1/2 inch/1 cm distal to patellar apex).

Breathing Instructions Normal respiration.

Example Exposure Techniques
Measure at CR and Use Chart (p.42)

Room	cm	kVp	mAs	mA	Sec	Beam	Film	Grid	1Ø3Ø
	7								
	8								
	9								
	10								
	11								
	12								
	13								
	14								
	15								
	16								

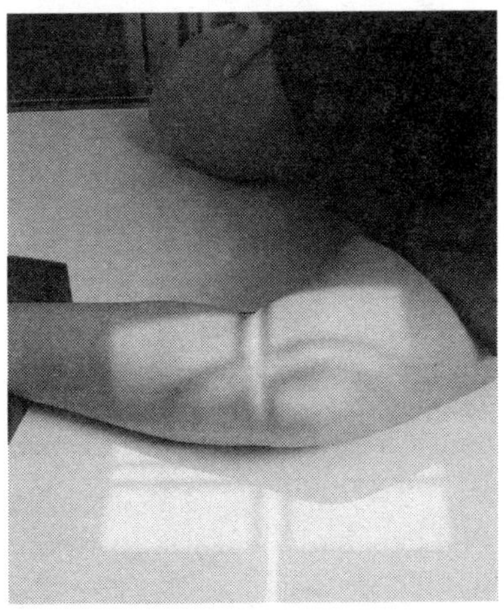

Evaluation Criteria

- Femoral condyles should be superimposed.
- Patella should be projected in profile.
- Femoropatellar space should be open.
- Fibular head and the tibia should be slightly superimposed.

Exam Rationale Structures demonstrated on the lateral projection of the knee include the distal femur, the proximal tibia and fibula, and the knee joint.

Tips

1. A support placed under the heel/ankle of the affected leg helps in maintaining the knee in true lateral position.
2. Non-grid method may be used for a knee that measures less than 11 cm.
3. In cases of patella fracture, the knee should be flexed no more than 15°.

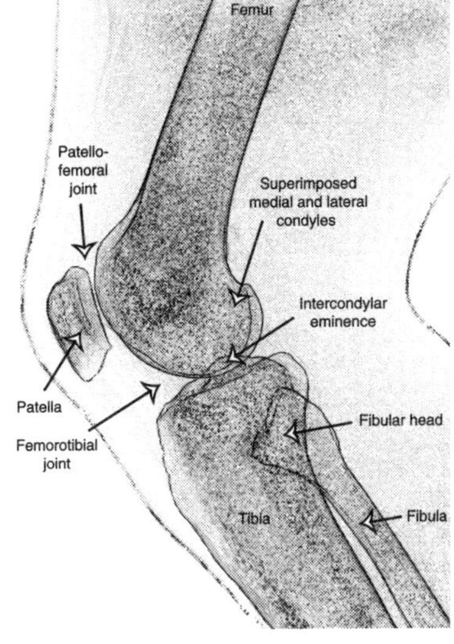

Technical Considerations

- Regular screen/film
- Grid
- kVp range: 60–70
- SID: 40 inch (100 cm)

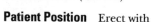

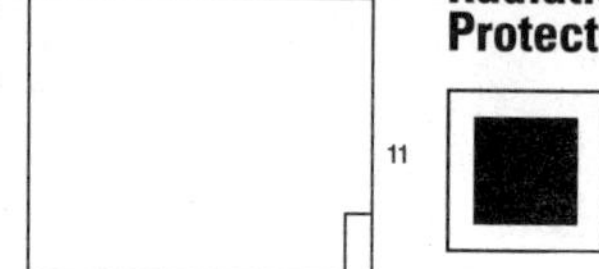

Patient Position Erect with the back toward a vertical grid device; the toes should be pointing forward and the feet separated sufficiently to achieve good balance (approximately 6– 8 inches [15–20 cm]); the patient should stand straight with the weight equally distributed on both feet; all potential artifacts from the distal femur down removed.

Part Position Center the patellar apices to the midline of the upright grid.

Central Ray Perpendicular to the film midway between the knees at the level of the patellar apices.

Breathing Instructions Normal respiration.

Example Exposure Techniques **Measure at CR and Use Chart (p.42)**									
Room	**cm**	**kVp**	**mAs**	**mA**	**Sec**	**Beam**	**Film**	**Grid**	**1Ø3Ø**
	8								
	9								
	10								
	11								
	12								
	13								
	14								
	15								
	16								

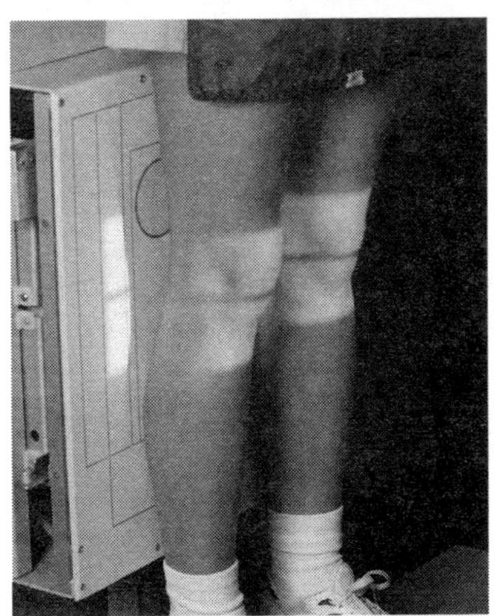

Evaluation Criteria

- Knees should not be rotated.
- Knee joint space should be centered to the exposed area of the film.

Exam Rationale Weight-bearing radiographic examination of the knee is commonly indicated in cases of degenerative joint disease. Structures demonstrated include the knee joint, the proximal tibia and fibula, and the distal femur.

Tip It is sometimes helpful in evaluating joint space narrowing to do a PA projection with the knees completely extended or with them flexed from 30° to 60°.

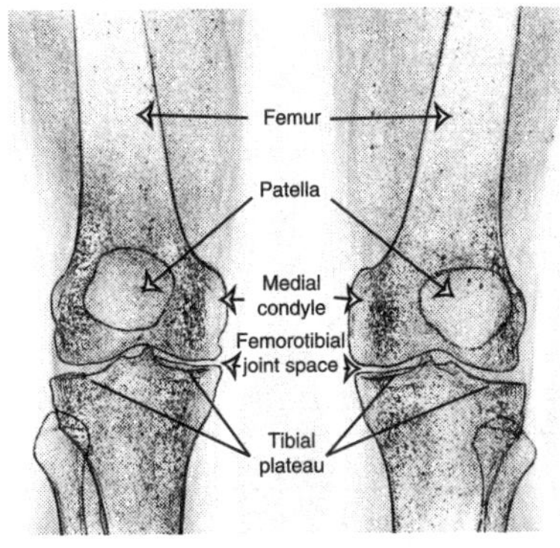

Technical Considerations

- Regular screen/film
- Grid
- kVp range: 60–70
- SID: 40 inch (100 cm)

10

12

Radiation Protection

AEC (Phototiming)

N DENSITY

Patient Position Seated or supine on the table with the knee extended; all potential artifacts from the distal femur down removed.

Part Position With the knee centered to the midline of the table, rotate the affected leg 45° externally.

Central Ray 5° cephalic to the knee joint (1/2 inch/1 cm distal to patellar apex).

Breathing Instructions Normal respiration.

Evaluation Criteria

- Fibula should be nearly completely superimposed by the lateral tibia.
- Medial condyles of the femur and tibia should be visualized.

Example Exposure Techniques
Measure at CR and Use Chart **(p.42)**

Room	cm	kVp	mAs	mA	Sec	Beam	Film	Grid	1Ø3Ø
	8								
	9								
	10								
	11								
	12								
	13								
	14								
	15								
	16								

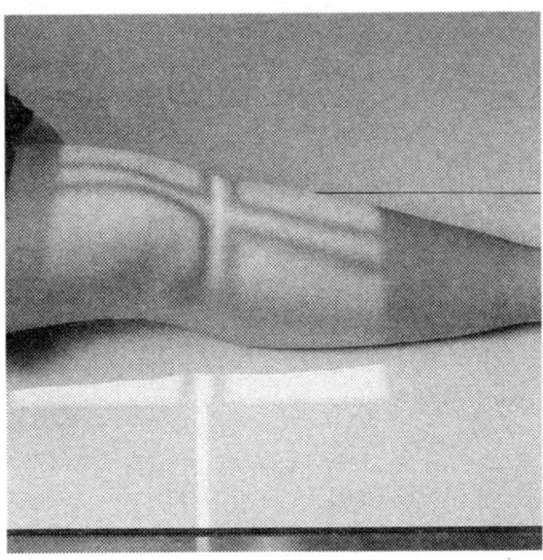

- Knee joint should be open.
- Both tibial plateaus should be visualized.
- Lateral margin of the patella should be projected slightly beyond the lateral margin of the femur.

Exam Rationale The oblique is an alternative position of the knee that is used to provide a different perspective from that of the AP and lateral. Structures demonstrated include the proximal tibia and fibula, the distal femur, and the knee joint. The external oblique demonstrates the medial femoral and tibial condyles and the lateral tibial plateau.

Tip Non-grid method may be used for a knee that measures less than 11 cm.

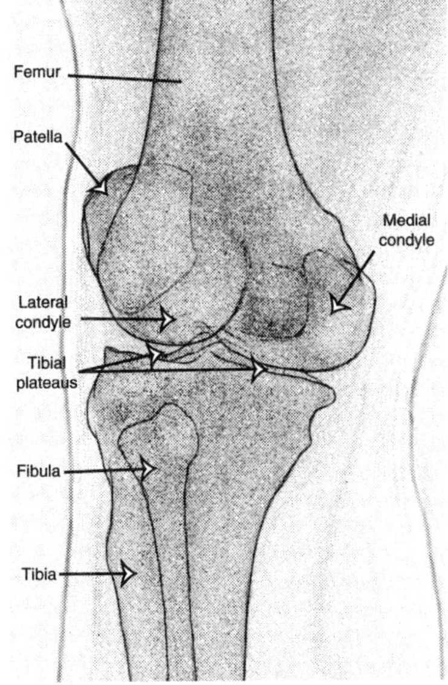

Technical Considerations
- Regular screen/film
- Grid
- kVp range: 60–70
- SID: 40 inch (100 cm)

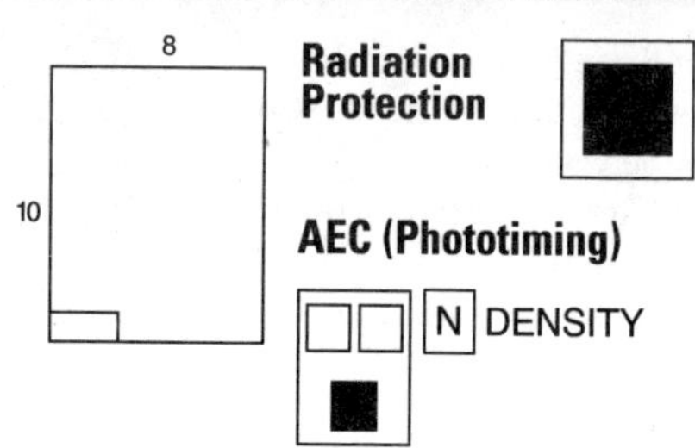

Patient Position Prone on the table with the knee extended; all potential artifacts from the distal femur down removed.

Part Position Center the patella to the midline of the table and adjust it so the patella is parallel with the plane of the film; this usually requires a 5° to 10° lateral rotation of the heel.

Central Ray Perpendicular to the knee joint (1/2 inch/1 cm distal to patellar apex).

Breathing Instructions Normal respiration.

Evaluation Criteria
- Femorotibial joint space should be open.
- Femur and tibia should not be rotated.

Example Exposure Techniques **Measure at CR and Use Chart (p.42)**									
Room	**cm**	**kVp**	**mAs**	**mA**	**Sec**	**Beam**	**Film**	**Grid**	**1Ø3Ø**
	8								
	9								
	10								
	11								
	12								
	13								
	14								
	15								

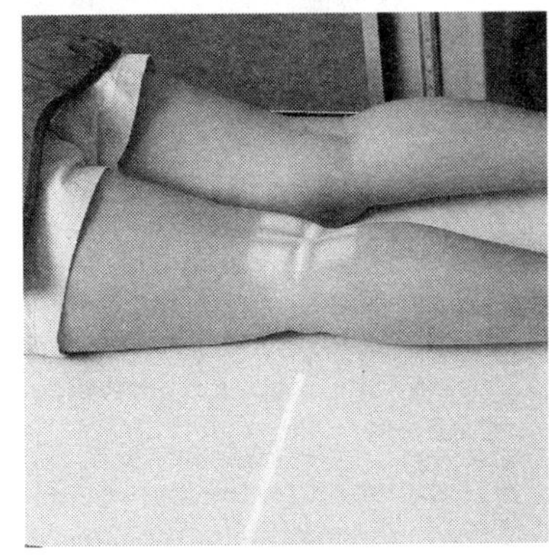

- The head of the fibula should be slightly overlapped by the proximal tibia.
- Patella should be completely superimposed over the femur.
- In a normal knee, the femorotibial joint space should be equal on both sides.
- Density should be sufficient for the patella to be visualized.

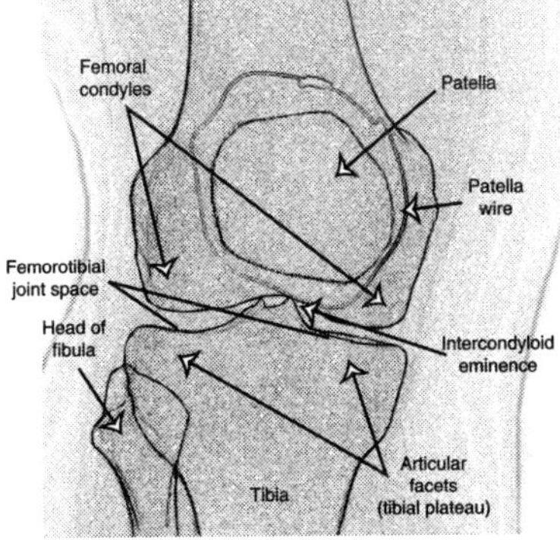

Exam Rationale

Radiographic examination of the patella is indicated in cases of trauma. Structures demonstrated include the proximal tibia and fibula, the distal femur, the knee joint, and the patella. The PA projection provides better detail than the routine AP projection of the knee.

Tip Non-grid method may be used for a knee that measures less than 11 cm.

Technical Considerations

- Regular screen/film
- Grid
- kVp range: 60–70
- SID: 40 inch (100 cm)

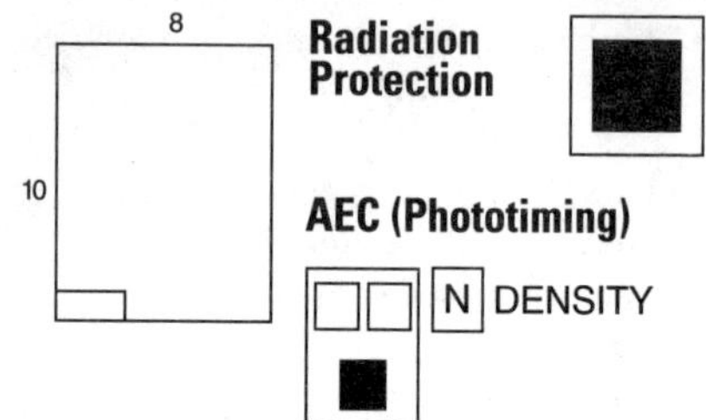

Patient Position Lateral recumbent on the affected side with the unaffected leg behind the affected leg; all potential artifacts from the distal femur down removed.

Part Position Rest the knee on its lateral surface and center the patella to the midline of the table; flex the knee 5° to 10° and adjust it so the interepicondylar plane is perpendicular to the cassette.

Central Ray Perpendicular to the femoropatellar joint space.

Breathing Instructions Normal respiration.

Evaluation Criteria

- Femoral condyles should be superimposed.
- Patella should be projected in profile.

Example Exposure Techniques
Measure at CR and Use Chart (p.42)

Room	cm	kVp	mAs	mA	Sec	Beam	Film	Grid	1Ø3Ø
	3								
	4								
	5								
	6								
	7								
	8								
	9								

- Femoropatellar space should be open.
- Fibular head and tibia should be slightly superimposed.

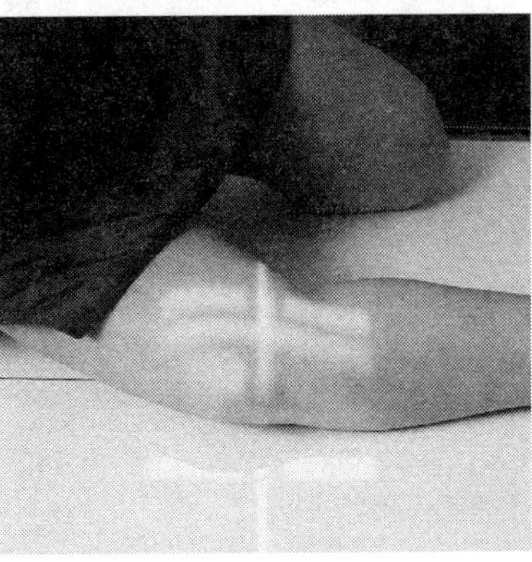

Exam Rationale Structures demonstrated on the lateral projection of the patella include the distal femur, the proximal tibia and fibula, the knee joint, and the patella in profile.

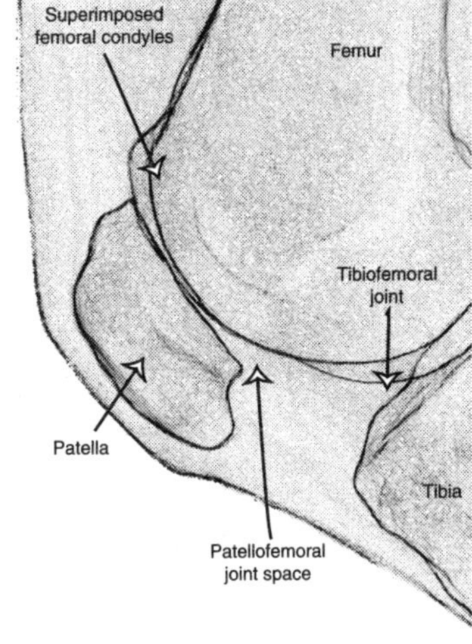

Tips

1. A support placed under the heel/ankle of the affected leg helps in maintaining the knee in true lateral position.
2. Non-grid method may be used for a knee that measures less than 11 cm.

Technical Considerations

- Extremity screen/film
- Non-grid
- kVp range: 55–60
- SID: 40 inch (100 cm)

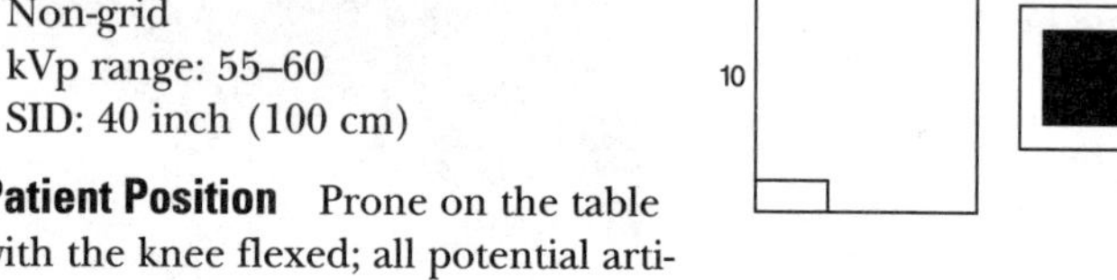

Radiation Protection

Patient Position Prone on the table with the knee flexed; all potential artifacts from the distal femur down removed.

Part Position Center the patella 2 to 3 inches from the lower edge of the cassette; slowly flex the knee until the patella is perpendicular to the cassette (approximately 100°).

Central Ray Perpendicular to the space between the patella and the femoral condyles; the degree of angulation will depend on the degree of flexion of the knee.

Breathing Instructions Normal respiration.

Evaluation Criteria

- Patellofemoral interspace should be open.
- Patella should be seen in profile.
- Femoral condyles should be visualized.

Example Exposure Techniques **Measure at CR and Use Chart (p.42)**									
Room	**cm**	**kVp**	**mAs**	**mA**	**Sec**	**Beam**	**Film**	**Grid**	**1Ø3Ø**
	3								
	4								
	5								
	6								
	7								
	8								
	9								

Exam Rationale Tangential positions of the patella are used to demonstrate patellar fracture or subluxation. Because of the danger of separation of fractured segments of the patella, this position should not be attempted until a lateral projection has been done to rule out a transverse fracture. This position is used to demonstrate vertical fractures and to evaluate the articulating surfaces of the femur and patella.

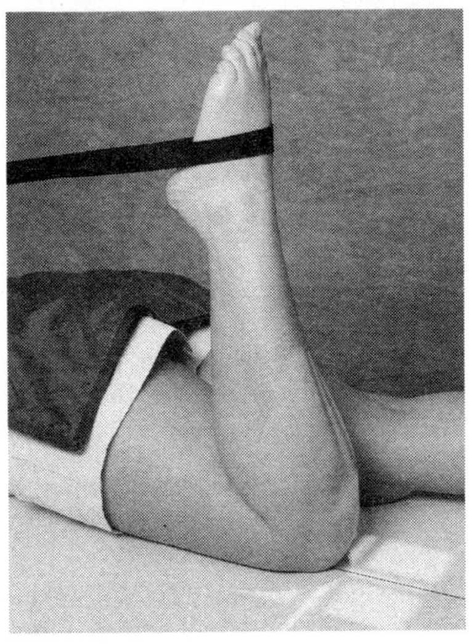

Tips

1. A gauze strip may be looped around the ankle and used to achieve/maintain the necessary flexion.
2. It is possible to obtain a similar radiograph with the patient in the supine, seated, or lateral position as long as the same part-film and tube-film relationships are maintained.

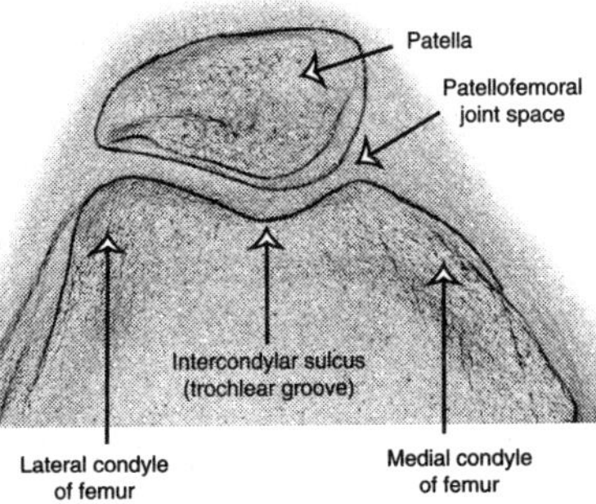

Technical Considerations

- Extremity screen/film
- Non-grid
- kVp range: 55–60
- SID: 40 inch (100 cm)

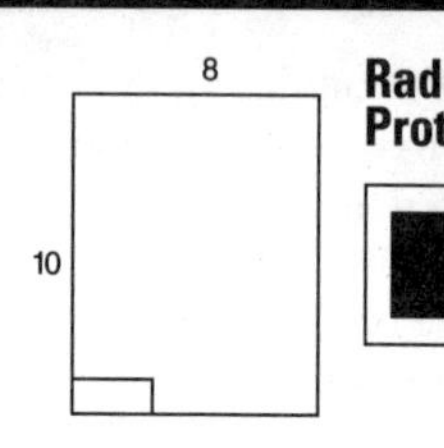

Radiation Protection

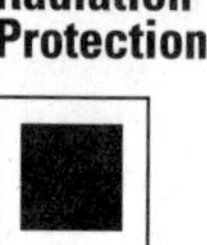

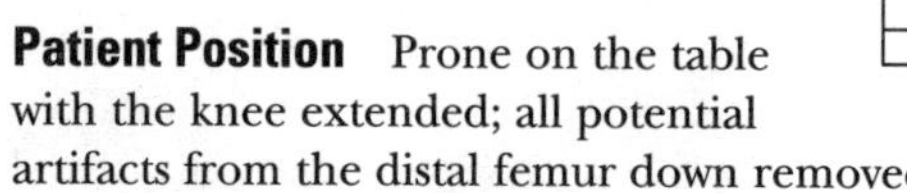

Patient Position Prone on the table with the knee extended; all potential artifacts from the distal femur down removed.

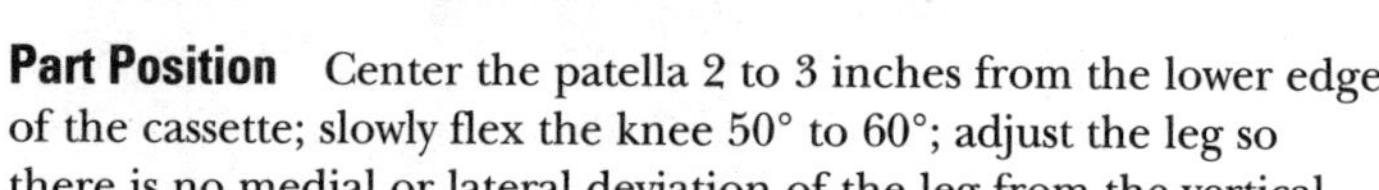

Part Position Center the patella 2 to 3 inches from the lower edge of the cassette; slowly flex the knee 50° to 60°; adjust the leg so there is no medial or lateral deviation of the leg from the vertical.

Central Ray 45° cephalic to the patellofemoral joint.

Breathing Instructions Normal respiration.

Evaluation Criteria

- Patellofemoral interspace should be open.
- Patella should be seen in profile.
- Femoral condyles should be visualized.

Example Exposure Techniques
Measure at CR and Use Chart (p.42)

Room	cm	kVp	mAs	mA	Sec	Beam	Film	Grid	1Ø3Ø
	3								
	4								
	5								
	6								
	7								
	8								
	9								

Exam Rationale Tangential positions of the patella are used to demonstrate patellar fracture or subluxation. This position demonstrates the patella; Hughston recommends that both knees be examined for comparison.

Tip The foot may be rested on the tube head for support but care must be taken that the surface is not too hot for patient comfort or safety.

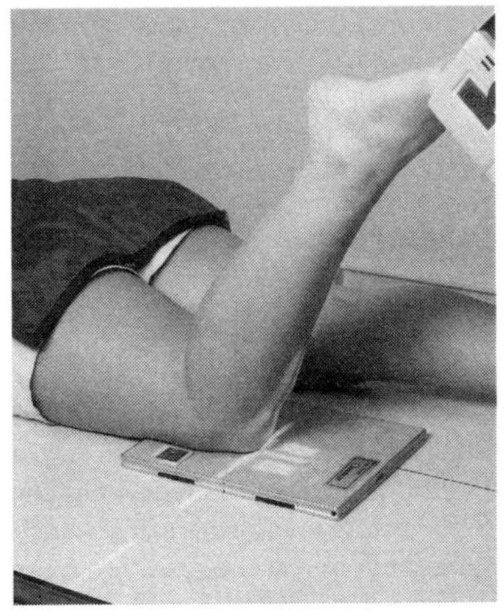

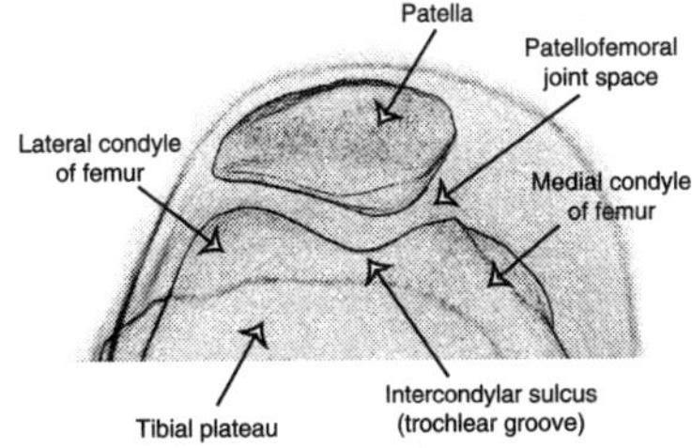

Technical Considerations

- Extremity screen/film
- Non-grid
- kVp range: 60–65
- SID: 72 inch (180 cm)

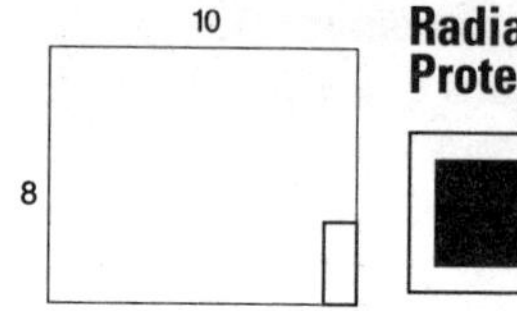

Patient Position Supine on the table with the knees flexed and the lower legs hanging off the end of the radiographic table; a special cassette holding device is required; all artifacts from the distal femur down removed.

Part Position Place the femora parallel to the table top by elevating the knees approximately 2 inches and flex the knees 45°; strap the legs together at the calf level to control rotation and help eliminate motion; rest the cassette on the shins perpendicular to them and approximately 1 foot distal to the patellae.

Central Ray Perpendicular to the cassette midway between the patellae at level of the patellofemoral joint.

Breathing Instructions Normal respiration.

Example Exposure Techniques
Measure at CR and Use Chart (p.42)

Room	cm	kVp	mAs	mA	Sec	Beam	Film	Grid	1Ø3Ø
	3								
	4								
	5								
	6								
	7								
	8								
	9								

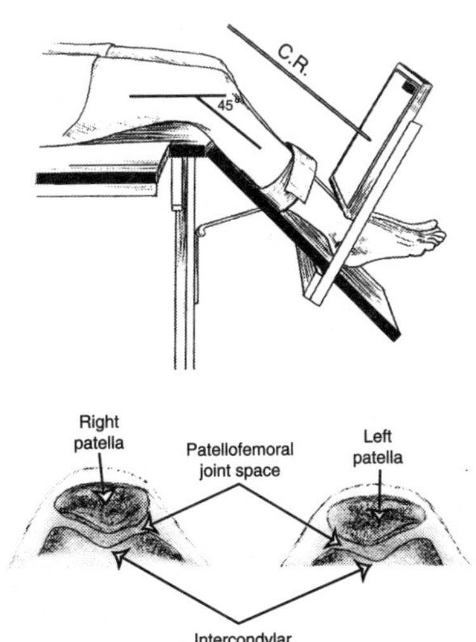

Evaluation Criteria

- Patellofemoral interspace should be open.
- Patella should be seen in profile.
- Femoral condyles should be visualized.

Exam Rationale Tangential positions of the patella are used to demonstrate patellar fracture or subluxation. This bilateral method demonstrates the patellae in profile and the patellofemoral joints.

Tips

1. Relaxation of the quadriceps femoris is important for accurate diagnosis because tightened muscles may pull the patella into the intercondylar sulcus, giving a false normal appearance.
2. The angle of flexion of the knee should be recorded so it can be reproduced in follow-up films because of the tendency of patellar subluxation to vary with variance in the angle of knee flexion.

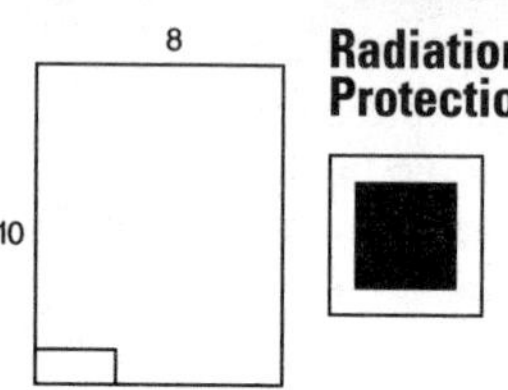

Radiation Protection

Technical Considerations
- Extremity screen/film
- Non-grid
- kVp range: 55–65
- SID: 40 inch (100 cm)

Patient Position Kneeling on the table with the knee flexed; all potential artifacts from the distal femur down removed.

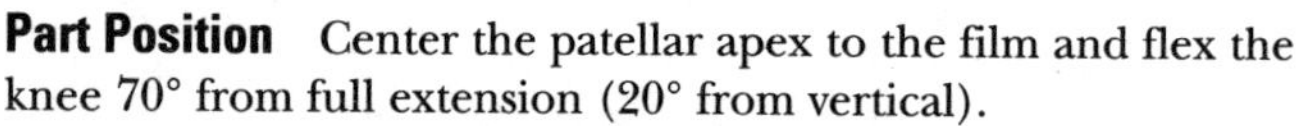

Part Position Center the patellar apex to the film and flex the knee 70° from full extension (20° from vertical).

Central Ray Perpendicular to the midpoint of the film.

Breathing Instructions Normal respiration.

Evaluation Criteria
- Fossa should be open and visualized.
- Apex of the patella should not be projected in the fossa.
- Posterior surface of the femoral condyles should be visualized.
- Leg should not be rotated as evidenced by slight overlap of the proximal tibia and fibula.

Example Exposure Techniques **Measure at CR and Use Chart (p.42)**									
Room	**cm**	**kVp**	**mAs**	**mA**	**Sec**	**Beam**	**Film**	**Grid**	**1Ø3Ø**
	8								
	9								
	10								
	11								
	12								
	13								
	14								
	15								
	16								

INTERCONDYLAR FOSSA—AXIAL PA PROJECTION (HOLMBLAD METHOD)

Exam Rationale

Radiographic examination of the intercondylar fossa is indicated in the evaluation of loose bodies in the joint and cartilage abnormalities. This position demonstrates the intercondylar fossa of the femur and the tibial spine.

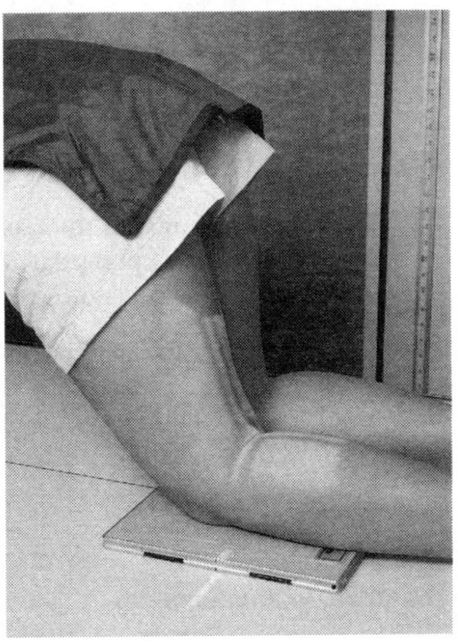

Tips

1. It is possible to obtain a similar view with the patient standing and resting the flexed knee on the cassette on stool or with patient standing with the flexed knee in contact with the film in front of the knee.
2. It is also possible to flex the knee at a 90° angle and use a 20° cephalic angle.

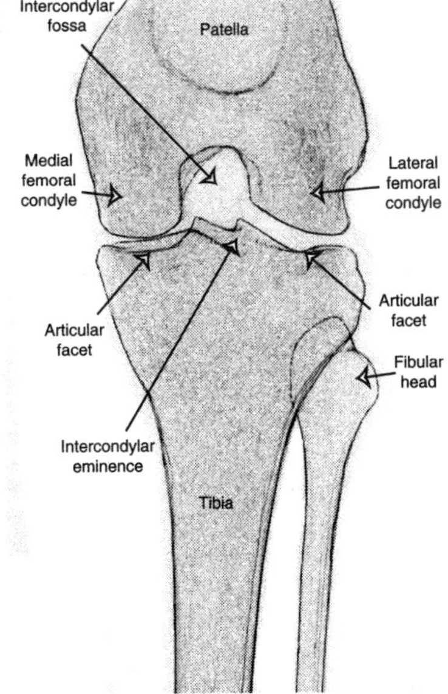

Technical Considerations
- Extremity screen/film
- Non-grid
- kVp range: 55–60
- SID: 40 inch (100 cm)

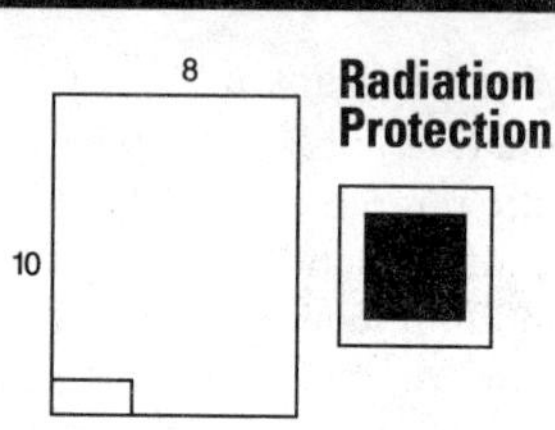

Patient Position Prone on the table with the knee flexed; all potential artifacts from the distal femur down removed.

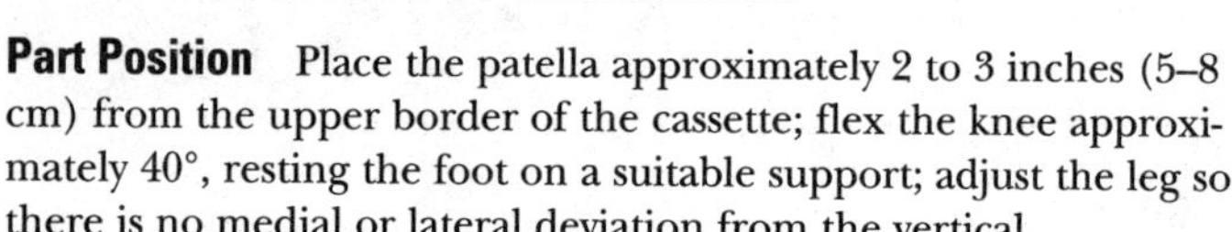

Part Position Place the patella approximately 2 to 3 inches (5–8 cm) from the upper border of the cassette; flex the knee approximately 40°, resting the foot on a suitable support; adjust the leg so there is no medial or lateral deviation from the vertical.

Central Ray Perpendicular to the long axis of the lower leg to the popliteal depression (50° caudad).

Breathing Instructions Normal respiration.

Example Exposure Techniques
Measure at CR and Use Chart (p.42)

Room	cm	kVp	mAs	mA	Sec	Beam	Film	Grid	1Ø3Ø
	8								
	9								
	10								
	11								
	12								
	13								
	14								
	15								
	16								

Evaluation Criteria

- Fossa should be open and visualized.
- Apex of the patella should not be projected in the fossa.
- Posterior surface of the femoral condyles should be visualized.
- Leg should not be rotated as evidenced by slight overlap of the proximal tibia and fibula.

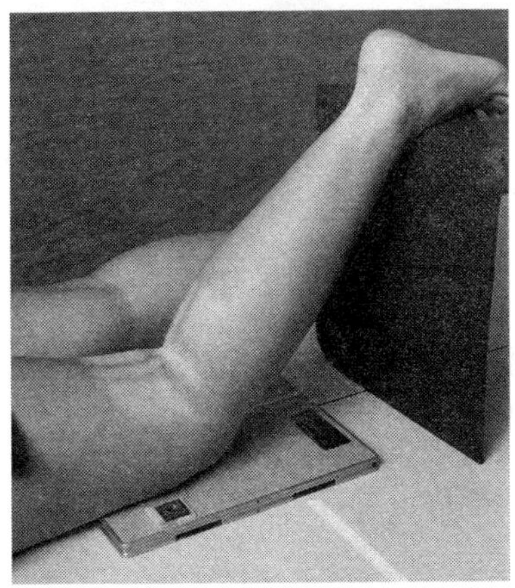

Exam Rationale

Radiographic examination of the intercondylar fossa is indicated in the evaluation of loose bodies in the joint and cartilage abnormalities. This position demonstrates the intercondylar fossa of the femur and the tibial spine.

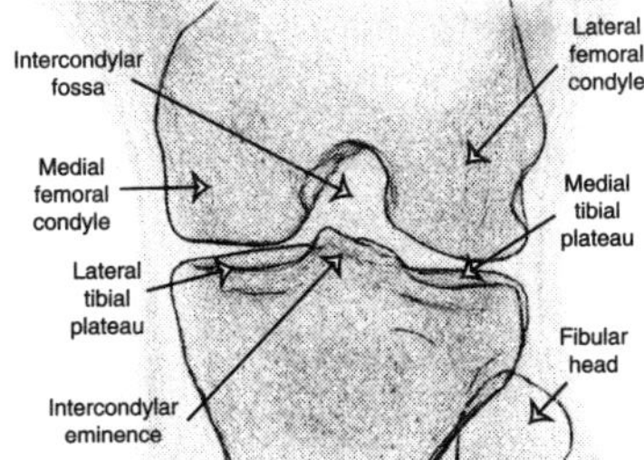

Technical Considerations

- Extremity screen/film
- A curved cassette is preferred to obtain closer part-film distance than is possible with a regular cassette.
- Non-grid
- kVp range: 55–65
- SID: 40 inch (100 cm)

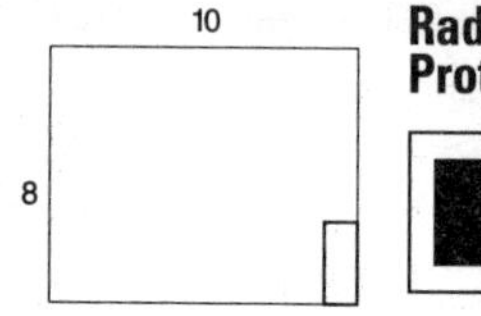

Patient Position Supine on the table with the knee flexed; all potential artifacts from the distal femur down removed.

Part Position Center the knee joint to the cassette; flex the knee enough to place the long axis of the femur at an angle of 60° to the long axis of the tibia.

Central Ray Perpendicular to the long axis of the lower leg to the knee joint.

Breathing Instructions Normal respiration.

Example Exposure Techniques **Measure at CR and Use Chart (p.42)**									
Room	**cm**	**kVp**	**mAs**	**mA**	**Sec**	**Beam**	**Film**	**Grid**	**1Ø3Ø**
	8								
	9								
	10								
	11								
	12								
	13								
	14								
	15								
	16								

Evaluation Criteria

- Fossa should be open and visualized.
- Apex of the patella should not be projected in the fossa.
- Posterior surface of the femoral condyles should be visualized.
- Leg should not be rotated as evidenced by slight overlap of the proximal tibia and fibula.

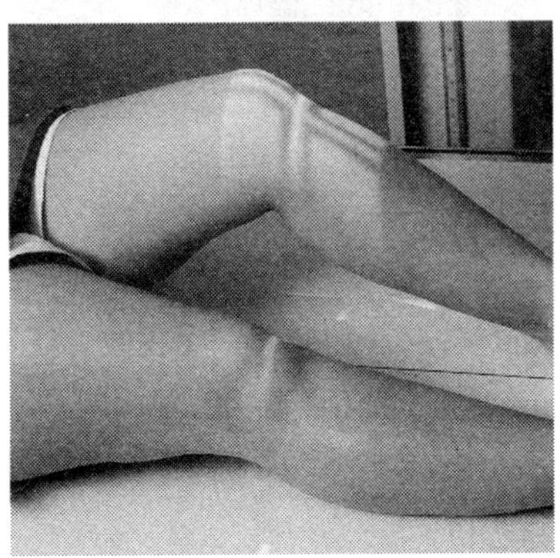

Exam Rationale

Radiographic examination of the intercondylar fossa is indicated in the evaluation of loose bodies in the joint and cartilage abnormalities. This position demonstrates the intercondylar fossa of the femur and the tibial spine.

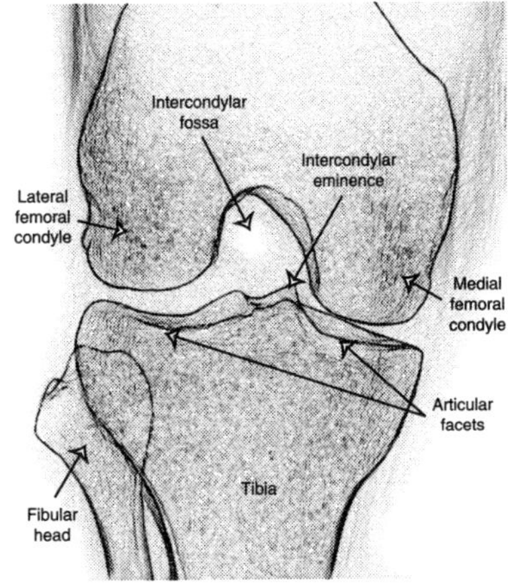

Technical Considerations
- Regular screen/film
- Grid
- kVp range: 70–80
- SID: 40 inch (100 cm)

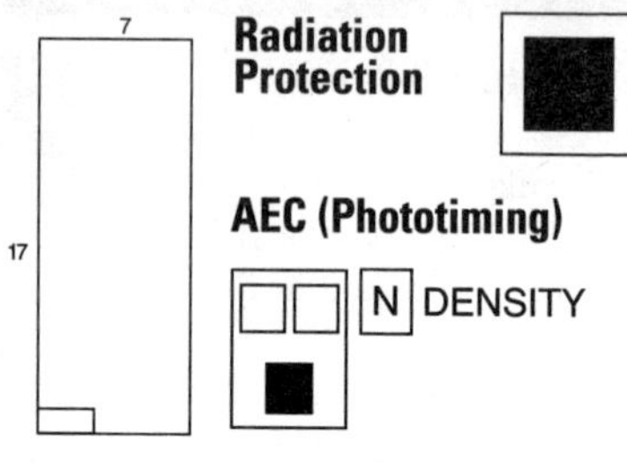

Patient Position Supine on the table with the knee extended; the patient should be dressed in a patient gown with all clothing from waist down removed.

Part Position Center the thigh to the midline of the table and position it to include both joints when possible or, if not possible, the joint nearest the site of injury or suspected pathology; adjust the femur into the AP position, with the interepicondylar plane parallel to the film, and internally rotate the foot approximately 15°.

Central Ray Perpendicular to the midpoint of the femur.

Breathing Instructions Suspend on inspiration.

Example Exposure Techniques **Measure at CR and Use Chart (p.42)**									
Room	**cm**	**kVp**	**mAs**	**mA**	**Sec**	**Beam**	**Film**	**Grid**	**1Ø3Ø**
	12								
	13								
	14								
	15								
	16								
	17								
	18								
	19								
	20								
	21								

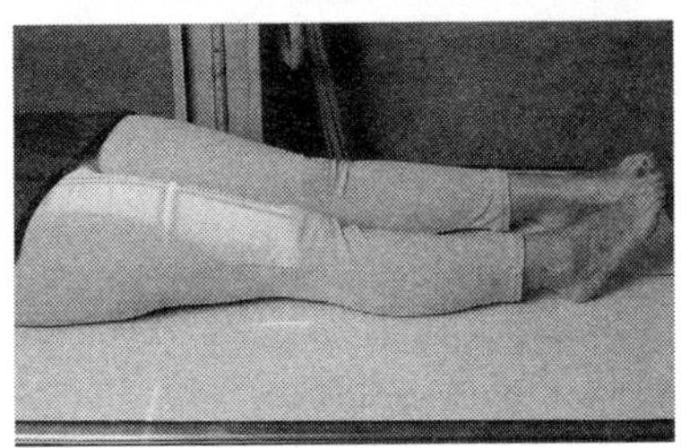

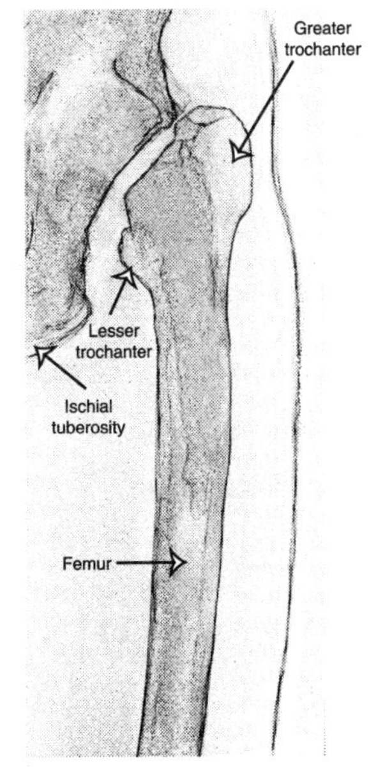

Evaluation Criteria

- Either the knee or hip joint (the one closest to the injury or suspected pathology) should be included; a separate AP of the other joint may be indicated.
- Little or none of the lesser trochanter should be visible beyond the medial edge of the femur.
- Any orthopedic appliance (e.g., surgical plate) should be seen in its entirety.

Exam Rationale The most common indication for an examination of the femur is trauma. Structures demonstrated on the AP projection include the entire length of the femur and the knee or hip joint or both.

Tip Automatic exposure control should not be used when an orthopedic appliance is in place.

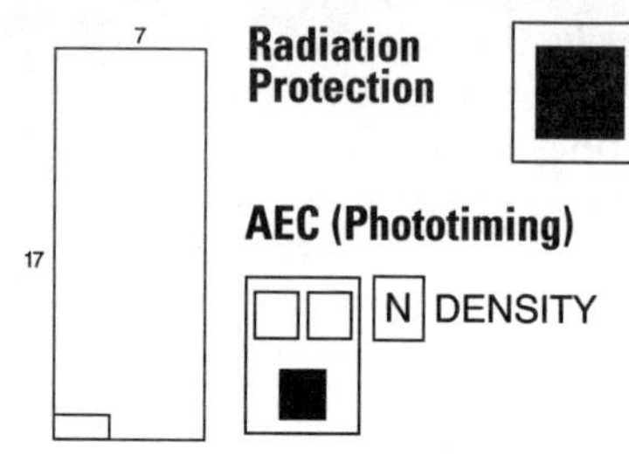

Technical Considerations
- Regular screen/film
- Grid
- kVp range: 70–80
- SID: 40 inch (100 cm)

Patient Position Lateral recumbent position on the affected side; if the proximal femur is the area of interest, the unaffected leg is placed behind the affected leg; if the distal femur is the area of interest, the unaffected leg is flexed and in front of the affected leg; the patient should be dressed in a patient gown with all clothing from waist down removed.

Part Position Flex the knee and center the thigh to the midline of the table and position it to include both joints when possible or, if not possible, the joint nearest the site of injury or suspected pathology; adjust the femur into the lateral position, with the interepicondylar plane perpendicular to film.

Central Ray Perpendicular to the midpoint of the femur.

Breathing Instructions Suspend on inspiration.

Example Exposure Techniques **Measure at CR and Use Chart (p.42)**									
Room	**cm**	**kVp**	**mAs**	**mA**	**Sec**	**Beam**	**Film**	**Grid**	**1Ø3Ø**
	11								
	12								
	13								
	14								
	15								
	16								
	17								
	18								
	19								
	20								

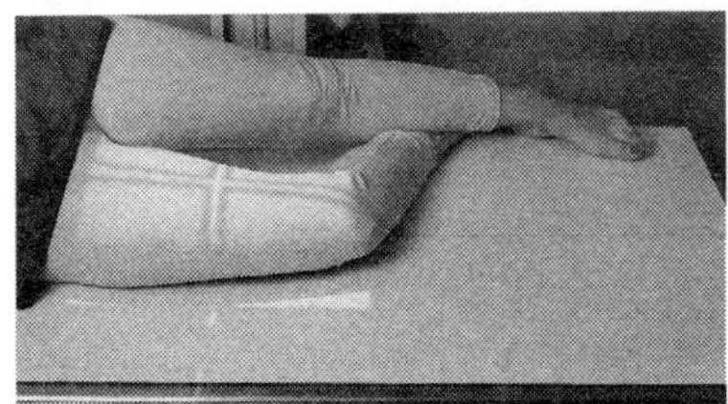

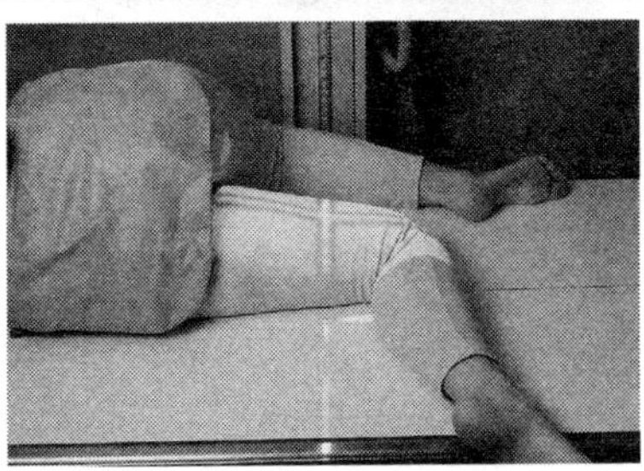

Evaluation Criteria

- Same joint(s) included on the AP should also be included on the lateral; a separate lateral of one joint may be indicated.
- Any orthopedic appliance (e.g., surgical plate) should be seen in its entirety.
- When the knee is included, it should meet the criteria identified in evaluating a lateral knee.
- When the hip is included, the thigh of the unaffected leg should not overlap the area of interest.

Exam Rationale Structures demonstrated on the radiograph include the entire length of the femur and the knee or hip joint or both.

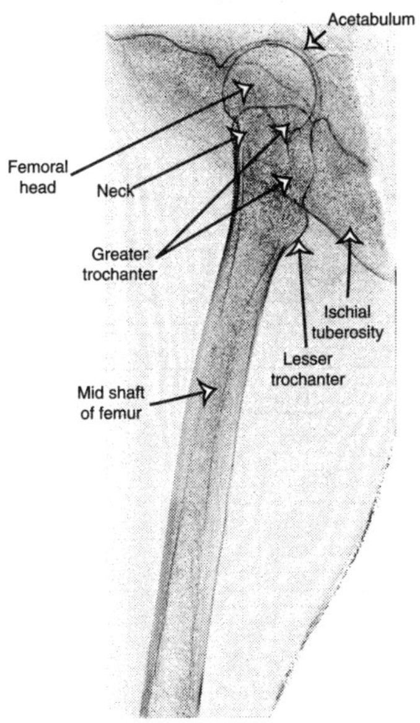

Tips

1. The regular lateral position should not be used when a fracture is suspected because of the possibility of displacing fragments; a translateral should be done instead.
2. Automatic exposure control should not be used when an orthopedic appliance is in place.

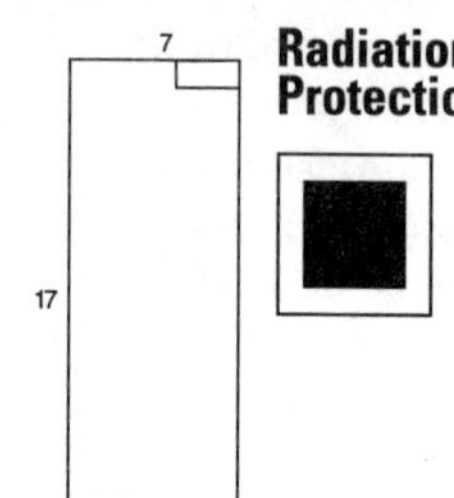

Technical Considerations

- Regular screen/film
- Non-grid
- kVp range: 70–80
- SID: 40 inch (100 cm)

Patient Position Supine on the table; the patient should be dressed in a patient gown with all clothing from the waist down removed; the cassette is placed on the lateral surface of the leg and the central ray directed horizontally from the medial side.

Part Position The knee of the affected leg should be extended.

Central Ray To the midpoint of the film.

Breathing Instructions Suspend on inspiration.

Evaluation Criteria

- Knee joint should be included.

Example Exposure Techniques
Measure at CR and Use Chart (p.42)

Room	cm	kVp	mAs	mA	Sec	Beam	Film	Grid	1Ø3Ø
	11								
	12								
	13								
	14								
	15								
	16								
	17								
	18								
	19								
	20								

Exam Rationale This lateral position of the femur is indicated when the patient's condition contraindicates turning the patient for a routine lateral. It demonstrates the length of the femur and the knee joint.

Tip If the proximal femur is the primary area of interest, it is necessary to do a superoinferior view of the hip joint.

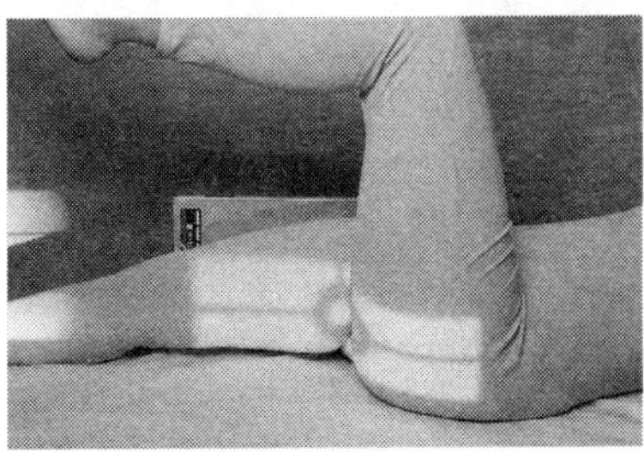

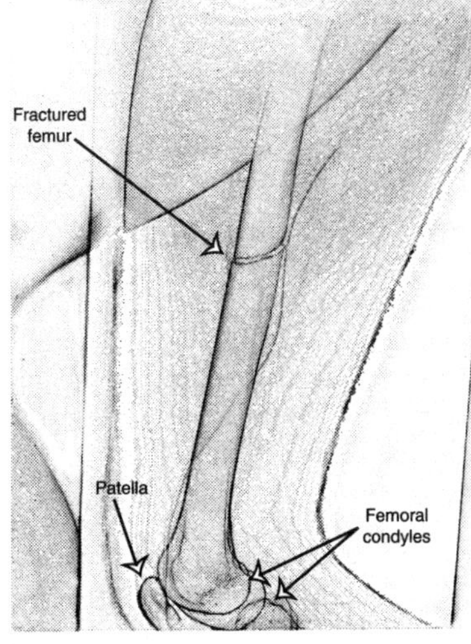

Technical Considerations

- Regular screen/film
- Grid
- kVp range: 85–90
- SID: 40 inch (100 cm)

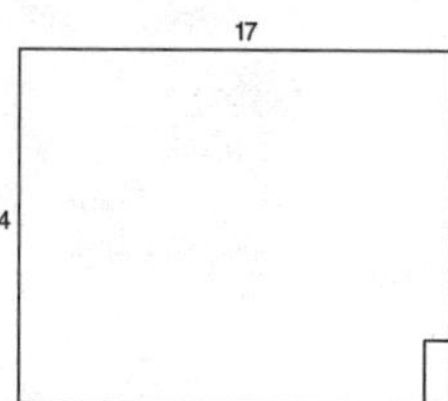

Radiation Protection

(for males). Gonadal shielding not possible for female patients.

AEC (Phototiming)

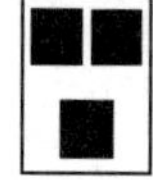

N DENSITY

Patient Position

Supine on the table; the patient should be dressed in a patient gown with clothing from the waist down removed.

Part Position The midsagittal plane of the body should be centered to the midline of the table; the shoulders should be adjusted to lie in the same transverse plane and the elbows should be flexed with the hands resting on the upper chest; the pelvis should be adjusted to that it is not rotated (distance from anterior superior iliac spine and table top is the same on both sides); the feet should be internally rotated approximately 15°; cassette should be positioned so that its upper border is 1 to 1 1/2 inches (3–4 cm) above the iliac crest.

Example Exposure Techniques **Measure at CR and Use Chart (p.24)**									
Room	**cm**	**kVp**	**mAs**	**mA**	**Sec**	**Beam**	**Film**	**Grid**	**1Ø3Ø**
	15								
	16								
	17								
	18								
	19								
	20								
	21								
	22								
	23								
	24								

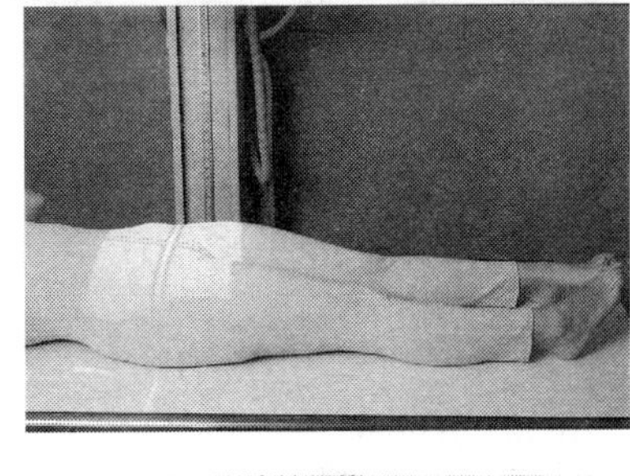

Central Ray Perpendicular to the midpoint of the film (approximately 2 inches superior to symphysis pubis).

Breathing Instructions
Suspend on inspiration.

Evaluation Criteria

- Entire pelvis and proximal femora should be visualized.
- Pelvis should not be rotated as evidenced by:
  —Symmetrical iliac alae
  —Symmetrical obturator foramina
  —Visualization of ischial spines equally on both sides
  —Sacrum and coccyx aligned with the symphysis pubis
- Little or none of the lesser trochanters should be visible beyond the medial edges of the femora.
- Greater trochanters should be fully visualized.
- Density should be sufficient for femoral heads to be demonstrated through acetabula.

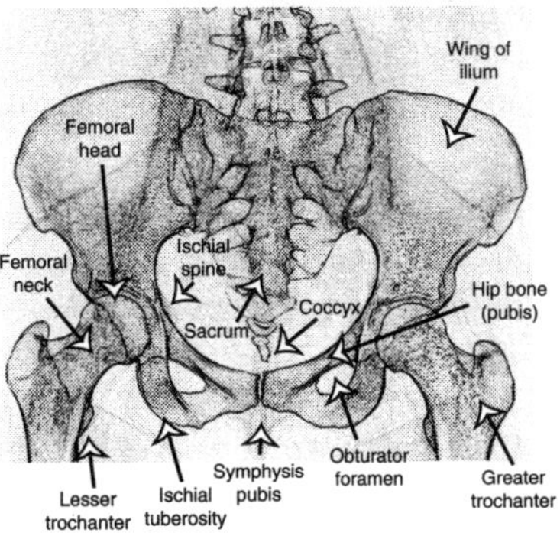

Exam Rationale This projection provides a general survey of the bones of the pelvis and the head, neck, and greater trochanter of each of the femora.

Technical Considerations

- Regular screen/film
- Grid
- kVp range: 85–90
- SID: 40 inch (100 cm)

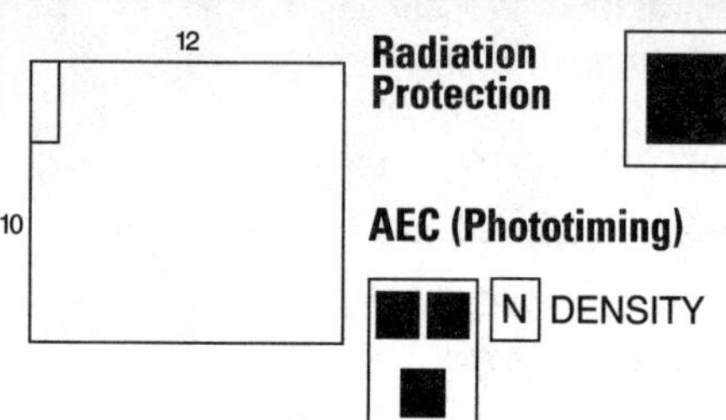

Patient Position

Supine on the table with the legs extended; the patient should be dressed in a patient gown with all clothing from the waist down removed.

Part Position The midsagittal plane of the body should be centered to the midline of the table; the shoulders should be adjusted to lie in the same transverse plane and the elbows should be flexed with the hands resting on the upper chest; the pelvis should be adjusted to that it is not rotated (distance from anterior superior iliac spine and table top is the same on both sides); the cassette should be positioned so that its midpoint will coincide with the central ray.

Example Exposure Techniques **Measure at CR and Use Chart (p.24)**									
Room	**cm**	**kVp**	**mAs**	**mA**	**Sec**	**Beam**	**Film**	**Grid**	**1Ø3Ø**
	15								
	16								
	17								
	18								
	19								
	20								
	21								
	22								
	23								
	24								

Central Ray Directed 2 inches (5 cm) distal to the upper border of the symphysis pubis at 25° (for males) and 40° (for females) cephalic angle.

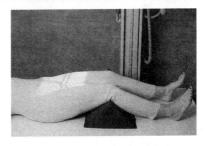

Breathing Instructions
Suspend on inspiration.

Evaluation Criteria

- Symmetrical obturator foramina.
- Pubic and ischial bones should be magnified and superimposed over the sacrum and coccyx.
- Hip joints should be included at the edges of the film.

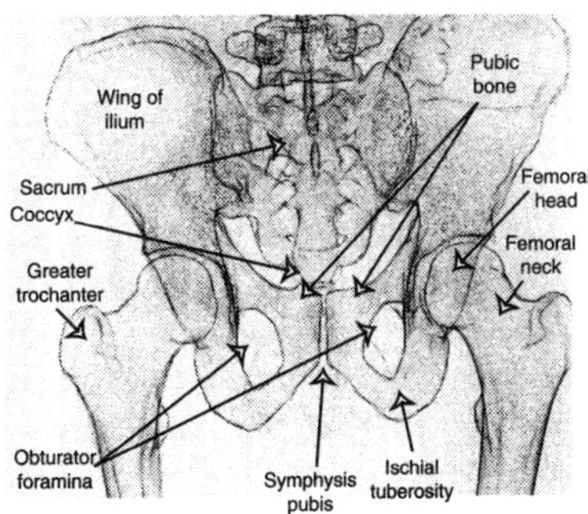

Exam Rationale This axial projection demonstrates the pubic and ischial rami elongated and magnified but free of superimposition.

Tip The most prominent lateral portion of the greater trochanter of the femur may be used to determine the level of the central ray.

Technical Considerations

- Regular screen/film
- Grid
- kVp range: 85–90
- SID: 40 inch (100 cm)

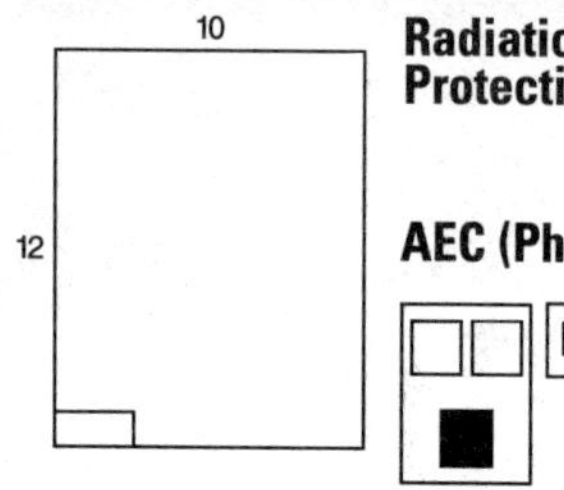

Radiation Protection

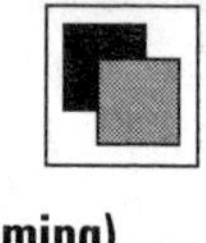

AEC (Phototiming)

N DENSITY

Patient Position

Supine on the table;
the patient should be dressed in a patient gown with all clothing from the waist down removed.

Part Position The sagittal plane 2 inches medial to the anterior superior iliac spine of the affected side should be centered to the midline of the table; the shoulders should be adjusted to lie in the same transverse plane and the elbows flexed with the hands resting on the upper chest; the pelvis should be adjusted to that it is not rotated (distance from anterior superior iliac spine and table top is the same on both sides); the foot should be internally rotated approximately 15°; the cassette should be centered to the upper limit of the greater trochanter.

Example Exposure Techniques **Measure at CR and Use Chart (p.24)**									
Room	**cm**	**kVp**	**mAs**	**mA**	**Sec**	**Beam**	**Film**	**Grid**	**1Ø3Ø**
	15								
	16								
	17								
	18								
	19								
	20								
	21								
	22								
	23								
	24								

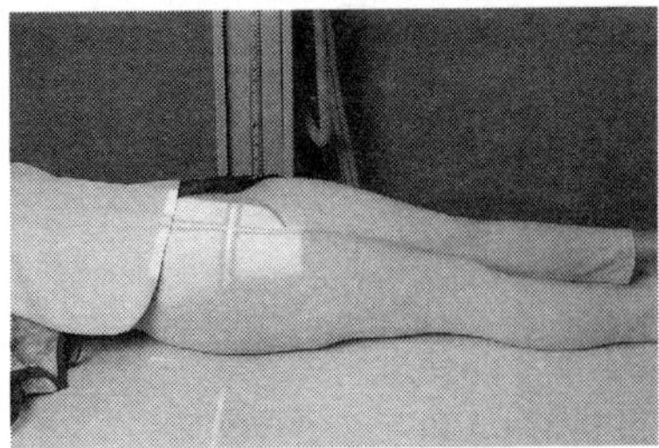

Central Ray Perpendicular to the midpoint of the film (approximately 2 inches medial to the ASIS of the affected side at a level just above the greater trochanter).

Breathing Instructions
Suspend on inspiration.

Evaluation Criteria

- Little or none of the lesser trochanter should be visible beyond the medial edge of the femur.
- Greater trochanters should be fully visualized.
- Density should be sufficient for the femoral head to be demonstrated through the acetabulum.

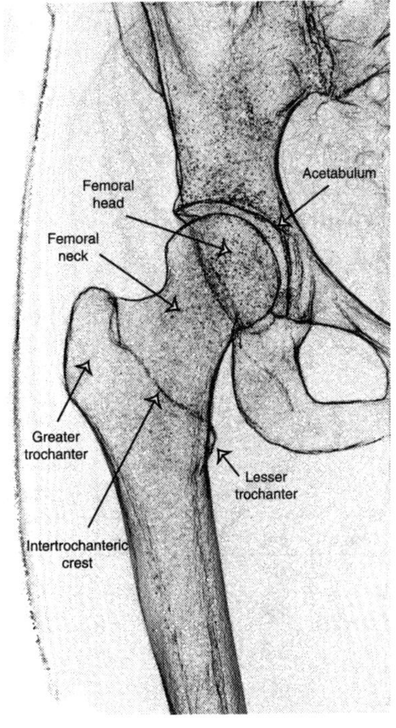

Exam Rationale Structures demonstrated include the head, neck, trochanter, and the proximal third of the femoral shaft.

Tips

1. In the initial examination of a hip, an AP pelvis is often done to demonstrate the entire pelvic girdle and both upper femora; follow-up studies are confined to the affected side.
2. If an orthopedic appliance is in place, automatic exposure control should not be used; it may also require a larger film to demonstrate the entire prosthesis.

Technical Considerations
- Regular screen/film
- Grid
- kVp range: 85–90
- SID: 40 inch (100 cm)

10

12

Radiation Protection

AEC (Phototiming)

N DENSITY

Patient Position
Supine on the table; the patient should be dressed in a patient gown with all clothing from the waist down removed.

Part Position Patient should flex the knee and turn slightly toward the affected side and abduct the leg to place the femur parallel to the film; center the hip (midway between ASIS and symphysis pubis) to the midline of the table; the unaffected leg should be extended behind the affected leg.

Central Ray Perpendicular to hip.

Breathing Instructions Suspend on inspiration.

Example Exposure Techniques
Measure at CR and Use Chart (p.24)

Room	cm	kVp	mAs	mA	Sec	Beam	Film	Grid	1Ø3Ø
	17								
	18								
	19								
	20								
	21								
	22								
	23								
	24								
	25								
	26								

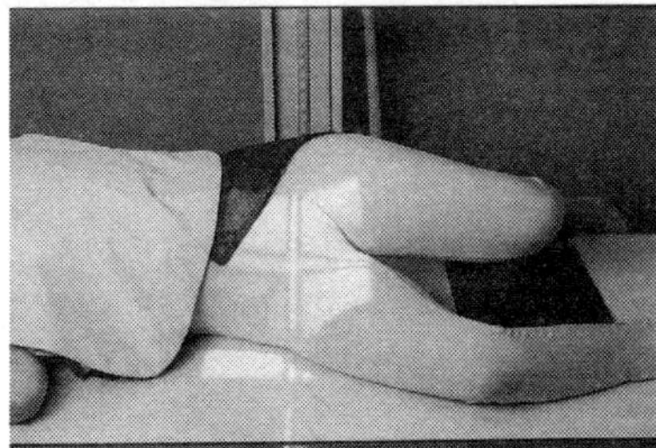

Evaluation Criteria

- Hip joint should be centered to exposed area.
- Any orthopedic appliance (e.g., surgical plate) should be seen in its entirety.

Exam Rationale Structures demonstrated on the radiograph include the proximal femur and the acetabulum. This position is contraindicated in patients with suspected fractures or pathologic hip disease.

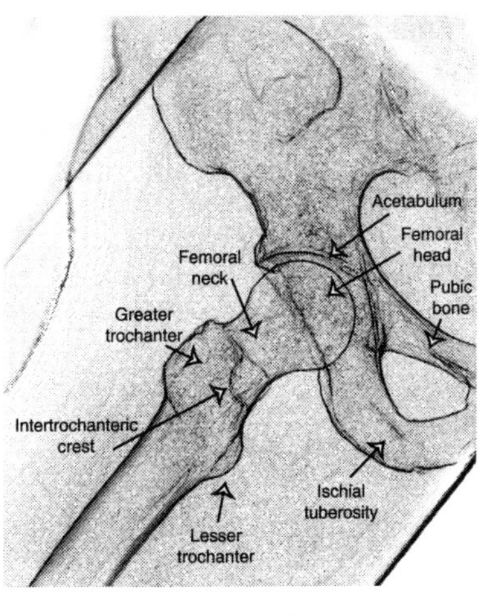

Tips

1. This position should not be used when a fracture is suspected because of the possibility of displacing fragments; a superoinferior projection should be done instead.
2. In the initial examination of a hip, a bilateral frog-leg pelvis is often done to demonstrate the entire pelvic girdle and lateral views of both upper femora; follow-up studies are confined to the affected side.

Technical Considerations

- Regular screen/film
- Grid
- kVp range: 85–90
- SID: 40 inch (100 cm)

17

14

Radiation Protection

(males) (females)

AEC (Phototiming)

N DENSITY

Patient Position Supine on the table; the patient should be dressed in a patient gown with all clothing from the waist down removed.

Part Position The midsagittal plane of the body should be centered to the midline of the table; the shoulders should be adjusted to lie in the same transverse plane and the elbows flexed with the hands resting on the upper chest; the pelvis should be adjusted to that it is not rotated (distance from anterior superior iliac spine and table top is the same on both sides); the knees and hips should be flexed and the feet drawn up as much as possible, allowing the femora to be abducted to approximately a 40° angle from the vertical.

Example Exposure Techniques
Measure at CR and Use Chart (p.24)

Room	cm	kVp	mAs	mA	Sec	Beam	Film	Grid	1Ø3Ø
	16								
	17								
	18								
	19								
	20								
	21								
	22								
	23								
	24								
	25								

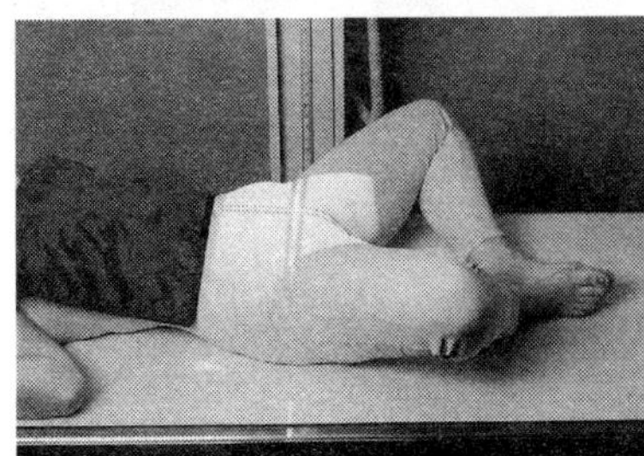

Central Ray Perpendicular to a point 1 inch (2.5 cm) superior to the symphysis pubis.

Breathing Instructions Suspend on inspiration.

Evaluation Criteria

- Should include acetabula, femoral heads, and necks.
- Pelvis should not be rotated as evidenced by:
  —Symmetrical iliac alae
  —Visualization of ischial spine equally on both sides
  —Sacrum and coccyx aligned with symphysis pubis
- Lesser trochanter should be projected on the medial side of the femur.

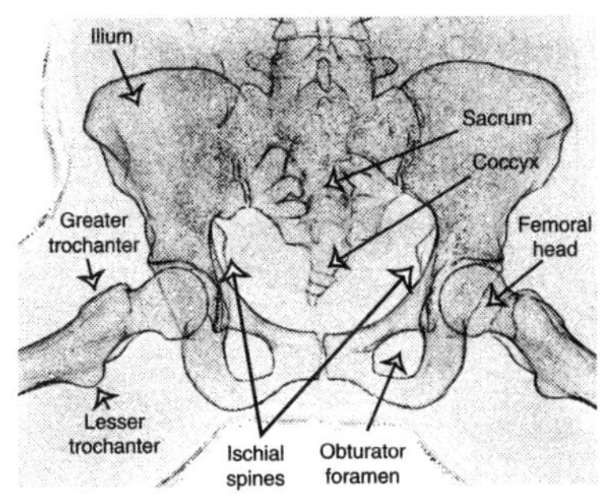

Exam Rationale This exam is commonly indicated for investigation of congenital hip disease. It is contraindicated in patients with suspected fractures or pathologic hip disease.

Tip This is a modification of the original Cleaves method, which called for cephalic angulation to parallel the long axis of the femora.

Technical Considerations

- Regular screen/film
- Grid: stationary
- kVp range: 90–95
- SID: 40 inch (100 cm)

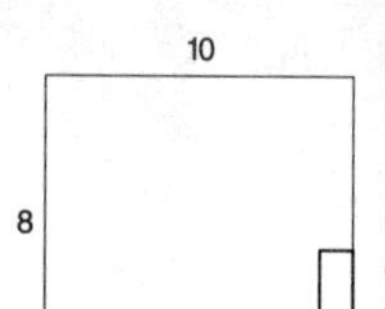

Radiation Protection

(for females). Gonadal dhielding not possible for males.

Patient Position Supine on the table; the patient should be dressed in a patient gown with all clothing from the waist down removed.

Part Position The knee of the affected leg should be extended; unless contraindicated, internally rotate the foot of the affected side 15°; flex the knee and hip of the unaffected side and raise the leg, using some suitable support for the leg. The top of the cassette should be at the top of the iliac crest and should be parallel to the femoral neck and perpendicular to the central ray.

Central Ray Horizontal, perpendicular to the hip (about 2 1/2 inches or 7 cm below the intersection of the localization points described below).

Breathing Instructions Suspend on inspiration.

Example Exposure Techniques
Measure at CR and Use Chart (p.24)

Room	cm	kVp	mAs	mA	Sec	Beam	Film	Grid	1Ø3Ø
	11								
	12								
	13								
	14								
	15								
	16								
	17								
	18								
	19								
	20								

Evaluation Criteria

- Proximal femur, hip joint, and acetabulum should be visualized.
- As much as possible of the femoral neck should be visualized.
- Only a small portion of lesser trochanter should be seen on anterior and posterior femur.

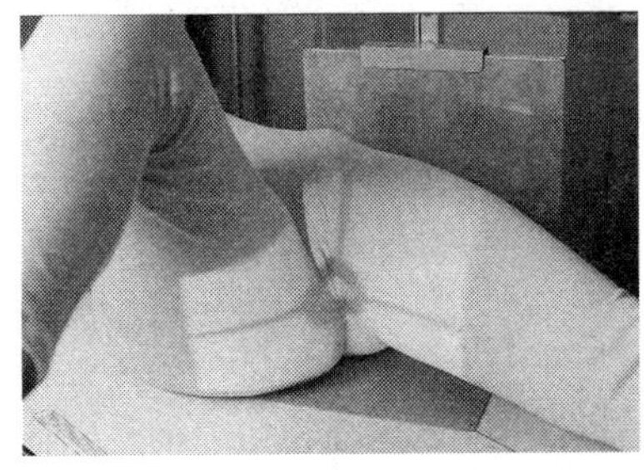

Exam Rationale This lateral projection of the hip is indicated when the patient cannot be positioned for a routine lateral.

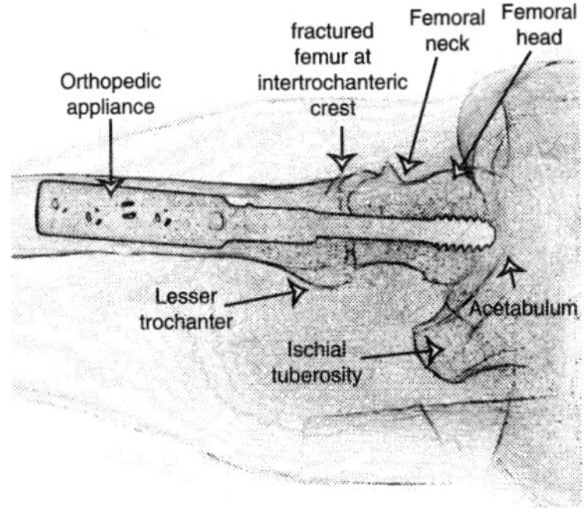

Tip To localize the long axis of the femoral neck, draw a line between the ASIS and the superior border of the symphysis pubis and note its center point; palpate the most prominent lateral protrusion of the greater trochanter and note a point 1 inch distal to it; a line drawn between these two points will parallel the long axis of the femoral neck.

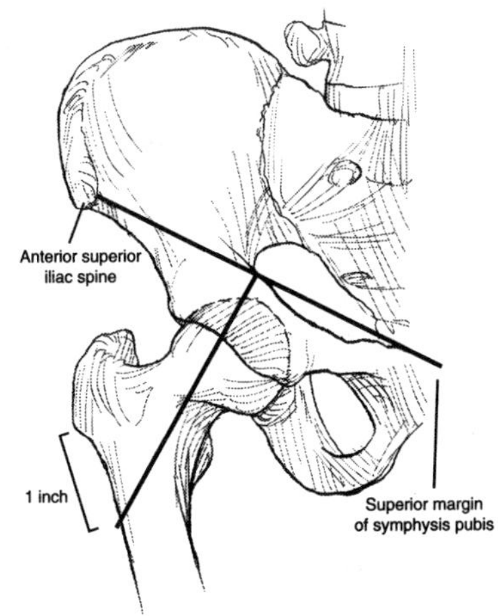

Technical Considerations

- Regular screen/film
- Grid: stationary
- kVp range: 85–95
- SID: 40 inch (100 cm)

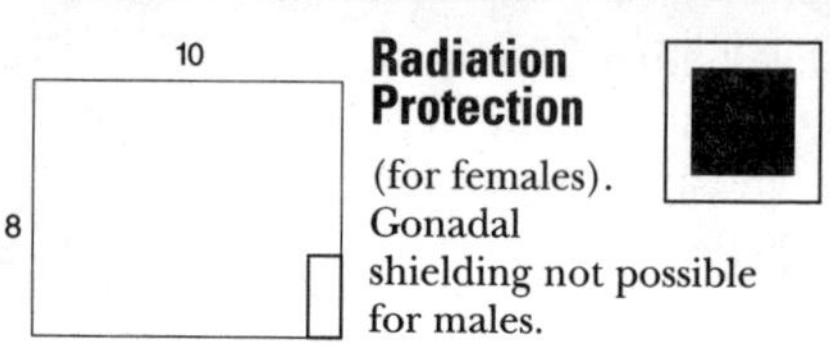

(for females). Gonadal shielding not possible for males.

Patient Position Supine, with affected side near the edge of the table, with both legs extended; patient should be dressed in a hospital gown with all clothing from the waist down removed.

Part Position Leg remains in neutral position. The cassette should rest on the extended Bucky tray and be placed so top of the cassette is at iliac crest; the cassette should be tilted 15° from the vertical, so it is parallel to the central ray.

Central Ray Aligned perpendicular to femoral neck at 15° posterior angle.

Breathing Instructions Suspend on inspiration.

Example Exposure Techniques
Measure at CR and Use Chart (p.24)

Room	cm	kVp	mAs	mA	Sec	Beam	Film	Grid	1Ø3Ø
	13								
	14								
	15								
	16								
	17								
	18								
	19								
	20								
	21								
	22								

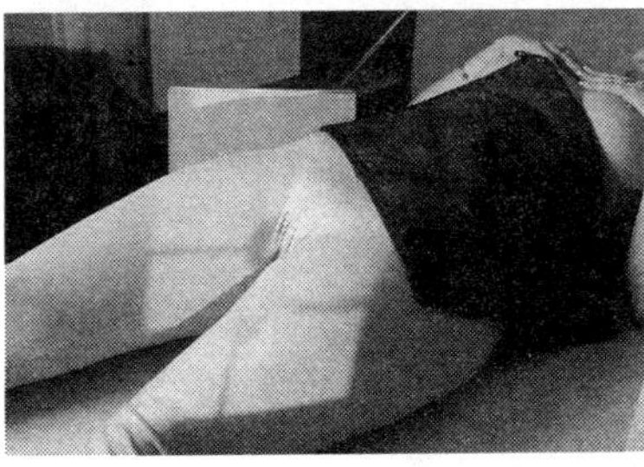

Evaluation Criteria

- Femoral head, neck, and trochanters should be centered to film area.
- Femoral head and neck should be seen in profile with minimal superimposition by greater trochanter.
- Lesser trochanter should be projected just below femoral shaft.

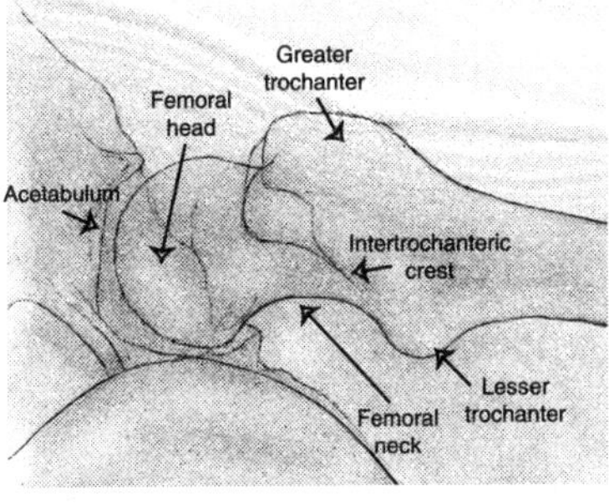

Exam Rationale This lateral projection of the hip is indicated when both a routine lateral and the axiolateral are contraindicated due to limited movement of both the affected and unaffected leg.

Tip Care must be taken that the grid is perpendicular to the central ray to prevent grid cutoff.

Technical Considerations

- Regular screen/film
- Grid
- kVp range: 85–95
- SID: 40 inch (100 cm)

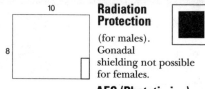

10

8

Radiation Protection

(for males). Gonadal shielding not possible for females.

AEC (Phototiming)

N DENSITY

Patient Position Supine on table with legs extended; patient should be dressed in hospital gown with all clothing from the waist down removed.

Part Position The midsagittal plane of the body should be centered to the midline of the table; shoulders should be adjusted to lie in same transverse plane and elbows should be flexed with hands resting on the upper chest; pelvis should be adjusted to that it is not rotated (distance from anterior superior iliac spine and table top is same on both sides).

Central Ray Directed to midline midway between level of ASIS and symphysis pubis at 30° to 35° cephalic angle.

Breathing Instructions Suspend on inspiration.

Example Exposure Techniques
Measure at CR and Use Chart (p.24)

Room	cm	kVp	mAs	mA	Sec	Beam	Film	Grid	1Ø3Ø
	15								
	16								
	17								
	18								
	19								
	20								
	21								
	22								
	23								
	24								

Evaluation Criteria

- Sacroiliac joints should be centered to collimation.
- Sacroiliac joint spaces should be open.

Exam Rationale This projection demonstrates the sacroiliac joints, the L5–S1 junction, and the majority of the sacrum.

Tip This may also be done in the prone position, with the central ray directed to the fourth lumbar segment at a 30° to 35° caudal angle at the level of the iliac crest; in the prone position, the obliquity of the sacroiliac joints more nearly parallels the divergence of the radiation beam.

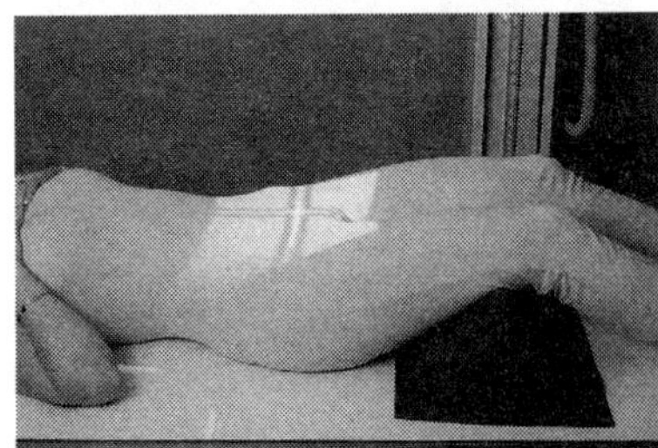

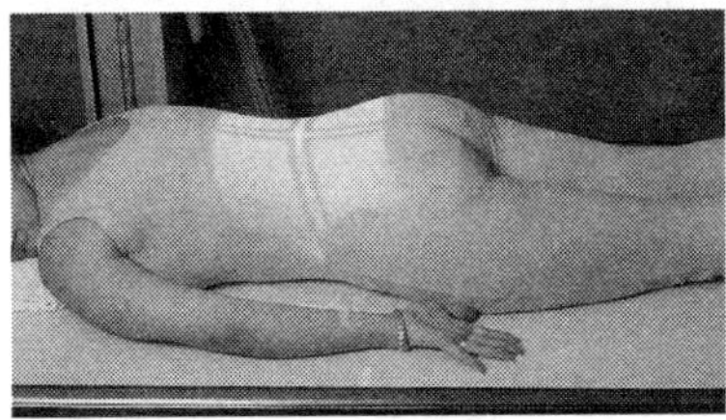

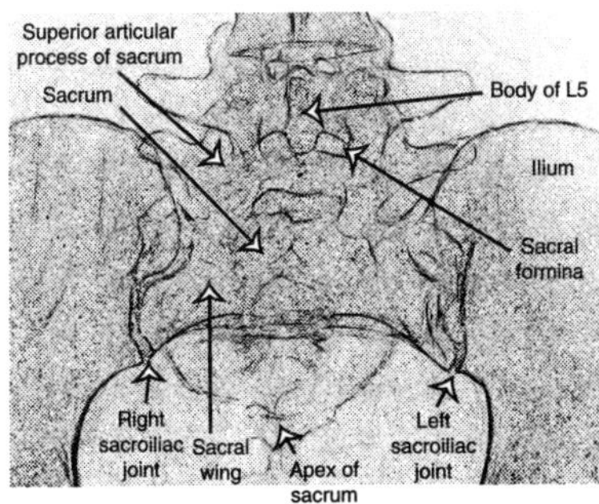

Technical Considerations

- Regular screen/film
- Grid
- kVp range: 85–95
- SID: 40 inch (100 cm)

Radiation Protection

(for males).
For females, gonadal shielding can be used only on the side not being examined.

AEC (Phototiming)

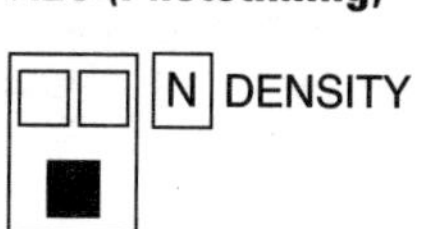

Patient Position

Supine on table; patient should be dressed in hospital gown with all clothing from the waist down removed.

Part Position Raise the side of interest 25° to 30° and center sacroiliac joint to midline of the table; both knees should be slightly flexed.

Central Ray Perpendicular to point 1 inch (2.5 cm) medial to elevated ASIS.

Breathing Instructions Suspend on inspiration.

Example Exposure Techniques
Measure at CR and Use Chart (p.24)

(p.24)

Room	cm	kVp	mAs	mA	Sec	Beam	Film	Grid	1Ø3Ø
	16								
	18								
	20								
	22								
	24								
	26								
	28								
	30								
	32								
	34								

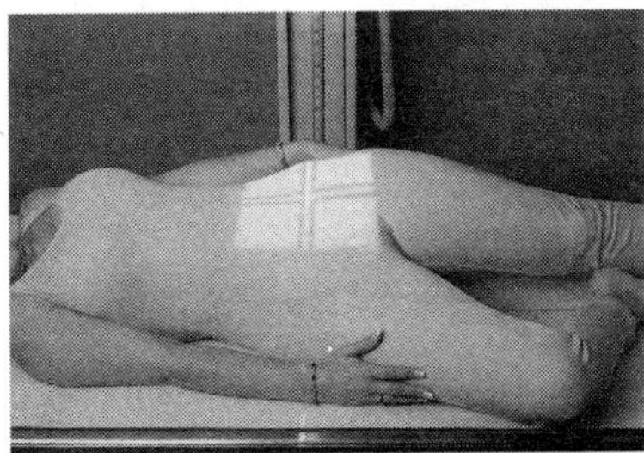

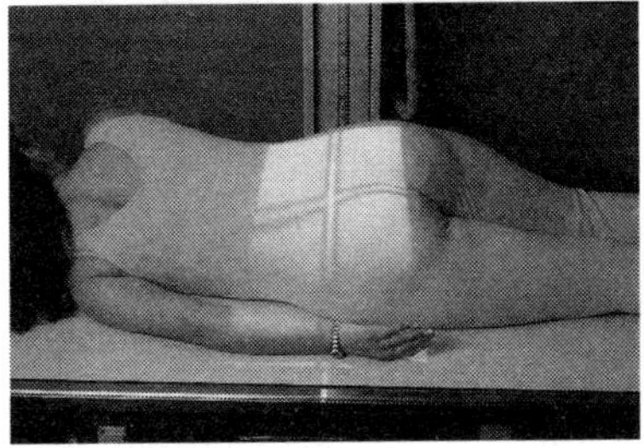

Evaluation Criteria

- There should be no overlap between the ala of the ilium and the sacrum, indicating the proper degree of obliquity.
- Elevated joint space should be open.

Exam Rationale In the supine position, the sacroiliac joint furthest from the film is demonstrated. Both sides are examined for comparison.

Tips

1. To demonstrate the distal portion of the joint more clearly, the central ray may be angled 15° to 20° cephalad.
2. This may also be done in the prone position, with the central ray directed to the vertebral spinous processes at the level of the ASIS; in the prone position, the downside joint will be visualized; to demonstrate the distal portion more clearly in the prone position, the central ray may be angled 15° to 20° caudad.

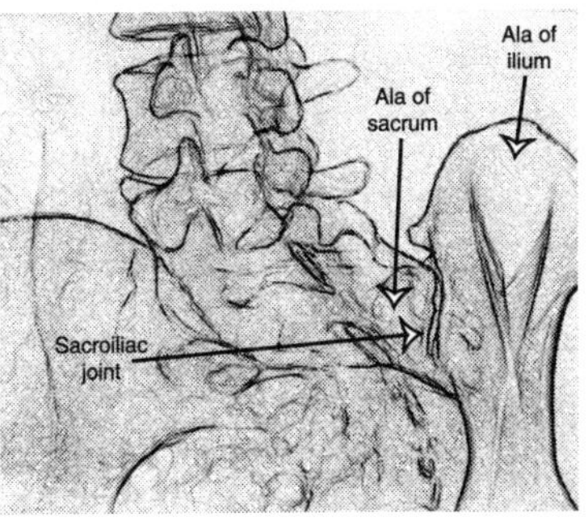

Pediatric Considerations When radiographing parts of the lower extremity on pediatric patients, the biggest challenge often comes from flailing arms and legs. Although immobilization may be a time-consuming process and is not always well received by the patient or the parents, immobilization of a patient who is unable or unwilling to cooperate by holding still is highly preferable to the need for repeated radiographs because of motion artifacts.

An effective method of immobilization is to use a mummy wrap on the torso and upper extremities. A heavy sandbag can be used to immobilize the unaffected extremity. The affected extremity can then be held by a parent or other individual (with appropriate radiation protection).

For radiography of the pelvis, the patient's legs can be immobilized with the table's compression band. The parent can hold the patient's humeri.

Geriatric Considerations The greatest difficulty in radiographing geriatric patients is the potential lack of flexibility. Patients should be assisted in assuming the various positions. Flexing or extending joints should be done slowly and gently and not forced.

RIBS AND STERNUM

ROUTINE POSITIONS/PROJECTIONS

Part	Routine	Page
Ribs	AP (above diaphragm)	200
	AP (below diaphragm)	202
	PA (above diaphragm)	204
	Oblique	206
Sternum	Right Anterior Oblique	208
	Lateral	210
Sternoclavicular joints	PA	212
	Oblique	214

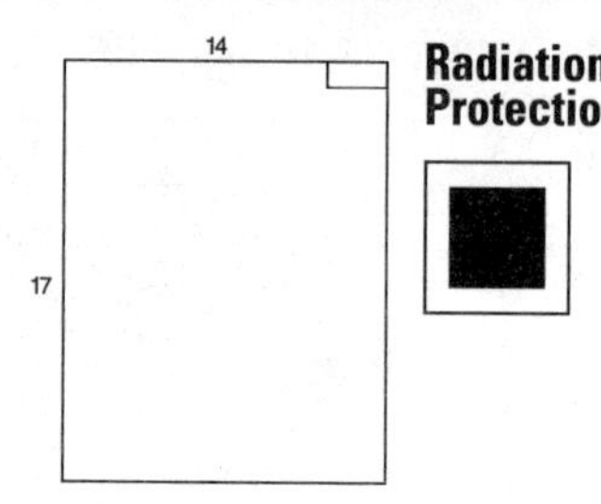

Technical Considerations

- Regular screen/film
- Grid
- kVp range: 65–70
- SID: 40 inch (100 cm)

Patient Position Erect with back against Bucky with all potential artifacts removed from area of interest.

Part Position Arms slightly abducted and weight equally distributed on both feet with no rotation; midsagittal plane aligned to midline of Bucky and perpendicular to the plane of the film; shoulders rotated anteriorly to reduce superimposition on the upper ribs.

Central Ray Upper border of cassette 2 inches (5 cm) above the upper border of the shoulders; central ray directed perpendicularly to the plane of the film at the level of the seventh thoracic vertebra.

Breathing Instructions Suspend at end of 2nd inspiration.

Example Exposure Techniques
Measure at CR and Use Chart (p.6)

Room	cm	kVp	mAs	mA	Sec	Beam	Film	Grid	1Ø3Ø
	14								
	16								
	18								
	20								
	22								
	24								
	26								
	28								
	30								
	32								

Evaluation Criteria

- First nine or ten pairs of posterior ribs inclusive of the axillary margin should be visualized with no evidence of motion or rotation.

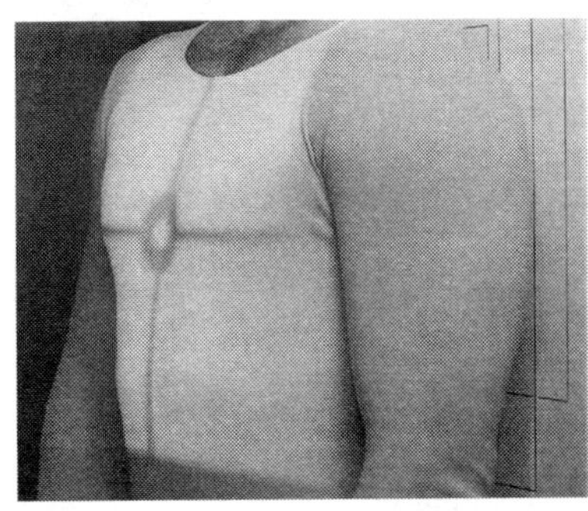

Exam Rationale Although the most common indication for radiographic examination of the ribs is trauma, rib projections may also be ordered for pathologic investigations. This position best demonstrates the upper, posterior ribs.

Tip The same procedure may be done with the patient in a recumbent position.

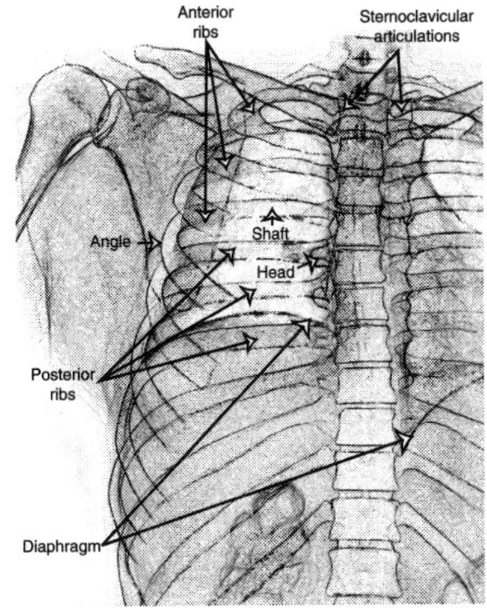

Technical Considerations

- Regular screen/film
- Grid
- kVp range: 75–80
- SID: 40 inch (100 cm)

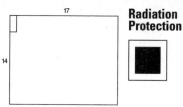

(may be lengthwise for smaller patients)

Patient Position Erect with back against Bucky with all potential artifacts removed from area of interest.

Part Position Arms slightly abducted and weight equally distributed on both feet with no rotation; midsagittal plane aligned to midline of Bucky and perpendicular to the plane of the film.

Central Ray Lower border of cassette 2 inches (5 cm) below the inferior rib margin; central ray directed perpendicularly to the plane of the film at the level of the twelfth thoracic vertebra for crosswise film placement or the tenth thoracic vertebra for lengthwise film placement.

Breathing Instructions Suspend on expiration.

Example Exposure Techniques **Measure at CR and Use Chart (p.6)**									
Room	cm	kVp	mAs	mA	Sec	Beam	Film	Grid	1Ø3Ø
	14								
	16								
	18								
	20								
	22								
	24								
	26								
	28								
	30								
	32								

Evaluation Criteria

- Eighth through twelfth pairs of posterior ribs inclusive of the axillary margins should be visualized with no evidence of motion or rotation.

Exam Rationale Because the lower ribs are superimposed by the diaphragm, it is necessary to expose the lower ribs using a darker density setting. The exposure is made on patient exhalation to allow the diaphragm excursion to be at its most superior extreme to demonstrate as many pairs of ribs as possible on the more dense setting.

Tips

1. Be sure lead shielding does not superimpose lower ribs.
2. The same procedure may be done with the patient in a recumbent position.

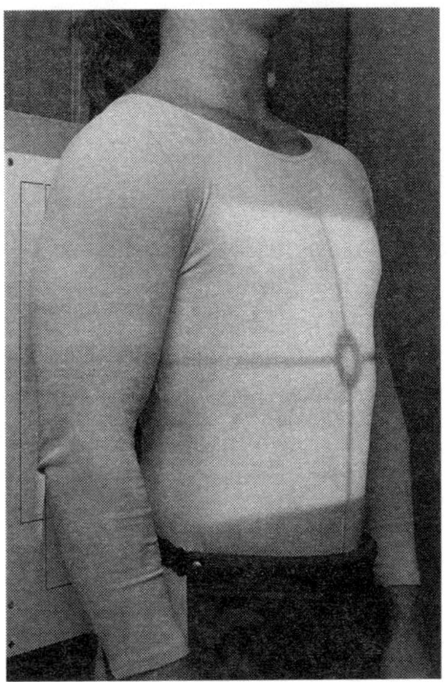

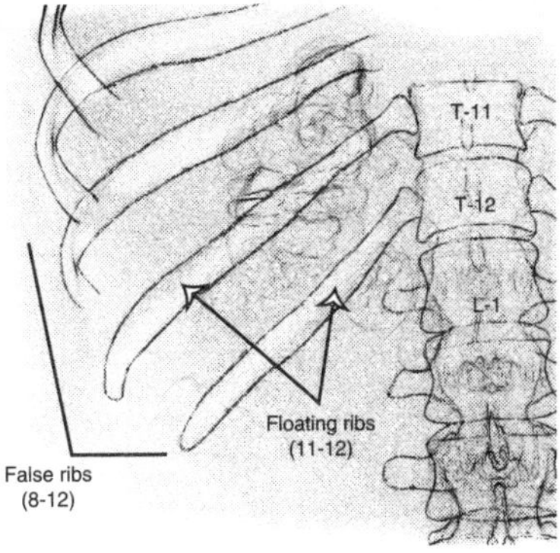

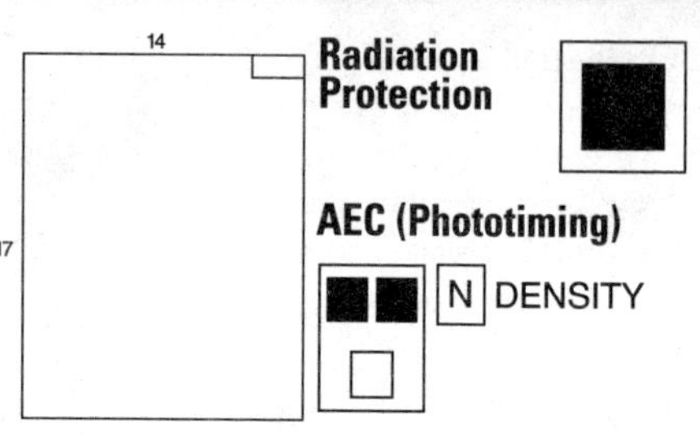

Technical Considerations

- Regular screen/film
- Grid
- kVp range: 65–70
- SID: 40 inch (100 cm)

Patient Position Erect facing Bucky with all potential artifacts removed from area of interest.

Part Position Arms slightly abducted and weight equally distributed on both feet with no rotation; midsagittal plane aligned to midline of Bucky and perpendicular to the plane of the film; shoulders rotated anteriorly to reduce superimposition on the upper ribs.

Central Ray Upper border of cassette 2 inches (5 cm) above the upper border of the shoulders; central ray directed perpendicularly to the plane of the film at the level of the seventh thoracic vertebra.

Breathing Instructions Suspend at end of 2nd inspiration.

Example Exposure Techniques
Measure at CR and Use Chart (p.6)

Room	cm	kVp	mAs	mA	Sec	Beam	Film	Grid	1Ø3Ø
	14								
	16								
	18								
	20								
	22								
	24								
	26								
	28								
	30								
	32								

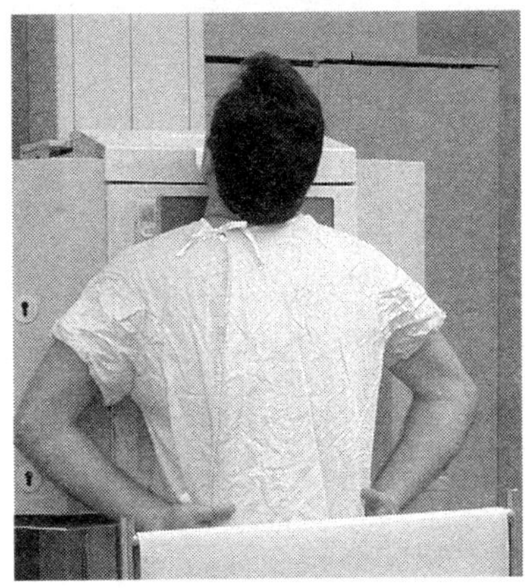

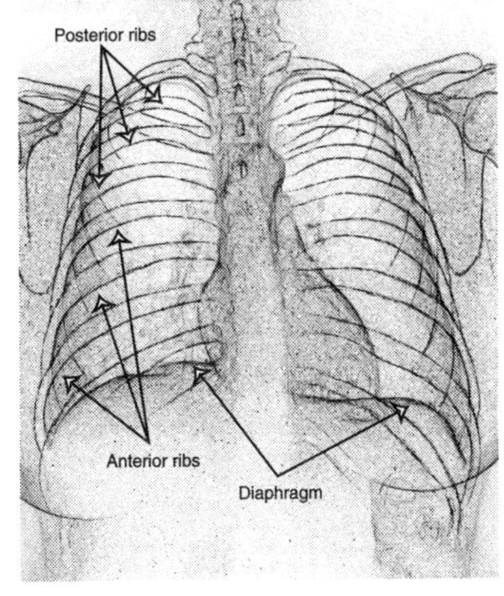

Evaluation Criteria

- First nine or ten pairs of anterior ribs inclusive of the axillary margins should be visualized with no evidence of motion or rotation.
- Should be no rotation as evidenced by the sternoclavicular articulations on each side being equidistant from the midsagittal plane.

Exam Rationale Although the most common indication for radiographic examination of the ribs is trauma, rib projections may also be ordered for pathologic investigations. This position best demonstrates the upper, anterior ribs.

Tips

1. The neck can be extended to lift the chin off the upper ribs.
2. The same procedure may be adapted for the patient in a recumbent position.

Technical Considerations

- Regular screen/film
- Grid
- kVp range: 65–70 (for ribs above diaphragm), 75–80 (for ribs below diaphragm)
- SID: 40 inch (100 cm)

14

17

Radiation Protection

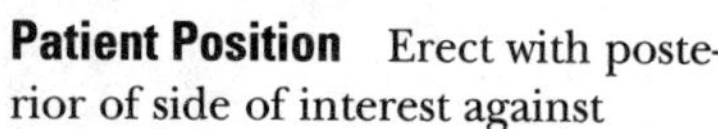

Patient Position Erect with posterior of side of interest against Bucky with all potential artifacts removed from area of interest.

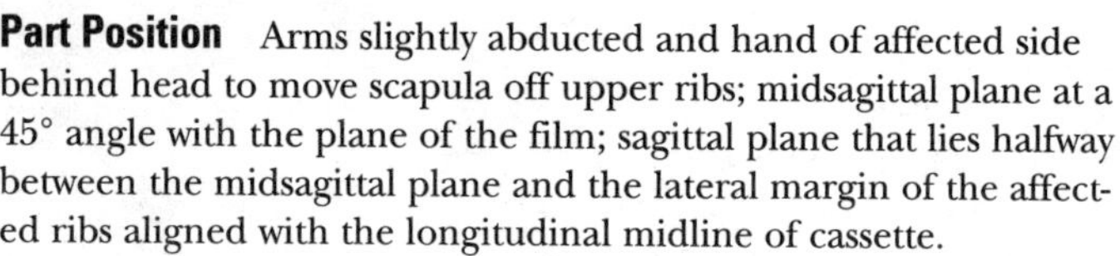

Part Position Arms slightly abducted and hand of affected side behind head to move scapula off upper ribs; midsagittal plane at a 45° angle with the plane of the film; sagittal plane that lies halfway between the midsagittal plane and the lateral margin of the affected ribs aligned with the longitudinal midline of cassette.

Central Ray

- Upper ribs: upper border of cassette 2 inches (5 cm) above the upper border of the shoulders; central ray directed perpendicularly to a sagittal plane halfway between the midsagittal plane and the lateral margin of the affected ribs at the level of the seventh thoracic vertebra.

Example Exposure Techniques
Measure at CR and Use Chart (p.6)

Room	cm	kVp	mAs	mA	Sec	Beam	Film	Grid	1Ø3Ø
	18								
	20								
	22								
	24								
	26								
	28								
	30								
	32								
	34								
	36								

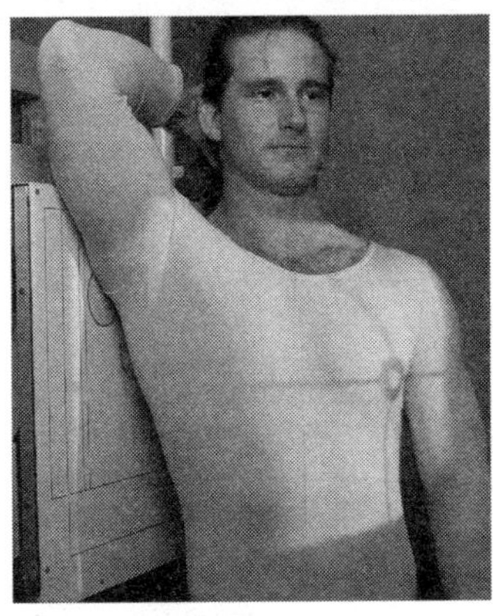

- Lower ribs: lower border of cassette 2 inches (5 cm) below inferior margin of the ribs; central ray directed perpendicularly to a sagittal plane halfway between the midsagittal plane and the lateral margin of the affected ribs at the level of the tenth thoracic vertebra.

Breathing Instructions Upper ribs: suspend on inspiration. Lower ribs: suspend on expiration.

Evaluation Criteria

- Upper ribs: first nine or ten pairs of ribs inclusive of the axillary margins should be visualized above the diaphragm with no evidence of motion; distance between the spine and the axillary margin of the affected side will appear to be double that of the distance between the same structures on the unaffected side.
- Lower ribs: eighth through the twelfth ribs inclusive of the axillary margins should be visualized below the diaphragm with no evidence of motion; distance between the spine and the axillary margin of the affected side wall will appear to be double that of the distance between the same structures on the unaffected side.

Exam Rationale Because the rib cage completely encircles the thoracic cavity, superimposition of the anterior and posterior ribs is always evident in AP or PA projections. It is necessary to oblique the thorax relative to the plane of the film to project the ribs free of superimposition and to demonstrate the axillary portion of the ribs. These projections/positions are selected in cases of trauma to the posterior or axillary aspects of the ribs.

Tips

1. Always rotate the spine away from side of interest.
2. Make sure the lead shield does not superimpose the lower ribs.
3. For a patient unable to stand, the same procedures may be adapted for the recumbent position.
4. The oblique may also be done in the PA projection. The patient begins in the erect position facing the Bucky and is rotated 45° away from the injured side.

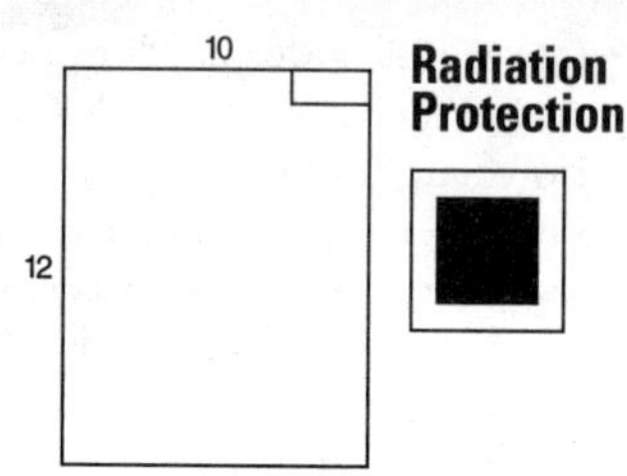

Technical Considerations
- Regular screen/film
- Grid
- kVp range: 65–70
- SID: 40 inch (100 cm)

Patient Position Erect facing Bucky with all potential artifacts removed from area of interest.

Part Position With the right anterior aspect of the patient's chest against the Bucky, rotate patient 15° to 20°; align long axis of sternum to long axis of cassette.

Central Ray Upper border of cassette 1 1/2 inches (4 cm) above manubrial notch; align central ray perpendicularly to the plane of the film at the level of the seventh thoracic vertebra (approximately 1 1/2 to 2 inches (4–5 cm) to the left of the midsagittal plane).

Breathing Instructions Slow, steady breathing.

Evaluation Criteria
- Entire sternum should be projected through the blurred heart shadow free of superimposition with the thoracic vertebrae.
- Lung markings and ribs should appear blurred.

Example Exposure Techniques
Measure at CR and Use Chart (p.6)

Room	cm	kVp	mAs	mA	Sec	Beam	Film	Grid	1Ø3Ø
	16								
	18								
	20								
	22								
	24								
	26								
	28								
	30								

Exam Rationale Because the sternum is a relatively thin, flat bone, it is completely obliterated by the superimposition of the thoracic vertebrae in a true PA projection. To obtain a PA projection of the sternum, it is necessary to slightly rotate the patient to move the thoracic vertebrae off the sternum. The RAO position is routinely selected because it projects the sternum through the heart shadow, which takes advantage of the more homogeneous anatomic density of the heart muscle to allow improved demonstration of the sternum relative to radiographic density.

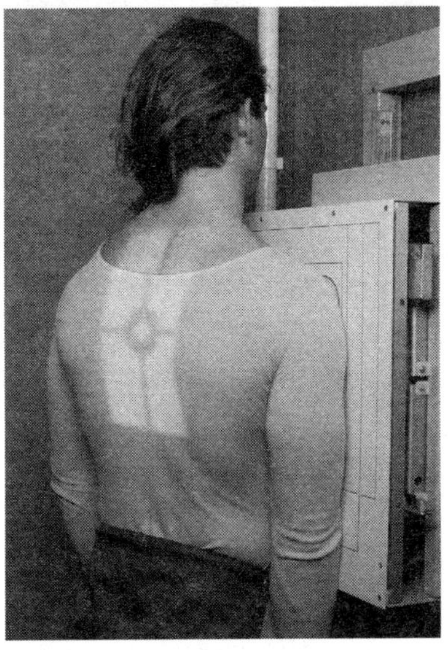

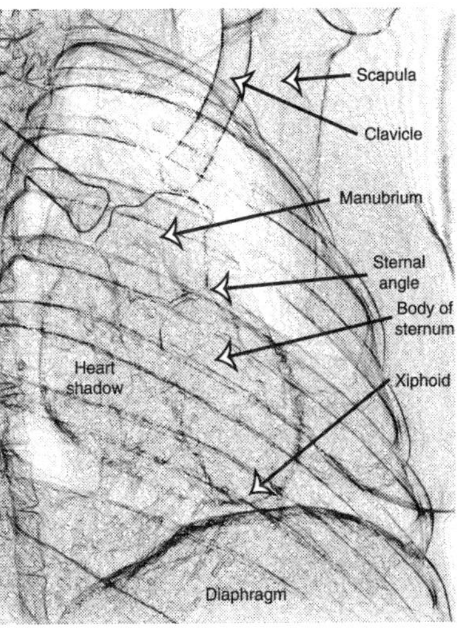

Tips

1. Palpate the thoracic vertebral spinous processes with one hand and the manubrial notch with the other when rotating patient. This will serve as a guide to ensure appropriate rotation of the thoracic spine away from the sternum.
2. A long exposure time (2–3 seconds) will ensure adequate blurring of ribs, pulmonary markings, and the heart shadow.
3. For a patient who is unable to stand, the patient may be examined in the recumbent position.

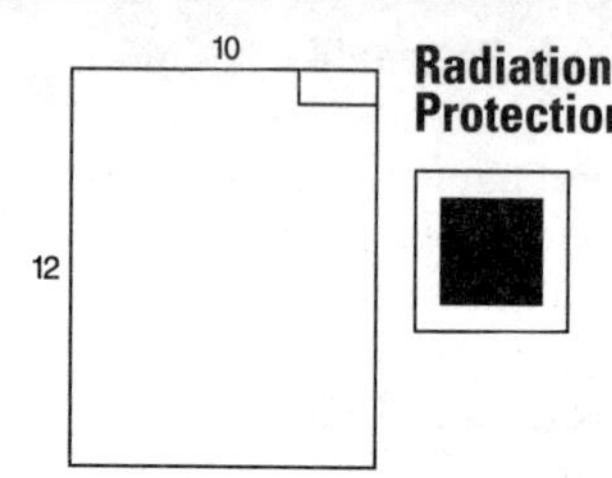

Technical Considerations

- Regular screen/film
- Grid
- kVp range: 70–75
- SID: 40 inch (100 cm)

Patient Position Erect right or left lateral with all potential artifacts removed from area of interest.

Part Position With midsagittal plane parallel to the plane of the film, align sternum to midline of cassette; have patient clasp hands behind back to move shoulders posteriorly and to project the sternum anteriorly.

Central Ray With upper border of cassette 1 1/2 inches above manubrial notch, align central ray perpendicularly to the lateral border of the sternum midway between the manubrial notch and the xiphoid process.

Breathing Instructions Suspend on inspiration.

Example Exposure Techniques **Measure at CR and Use Chart (p.6)**									
Room	**cm**	**kVp**	**mAs**	**mA**	**Sec**	**Beam**	**Film**	**Grid**	**1Ø3Ø**
	20								
	22								
	24								
	26								
	28								
	30								
	32								
	34								
	36								
	38								

Evaluation Criteria

- Entire sternum should be visualized with no evidence of rotation or motion.

Exam Rationale This position allows the sternum to be visualized in a lateral orientation that complements the RAO.

Tips

1. Be sure patient is in contact with Bucky but not leaning against it to ensure there is no forward or backward swaying during the exposure.
2. For female patients, it may be necessary to move the breasts to the side and secure them with a wide bandage to prevent superimposition of breast shadows over sternum.
3. For the patient who is unable to stand, this procedure may be done in the recumbent position.

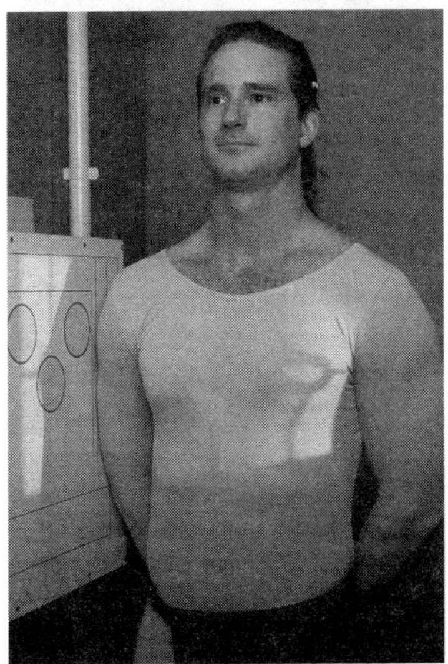

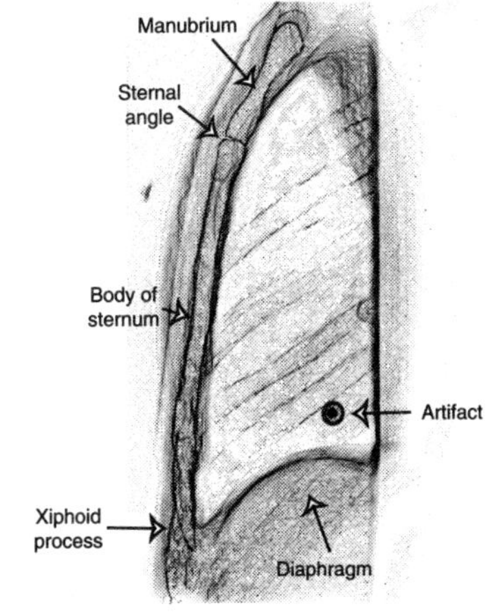

Technical Considerations

- Regular screen/film
- kVp range: 65–70
- SID: 40 inch (100 cm)

10

8

Radiation Protection

Patient Position Recumbent with MSP centered to midline of table and with all potential artifacts removed from area of interest.

Part Position Chin should be extended; adjust midsagittal plane perpendicular to plane of film.

Central Ray Perpendicular to the third thoracic vertebra.

Breathing Instructions Suspend on expiration.

Evaluation Criteria

- Sternoclavicular articulations should be visualized on either side of and equidistant from the midsagittal plane with no evidence of rotation or motion.

Example Exposure Techniques
Measure at CR and Use Chart (p.6)

Room	cm	kVp	mAs	mA	Sec	Beam	Film	Grid	1Ø3Ø
	14								
	16								
	18								
	20								
	22								
	24								
	26								
	28								
	30								
	32								

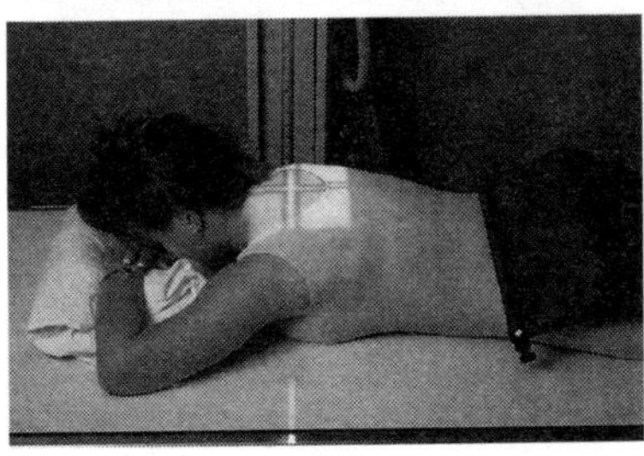

Exam Rationale

Occasionally, radiographic visualization of the sternoclavicular articulations may be desirable to demonstrate possible traumatic or pathologic (arthritic) changes.

Tips The same procedure may be adapted for the erect position.

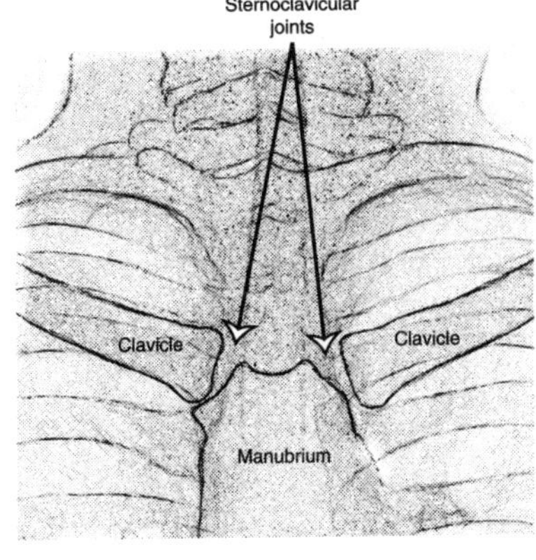

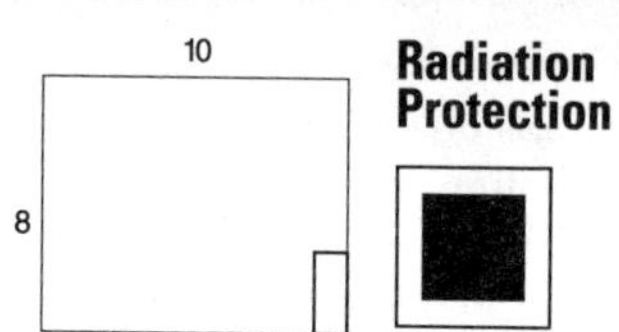

Technical Considerations

- Regular screen/film
- kVp range: 65–70
- SID: 40 inch (100 cm)

Patient Position Recumbent with all potential artifacts removed from area of interest.

Part Position Rotate patient 15° to place side of interest closest to Bucky; midsagittal plane forms 15° angle with plane of film.

Central Ray Perpendicular to the third thoracic vertebra.

Breathing Instructions Suspend on expiration.

Evaluation Criteria

- Sternoclavicular articulation, manubrium, and proximal clavicle should be demonstrated with the joint space "open" and free of superimposition with thoracic vertebrae.
- No evidence of rotation or motion.

Example Exposure Techniques
Measure at CR and Use Chart (p.6)

Room	cm	kVp	mAs	mA	Sec	Beam	Film	Grid	1Ø3Ø
	14								
	16								
	18								
	20								
	22								
	24								
	26								
	28								
	30								
	32								

Exam Rationale The oblique projections complement the PA projection by projecting the sternoclavicular articulations to one side of the thoracic vertebrae, which reduces superimposition and "opens" the joint space for better visualization. Both sides are examined for comparison.

Tips

1. Rotate the patient's head more than the patient's body to allow for patient comfort and to reduce magnification.
2. The same procedure may be adapted for the erect position.

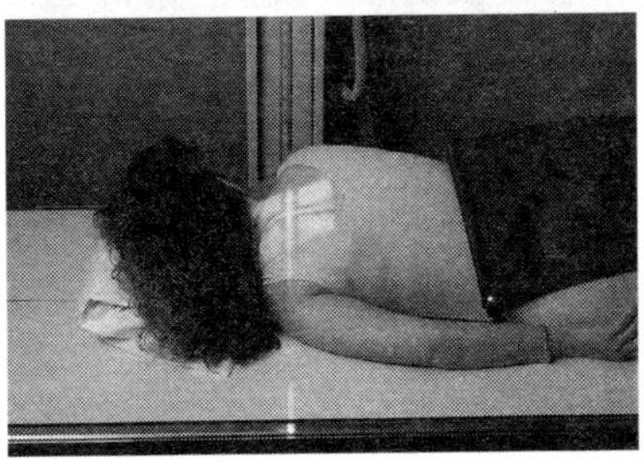

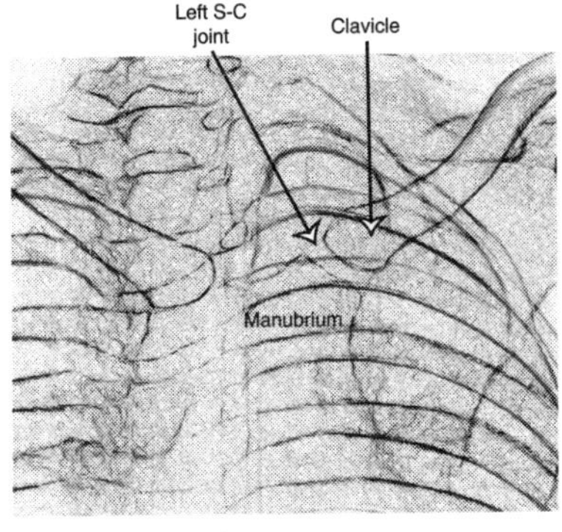

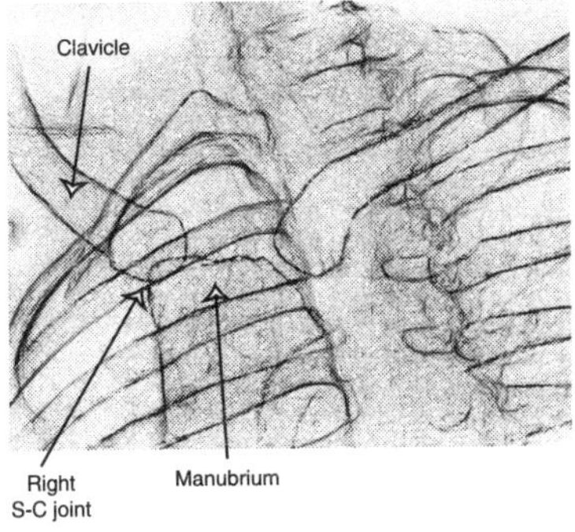

Trauma Considerations Injury to the ribs can be very painful due to the constant movement of respiration and, if severe enough, can be life-threatening. For this reason, perhaps the single most important radiograph in a rib examination series may be a routine, erect chest projection. If at all possible, it is important to radiograph the patient upright (or at least with some type of horizontal central projection) to rule out the possibility of **pneumothorax** (presence of air in the pleural cavity) or **hemothorax** (presence of blood in the pleural cavity) resulting from possible laceration of the lung tissue. It is more important to obtain this diagnostic information than to check for rib fractures. Once the patient is stabilized, a complete series of radiographs can be obtained.

Because rib and sternal injuries may be painful, it is generally more comfortable for the patient to stand in front of a Bucky than to lie on the painful injured side on the radiographic table. The area of interest is always placed closest to the recording medium (film). If the study is performed erect, the patient is not forced into uncomfortable positions. Because of the increased comfort in the erect position, improved patient cooperation helps realize improved radiographs studies (i.e., reduction of repeat radiographs, faster examinations, etc.).

Pediatric Considerations Because the bones of children are not fully **ossified** (changed to bone), children are not as susceptible to fractures resulting from trauma as are adults. This is particularly true in the thorax, which is designed for flexibility to facilitate the respiration process. Radiographic examinations of the ribs are rarely ordered for pediatric patients.

Geriatric Considerations Considerations when examining a geriatric patient are lack of mobility and flexibility. Patience and respect are the most important skills a radiographer can use to facilitate the examination. It is much more comfortable for the patient and quicker for the radiographer to radiograph the geriatric patient standing at the upright Bucky as opposed to examining the patient on a radiographic table.

CERVICAL SPINE

ROUTINE AND ALTERNATIVE POSITIONS/PROJECTIONS

Part	Routine	Page	Alternative	Page
Cervical spine	AP	218		
	AP open mouth	220	AP odontoid process (Fuchs)	226
	Oblique	220		
	Lateral	222	Flexion/extension laterals	224
			AP vertebral arch	228

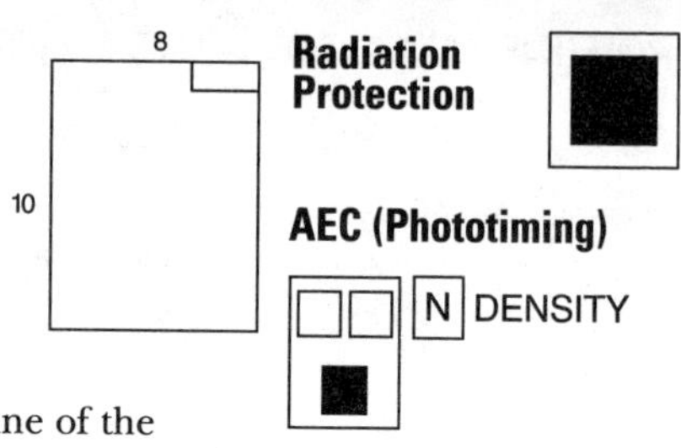

Technical Considerations
- Regular screen/film
- Grid
- kVp range: 75–80
- SID: 40 inch (100 cm)

Patient Position Supine with midsagittal plane (MSP) centered to the midline of the table.

Part Position Adjust so there is no rotation of the head or body; extend the neck so that a line from the lower edge of the upper incisors to the mastoid tips is perpendicular to the table.

Central Ray Directed to C5 (thyroid cartilage) at a 15° to 20° cephalic angle.

Breathing Instructions Normal respiration.

Example Exposure Techniques
Measure at CR and Use this Chart

Room	cm	kVp	mAs	mA	Sec	Beam	Film	Grid	1Ø3Ø
	9								
	10								
	11								
	12								
	13								
	14								
	15								
	16								
	17								
	18								

Evaluation Criteria

- Should include C3–T2.
- There should be no rotation as evidenced by equal distance from spinous processes to spinous border on each side.
- Intervertebral disk spaces should be open.
- Base of skull and mandible will overlap C1 and C2.

Exam Rationale

Examination of the cervical spine may be indicated in the investigation of degenerative disease or in cases of trauma.

Tip This projection may also be done with the patient in an erect position.

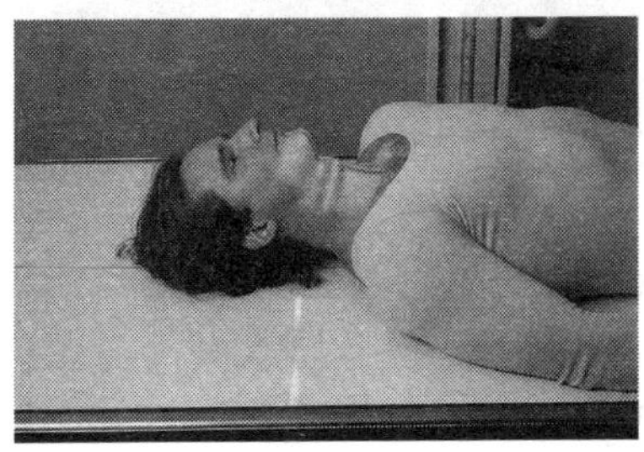

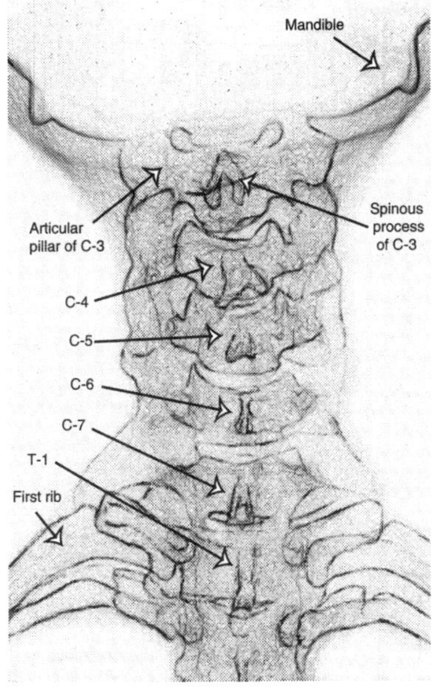

Technical Considerations
- Regular screen/film
- Grid
- kVp range: 70–75
- SID: 40 inch (100 cm)

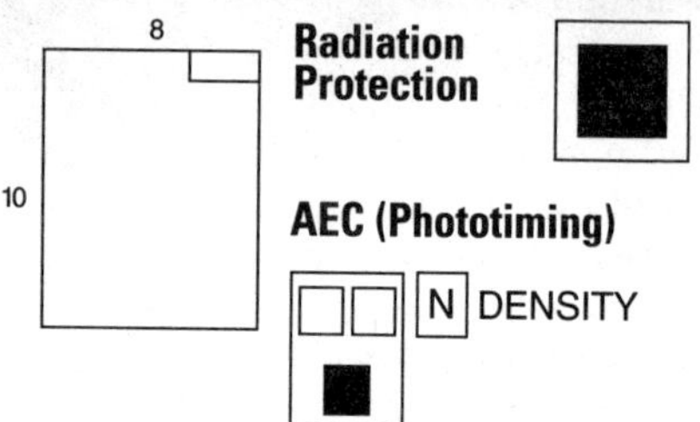

Patient Position Supine with MSP centered to the midline of the table.

Part Position Adjust so there is no rotation of the head or body; extend the neck so that a line from the lower edge of the upper incisors to the mastoid tips is perpendicular to the table; have the patient open mouth by lowering the lower mandible.

Central Ray Directed through the center of the open mouth.

Breathing Instructions Suspend respiration.

Evaluation Criteria
- C1 and C2 should be clearly demonstrated through the open mouth.
- C1–2 zygapophyseal joint should be clearly visible.

Example Exposure Techniques
Measure at CR and Use Chart (p.218)

Room	cm	kVp	mAs	mA	Sec	Beam	Film	Grid	1Ø3Ø
	13								
	14								
	15								
	16								
	17								
	18								
	19								
	20								
	21								
	22								

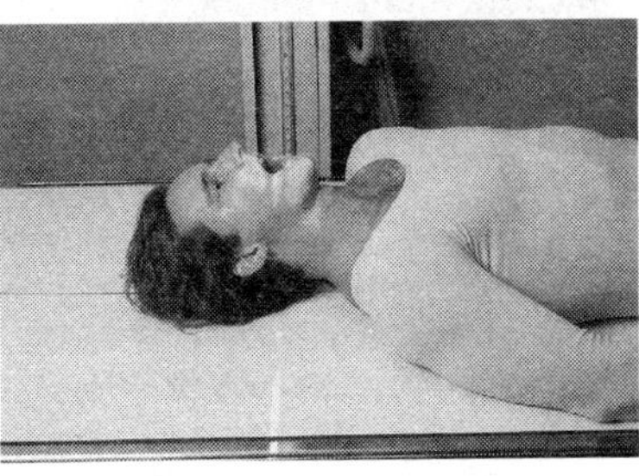

- If the lower edge of the upper incisors and the base of the skull are superimposed, the position cannot be improved.

Exam Rationale This projection demonstrates the first two cervical vertebrae free of superimposition.

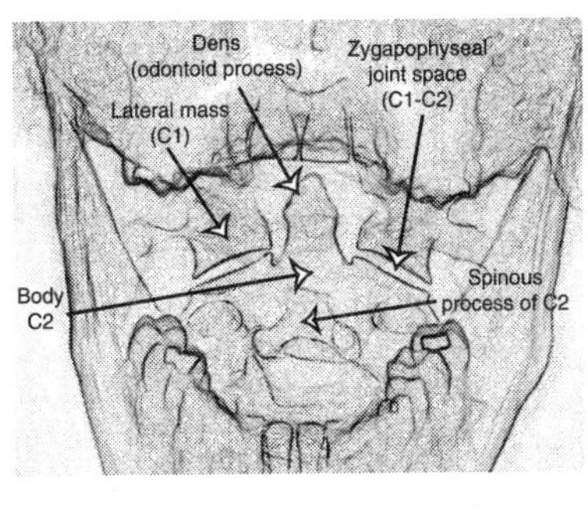

Tips

1. The patient should not open his mouth until just before the exposure is made because this position is somewhat uncomfortable and difficult to maintain.
2. Care must be taken that only the lower jaw is moved when the mouth is opened, maintaining the position of the spine.

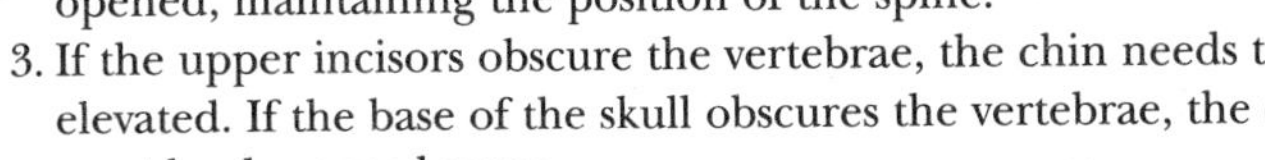

3. If the upper incisors obscure the vertebrae, the chin needs to be elevated. If the base of the skull obscures the vertebrae, the chin must be depressed more.
4. Take care that center AEC has full primary beam collimation.

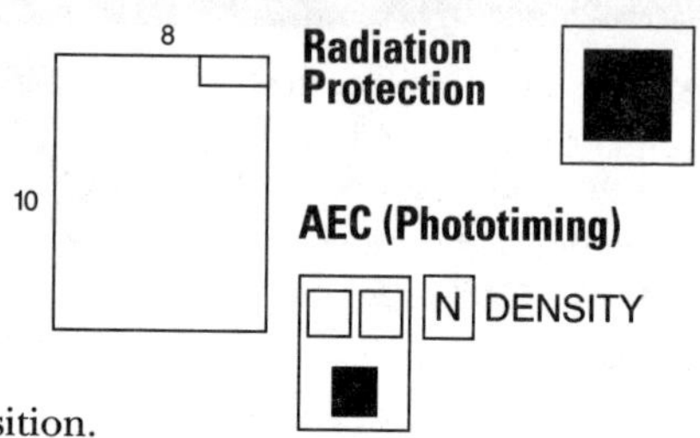

Technical Considerations
- Regular screen/film
- Grid
- kVp range: 75–80
- SID: 40 inch (100 cm)

Patient Position Erect or seated with the body at a 45° angle from the PA position.

Part Position Adjust so the whole body forms an angle of 45° with the plane of the film; the head should look straight ahead; chin should be extended slightly.

Central Ray Directed to C4 (upper margin of the thyroid cartilage) at 15 ° to 20° caudal angle.

Breathing Instructions Normal respiration.

Evaluation Criteria
- Intervertebral foramina and disk spaces should be open.
- All seven cervical vertebrae should be seen.
- Chin should be sufficiently elevated so the mandibular rami do not overlap C1.
- Cervical pedicles should be well demonstrated.

Example Exposure Techniques **Measure at CR and Use Chart (p.218)**									
Room	**cm**	**kVp**	**mAs**	**mA**	**Sec**	**Beam**	**Film**	**Grid**	**1Ø3Ø**
	9								
	10								
	11								
	12								
	13								
	14								
	15								
	16								
	17								
	18								

Exam Rationale This position demonstrates the open intervertebral foramina and pedicles closest to the film (the down side). Both sides are examined for comparison.

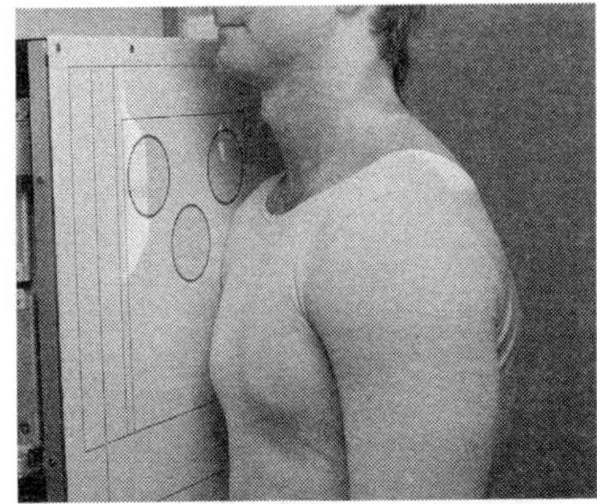

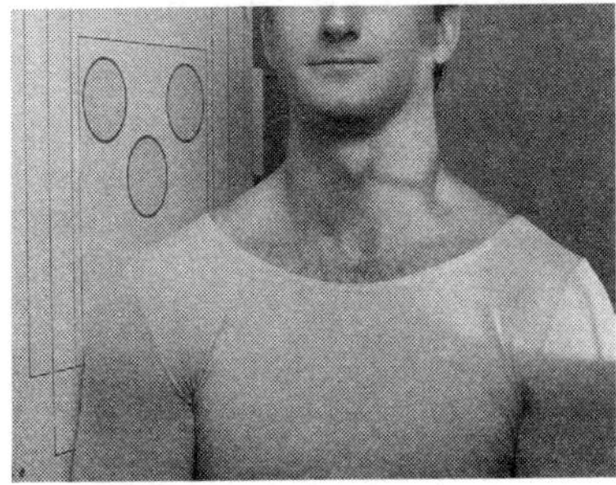

Tips

1. These projections may also be done with the patient in a recumbent position, although the erect or seated position is preferred.
2. These projections may also be done with the patient rotated 45° from the AP position; the central ray is then directed to C4 at a 15° to 20° cephalic angle.
3. Some department protocols call for these projections to be done at a 72-inch (180 cm) focus film distance (as with the lateral).
4. Take care that patient remains centered to AEC.

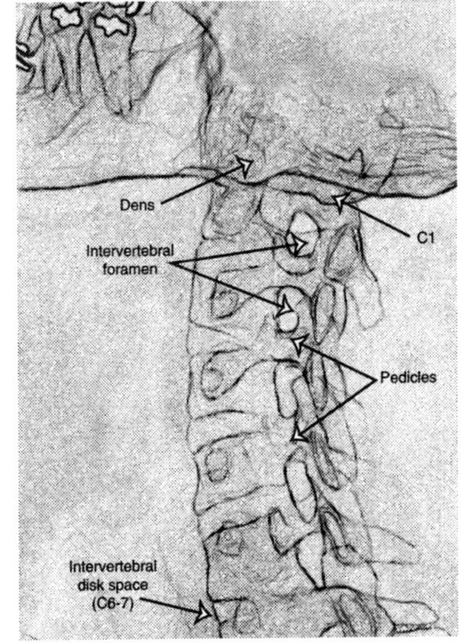

Technical Considerations

- Regular screen/film
- Grid
- kVp range: 75–80
- SID: 72 inch (180 cm)

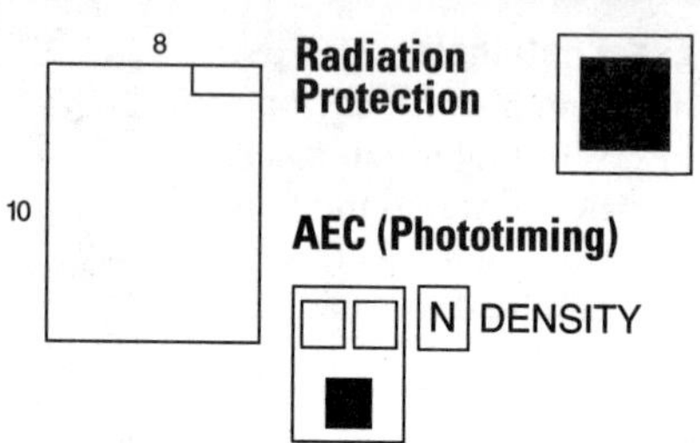

Patient Position Erect or seated with left side against film.

Part Position Center the midcoronal plane to the midline of the film; adjust the body so its MSP is parallel to the film; depress the shoulders; raise the chin slightly to prevent overlap of the mandibular rami on the upper vertebrae.

Central Ray Top of cassette should be placed about 2 inches (5 cm) above EAM; central ray is directed to center of film at the level of the upper margin of the thyroid cartilage.

Breathing Instructions Suspend on expiration.

Example Exposure Techniques **Measure at CR and Use Chart (p.218)**									
Room	**cm**	**kVp**	**mAs**	**mA**	**Sec**	**Beam**	**Film**	**Grid**	**1Ø3Ø**
	9								
	10								
	11								
	12								
	13								
	14								
	15								
	16								
	17								
	18								

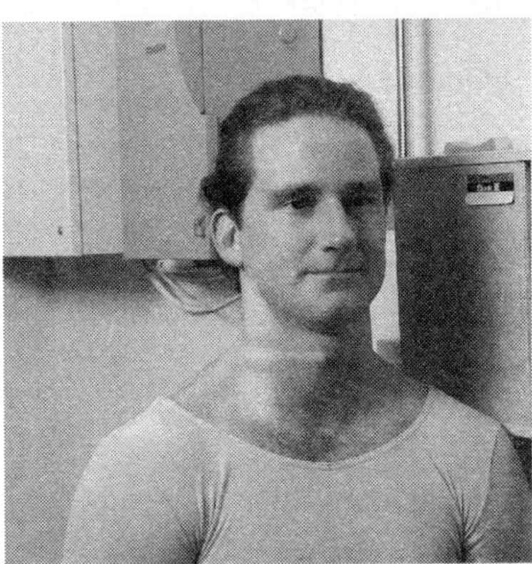

Evaluation Criteria

- Should include all seven cervical vertebrae.
- There should be no rotation as evidenced by superimposition or close approximation of the two mandibular rami.
- Mandibular rami should not be superimposed over upper cervical vertebrae.

Exam Rationale This position shows the vertebral bodies in a lateral position, the intervertebral joint spaces, the articular pillars, the spinous processes, and the articular facets of the lower five vertebrae.

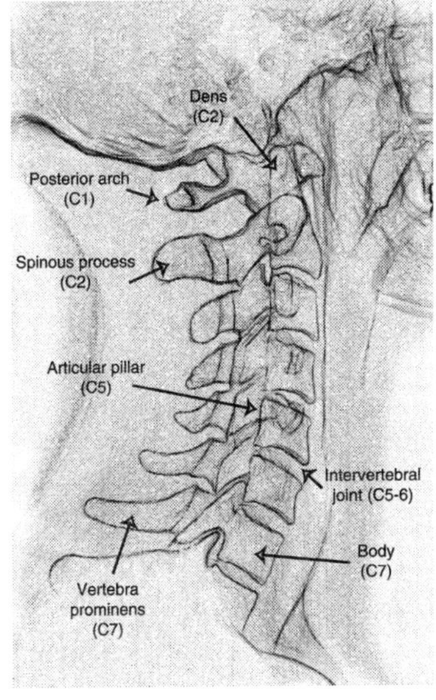

Tips

1. To help depress the shoulders, the patient can hold equal weights (sandbags) in each hand or pull up with both hands on a long strip of gauze under the feet.
2. If it is not possible to depress the shoulders sufficiently to visualize the lower cervical vertebrae, a separate swimmer's lateral should be done.

Technical Considerations

- Regular screen/film
- Grid
- kVp range: 75–80
- SID: 72 inch (180 cm)

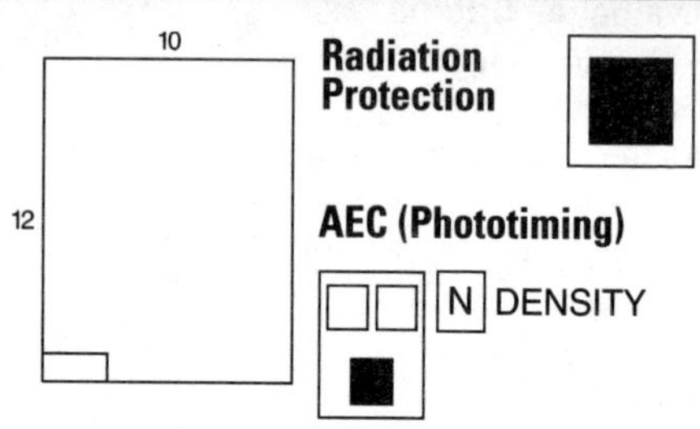

Patient Position Erect or seated with left side against film.

Part Position Center the midcoronal plane to the midline of the film; adjust the body so the MSP is parallel with the film; depress the shoulders.

- Exposure 1: the patient's head is dropped forward as close to the chest as possible.
- Exposure 2: the patient's head is leaned backward as much as possible.

Central Ray Top of cassette should be placed about 2 inches (5 cm) above EAM; central ray is directed to center of film at the level of the upper margin of the thyroid cartilage.

Example Exposure Techniques **Measure at CR and Use Chart (p.218)**									
Room	**cm**	**kVp**	**mAs**	**mA**	**Sec**	**Beam**	**Film**	**Grid**	**1Ø3Ø**
	9								
	10								
	11								
	12								
	13								
	14								
	15								
	16								
	17								
	18								

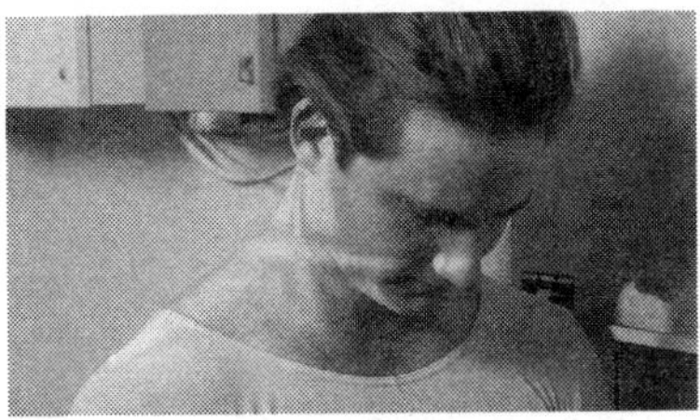

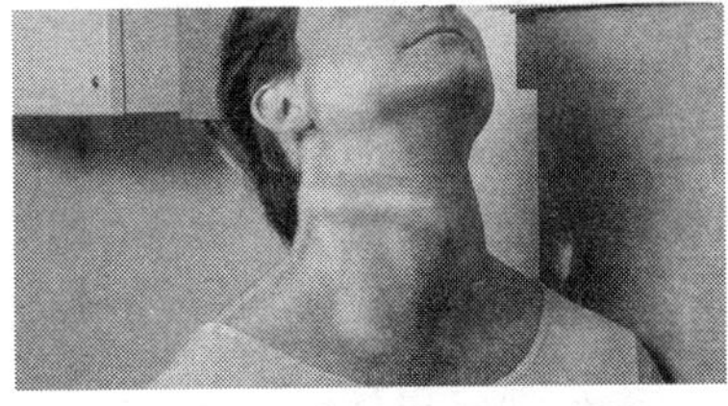

Breathing Instructions

Suspend on expiration.

Evaluation Criteria

- Should include all seven cervical vertebrae.
- There should be no rotation as evidenced by superimposition or close approximation of the two mandibular rami.

Exam Rationale These positions are functional studies to demonstrate the range of motion of the cervical vertebrae.

Tips

1. Care should be taken that only the head and neck are moved, not the shoulders or whole body.
2. These manipulations should not be done on any patient without first ruling out fracture.

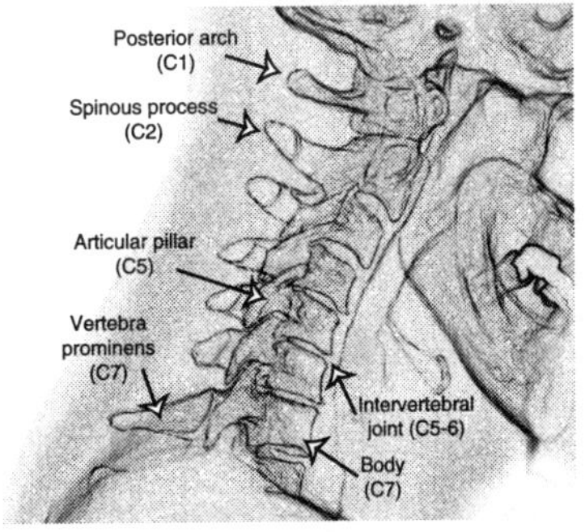

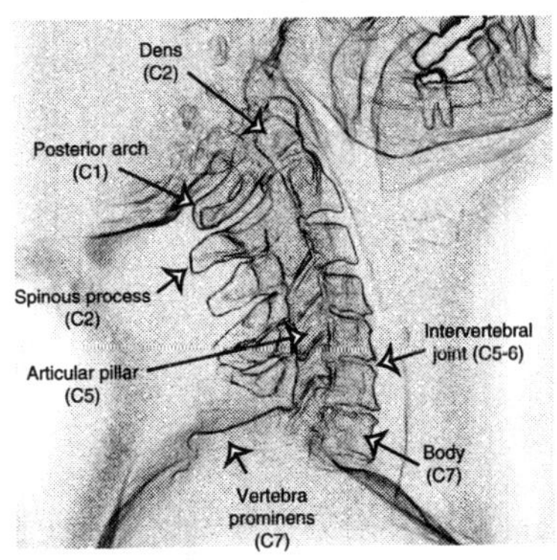

Technical Considerations

- Regular screen/film
- Grid
- kVp range: 75–80
- SID: 40 inch (100 cm)

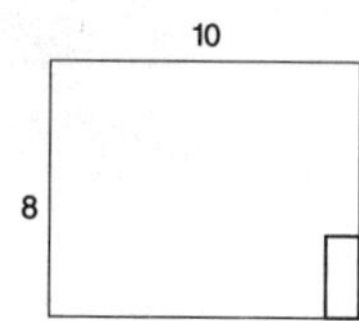

Radiation Protection

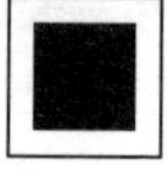

AEC (Phototiming)

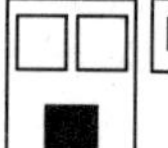

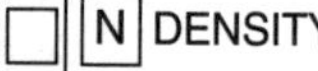

Patient Position

Supine with MSP centered to the midline of the table.

Part Position Adjust so there is no rotation of the head or body; extend the neck so that a line from the chin to the mastoid tips is perpendicular to the table.

Central Ray Center the cassette to the mastoid tips; the central ray is directed to the center of the film, entering the neck just distal to the chin.

Breathing Instructions Normal respiration.

Example Exposure Techniques **Measure at CR and Use Chart (p.218)**									
Room	**cm**	**kVp**	**mAs**	**mA**	**Sec**	**Beam**	**Film**	**Grid**	**1Ø3Ø**
	13								
	14								
	15								
	16								
	17								
	18								
	19								
	20								
	21								
	22								

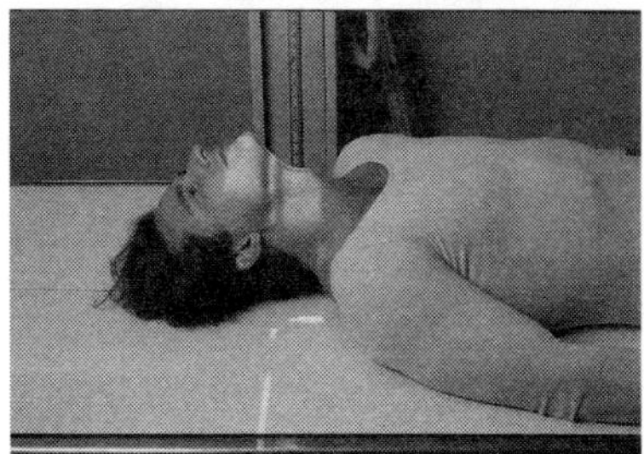

Evaluation Criteria

- Odontoid process should be seen in the foramen magnum.
- There should be no rotation of head or neck.

Exam Rationale This method demonstrates the odontoid process projected within the foramen magnum.

Tip This position should not be attempted with a patient who has a suspected fracture or degenerative disease.

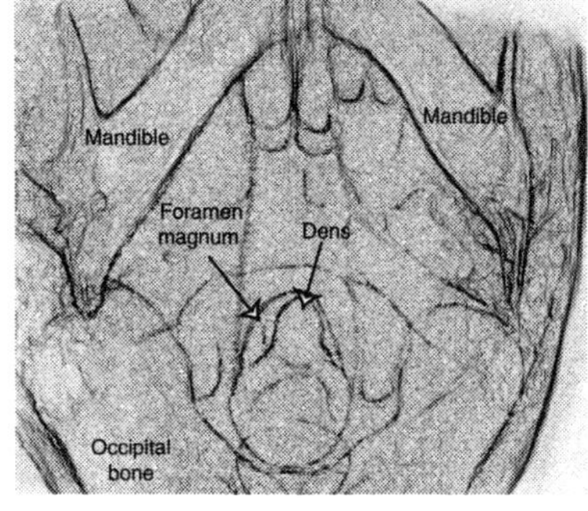

Technical Considerations
- Regular screen/film
- Grid
- kVp range: 75–80
- SID: 40 inch (100 cm)

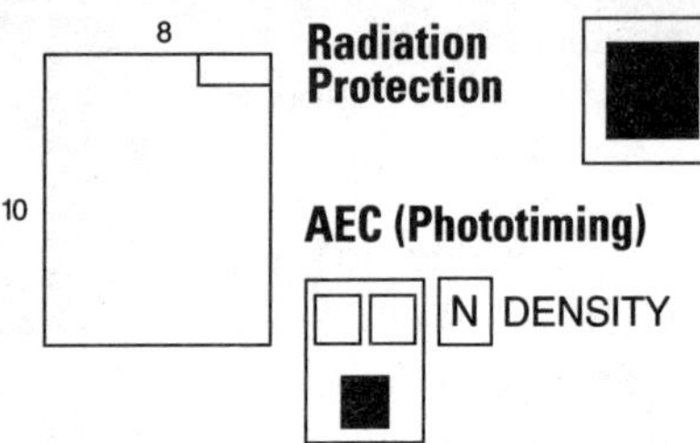

Patient Position Supine with MSP centered to the midline of the table.

Part Position Adjust so there is no rotation of the head or body; hyperextend the neck; a long strip of bandage should be looped around the patient's feet with the knees flexed; the patient should grasp both ends of the bandage and extend the knees, depressing the shoulders.

Central Ray Directed to C5 (thyroid cartilage) at a 25° caudal angle.

Breathing Instructions Normal respiration.

Example Exposure Techniques
Measure at CR and Use Chart (p.218)

Room	cm	kVp	mAs	mA	Sec	Beam	Film	Grid	1Ø3Ø
	11								
	12								
	13								
	14								
	15								
	16								
	17								
	18								
	19								
	20								

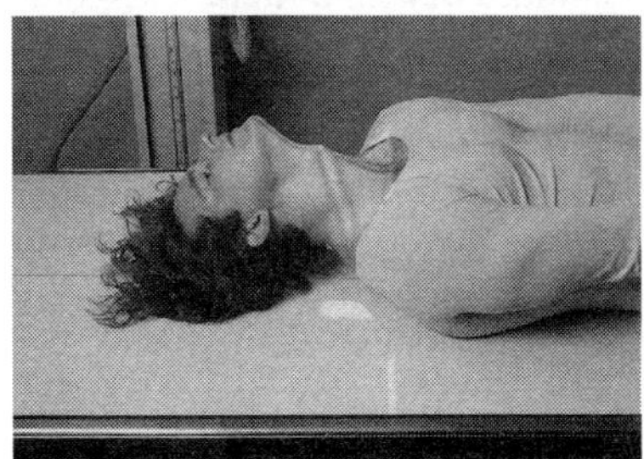

Evaluation Criteria

- Vertebral arches should be seen without superimposition from the vertebral bodies or transverse processes.
- The zygapophyseal joints should be open.

Exam Rationale This projection, sometimes also referred to as the pillar projection, demonstrates the posterior elements of the cervical and upper thoracic spine, including the lateral masses, the zygapophyseal joints, the articular pillars and facets, and the spinous processes.

Tip A patient with greater or lesser cervical lordosis may require more or less angulation of the central ray to achieve the goal of making it parallel with the plane of the articular facets.

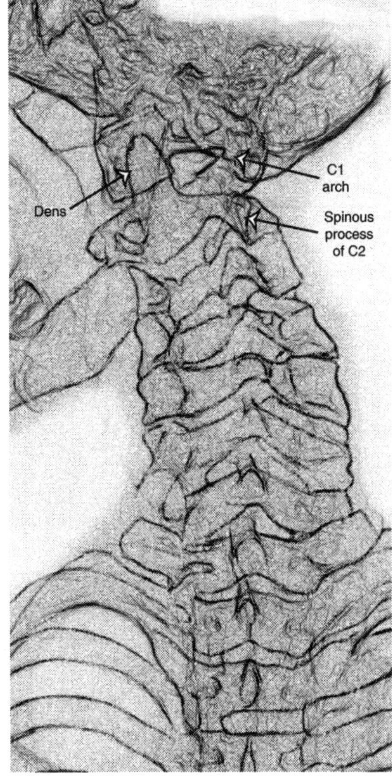

Pediatric Considerations Although cervical spine films are seldom done on young children, they are occasionally required. With children too young to hold very still, it is easier to do all of them, including the lateral, with the patient in the recumbent position. The lateral, difficult to obtain on adults in the recumbent position, is easier with children due to their greater flexibility. With the patient's torso and extremities in a mummy wrap, it is then necessary to only immobilize the child's head and neck.

THORACIC SPINE

ROUTINE AND ALTERNATIVE POSITIONS/PROJECTIONS

Part	Routine	Page	Alternative	Page
Thoracic spine	AP	234		
	Lateral	236	Swimmer's lateral	240
			Oblique	238

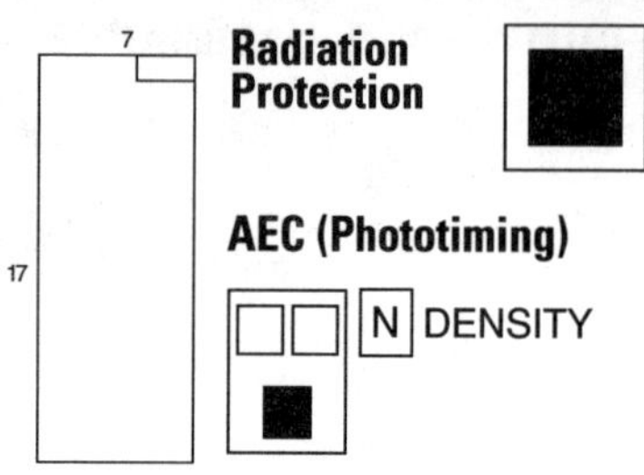

Technical Considerations

- Regular screen/film
- Grid
- kVp range: 75–80
- SID: 40 inch (100 cm)

Patient Position Supine with the MSP centered to the midline of the table; arms are placed at the patient's sides.

Part Position Scapulae and upper spine are flat on table with no rotation; knees may be flexed to bring the spine in closer contact with the table.

Central Ray Perpendicular and directed 3 to 4 inches (8–10 cm) below the jugular notch to the sixth thoracic vertebra. The top of the film should be 1 to 2 inches (3–5 cm) above the top of the shoulder.

Breathing Instructions Suspend on expiration.

Evaluation Criteria

- Must include all thoracic vertebrae.
- Transverse processes, pedicles, vertebral bodies, and intervertebral disk spaces should be demonstrated.
- Although visible, the transverse processes are normally superimposed on the heads of the ribs.

Example Exposure Techniques
Measure at CR and Use Chart (p.218)

Room	cm	kVp	mAs	mA	Sec	Beam	Film	Grid	1Ø3Ø
	14								
	16								
	18								
	20								
	22								
	24								
	26								
	28								

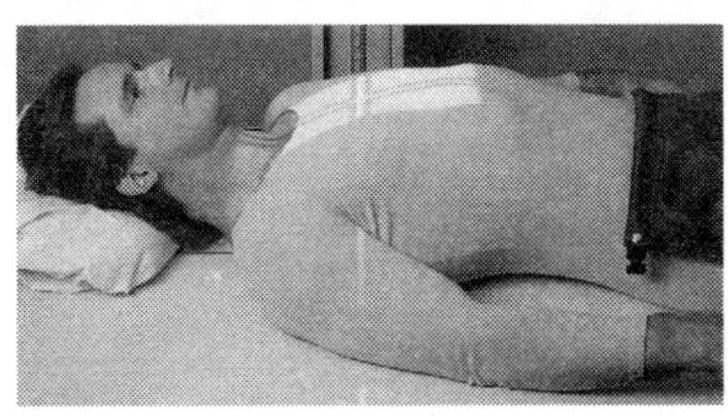

- Rotation, as evidenced by the asymmetrical appearance of the transverse processes or pedicles, should not be observed.
- Spinous processes should be in the midline.

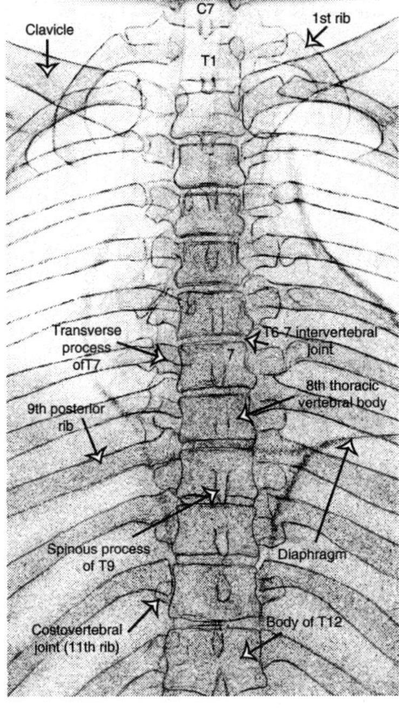

Exam Rationale The most common indications for thoracic spine examinations are trauma and degenerative disease. Structures best demonstrated on the AP include the vertebral bodies, transverse processes, pedicles, and intervertebral disk spaces.

Tips

1. Patients with severe kyphosis may be examined prone, with a PA projection.
2. Some department protocols require collimation to the edge of the transverse processes; others prefer the collimator to be left open to view the entire thorax, on a 14 × 17 inch film.
3. Radiographic densities in the thoracic region vary considerably. The air-filled trachea overlies the upper vertebrae; the fluid-filled heart overlies the mid and lower vertebrae. A wedge filter or the anode-heel effect may be used to help maintain even levels of density from T1–T12.
4. Care should be taken not to elevate the head too much because the chin may overlie vertebral bodies.
5. If a pillow is used, care must be taken not to place it under the thoracic vertebra.

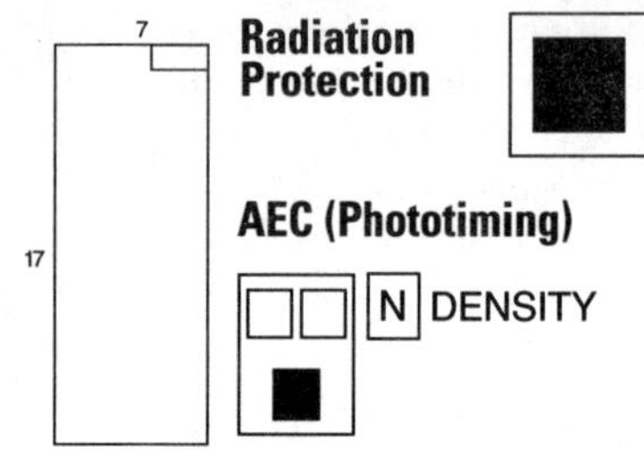

Technical Considerations
- Regular screen/film
- Grid
- kVp range: 75–80
- SID: 40 inch (100 cm)

Patient Position Recumbent left lateral with knees and hips flexed for comfort; arms are drawn forward at right angles to the body to prevent the scapulae from superimposing on the thoracic spine.

Part Position Place the long axis of the spine parallel to the table; the sagittal plane should be parallel and the coronal plane perpendicular to the table. The midaxillary line should be centered to the table.

Central Ray Perpendicular and directed 4 inches (10 cm) below the jugular notch to the seventh thoracic vertebra. The top of the film should be 1/2 to 1 inch (1–3 cm) above the top of the shoulder.

Breathing Instructions Normal respiration. The patient is allowed to continue normal breathing during the exposure, as this will blur thorax shadows, which frequently obscure bony detail. At least 2 seconds of exposure time is needed to accommodate the breathing technique.

Example Exposure Techniques **Measure at CR and Use Chart (p.218)**									
Room	**cm**	**kVp**	**mAs**	**mA**	**Sec**	**Beam**	**Film**	**Grid**	**1Ø3Ø**
	20								
	22								
	24								
	26								
	28								
	30								
	32								
	34								

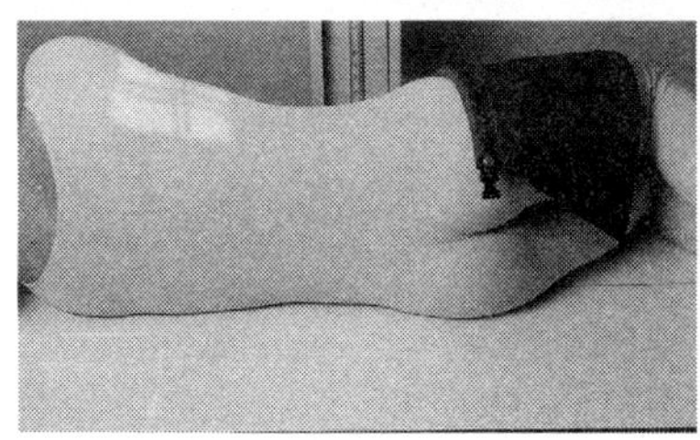

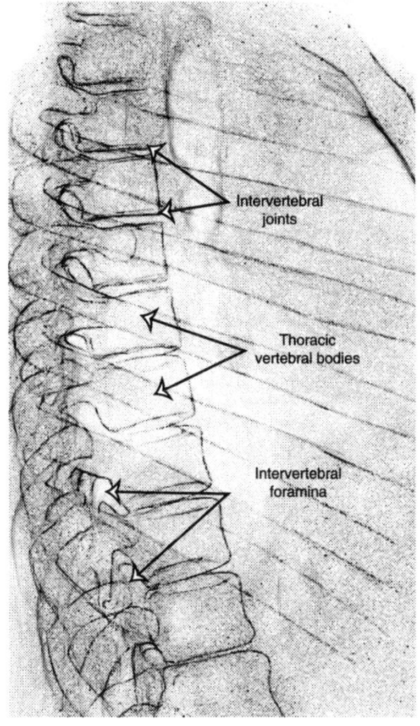

Evaluation Criteria

- Must include at least T4–T12.
- The posterior ribs should be mostly superimposed, indicating minimal rotation.
- Intervertebral disk spaces and intervertebral foramina should be clearly demonstrated.

Exam Rationale The lateral is taken at 90° to the AP. Structures best demonstrated include the vertebral bodies, intervertebral disk spaces, and intervertebral foramina. The spinous processes are not well visualized due to their superimposition on ribs. The upper three to four vertebrae are not visualized due to superimposition from shoulder structures.

Tips

1. If a visible downward sag is present in the spine after placing the patient into a lateral position, a small radiolucent sponge should be placed under the thoracolumbar area to make the spine parallel to the table.
2. To visualize the upper three to four vertebrae, a swimmer's lateral must be taken.
3. If a pillow is used, care must be taken not to place it under the thoracic vertebra.
4. If the patient is unable to lie on the left side, a right lateral may be substituted.

Technical Considerations
- Regular screen/film
- Grid
- kVp range: 75–80
- SID: 40 inch (100 cm)

7

17

Radiation Protection

AEC (Phototiming)

N DENSITY

Patient Position Semi-supine, RPO/LPO.

Part Position Place the spine at a 70° to 75° angle to the film (15–20° from the true lateral); center the spine to the midline of the table.

Central Ray Perpendicular and directed 3 inches (8 cm) below the jugular notch to the sixth thoracic vertebra. The top of the film should be 1 to 2 inches (3–5 cm) above the top of the shoulder.

Breathing Instructions Suspend on expiration.

Evaluation Criteria
- Must include all thoracic vertebrae.
- In the RPO and LPO positions, the zygapophyseal joints on the side farthest from the table should be clearly opened (this is the

Example Exposure Techniques **Measure at CR and Use Chart (p.218)**									
Room	**cm**	**kVp**	**mAs**	**mA**	**Sec**	**Beam**	**Film**	**Grid**	**1Ø3Ø**
	20								
	24								
	26								
	28								
	30								
	32								
	34								
	36								
	38								
	40								

same as cervical spine obliques, but differs from lumbar spine obliques).

- Superior and inferior articulating processes, pedicles, laminae, pars interarticularis, vertebral bodies, and disk spaces should be demonstrated.

Exam Rationale Oblique projections of the thoracic spine are usually done to demonstrate the zygapophyseal joints. They are occasionally done to demonstrate mediastinal structures or to remove mediastinal shadows from obscuring thoracic spine anatomy. Both right and left obliques are done.

Tips

1. If the patient cannot be placed supine, oblique PA projections may be performed with the patient semiprone (RAO/LAO); in the RAO/LAO positions, the zygapophyseal joint visualized is the one nearest the table.
2. To demonstrate the inferior zygapophyseal joints of T12, a 45° patient rotation is required.
3. Kyphosis or scoliosis of the thoracic spine requires varying patient rotation to demonstrate the zygapophyseal joints.

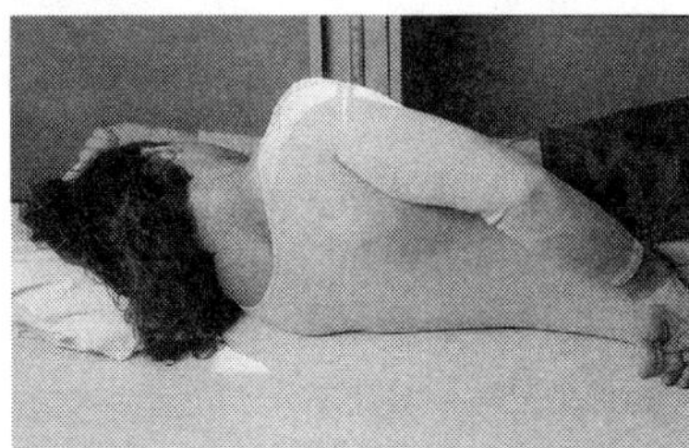

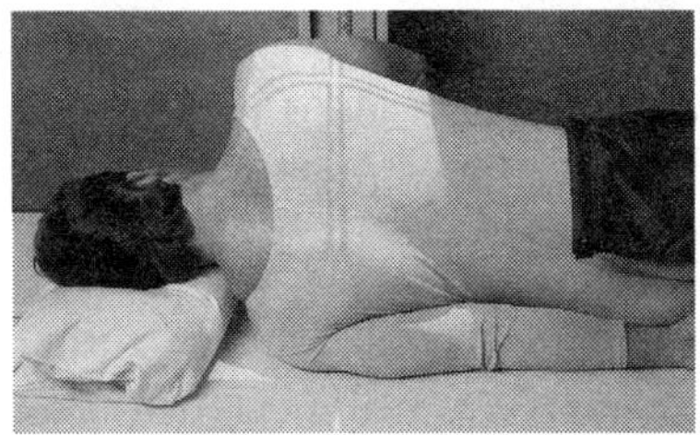

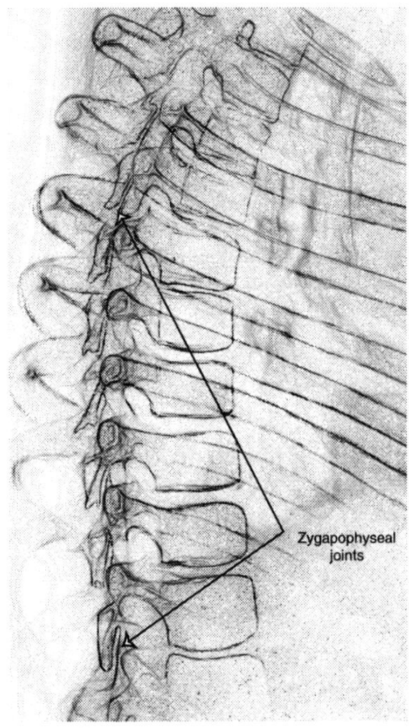

Technical Considerations
- Regular screen/film
- Grid
- kVp range: 80–90
- SID: 40 inch (100 cm)

Patient Position Left lateral recumbent.

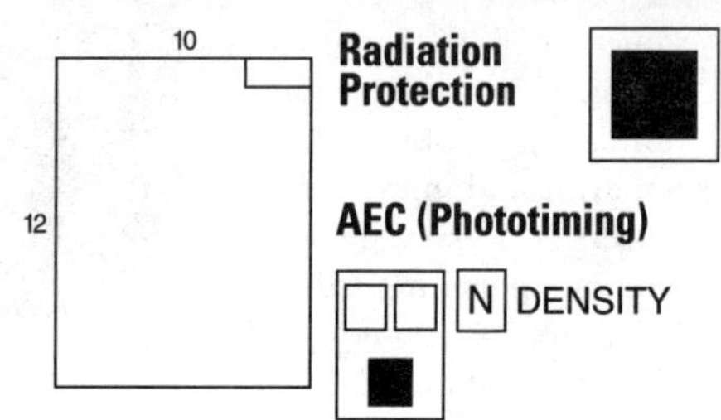

Part Position True lateral position with the MSP parallel to the table; the arm closest to the table is abducted far above the head while the shoulder farthest from the film should be depressed as much as possible; rotate the depressed shoulder forward slightly and the raised shoulder backward slightly to prevent superimposition of the humeral heads on the vertebral bodies.

Central Ray Directed at a 5° to 10° caudal angle to the level of T1–T2.

Breathing Instructions Suspend on expiration.

Example Exposure Techniques
Measure at CR and Use Chart (p.218)

Room	cm	kVp	mAs	mA	Sec	Beam	Film	Grid	1Ø3Ø
	16								
	18								
	20								
	22								
	24								
	26								
	28								
	30								
	32								
	34								

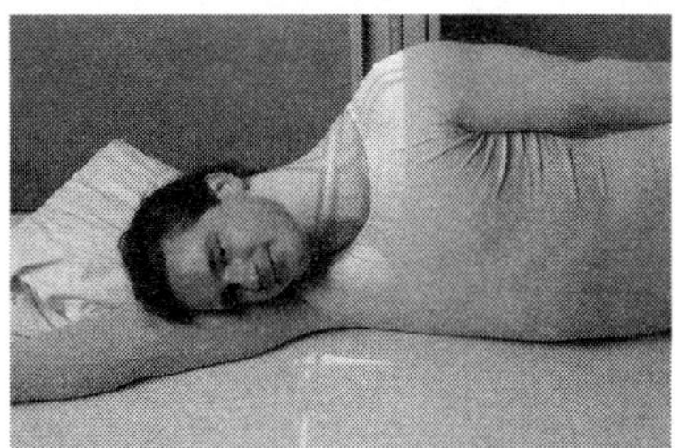

Evaluation Criteria

- The disk space between C7 and T1 and the first three to four thoracic vertebrae must be visualized.
- The humeral heads should not be superimposed on the vertebral bodies.

Exam Rationale The most common indication for the swimmer's lateral is trauma to the upper thoracic or lower cervical vertebra. The swimmer's lateral will demonstrate the junction between C7 and T1 and the first three to four thoracic vertebrae, which are not visualized on routine lateral thoracic spine radiographs.

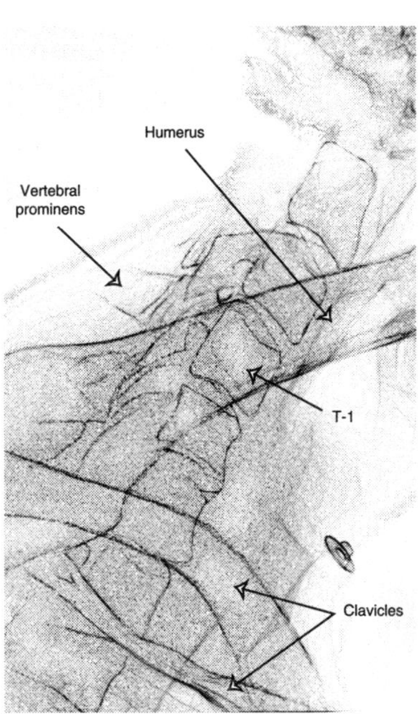

Tips

1. A pillow or sponge should be placed under the patient's head to prevent it from tilting toward the table.
2. The patient may be allowed to continue normal breathing during the exposure because this will blur thorax shadows, which frequently obscure bony detail.

Geriatric Considerations Several major degenerative diseases affect the spine of geriatric patients. These diseases reduce the patient's flexibility and mobility. To obtain optimum films, the radiographer needs to adapt routines to compensate for this loss of vertebral motion.

LUMBAR SPINE, SACRUM, AND COCCYX

ROUTINE AND ALTERNATIVE POSITIONS/PROJECTIONS

Technical Considerations

- Regular screen/film
- Grid
- kVp range: 75–80
- SID: 40 inch (100 cm)

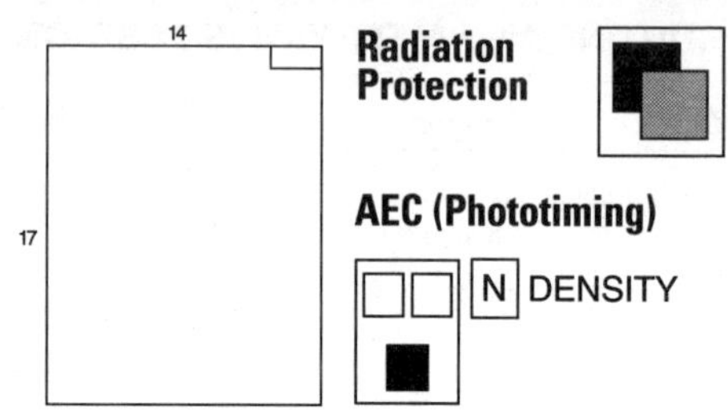

Patient Position

Supine with the MSP centered to the midline of the table; arms are placed at the patient's sides or high on the chest.

Part Position Flex the knees to place the small of the back in contact with the surface of the table and to help reduce rotation.

Central Ray Perpendicular and centered at the level of the iliac crest.

Breathing Instructions Suspend on expiration.

Evaluation Criteria

- Must include all lumbar vertebrae and part of the sacrum.
- Rotation, as evidenced by the asymmetrical appearance of the

Example Exposure Techniques
Measure at CR and Use Chart (p.218)

Room	cm	kVp	mAs	mA	Sec	Beam	Film	Grid	1Ø3Ø
	10								
	14								
	18								
	22								
	26								
	30								
	34								
	38								
	42								
	46								

sacroiliac joints, pedicles, or transverse processes, should not be observed.

- Transverse processes, pedicles, vertebral bodies, and intervertebral disk spaces should be demonstrated.
- Spinous processes should be in the midline.

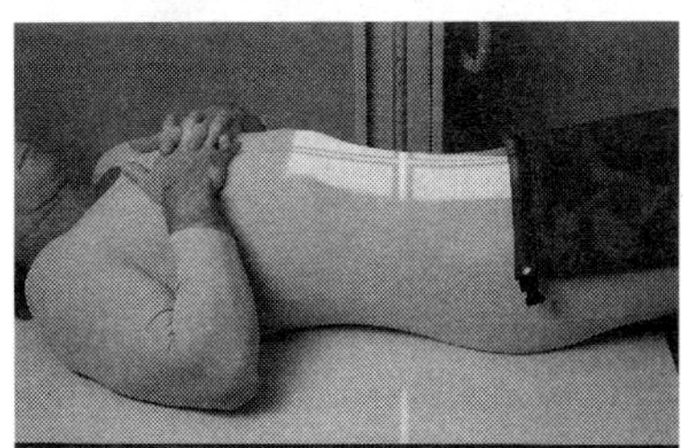

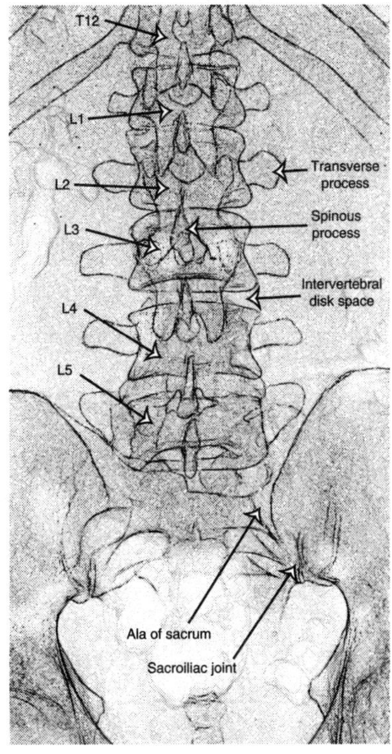

Exam Rationale The most common indications for lumbar spine examinations are trauma and degenerative disease. Structures best demonstrated on the AP include the vertebral bodies, transverse processes, pedicles, and intervertebral disk spaces.

Tips

1. If the patient cannot be placed supine, the PA projection may be performed with the patient prone. The PA will result in more magnification but may more clearly demonstrate the intervertebral disk spaces.
2. Some department protocols require collimation to the edge of the transverse processes, whereas others prefer the collimator to be left open to view the entire abdomen.

Technical Considerations

- Regular screen/film
- Grid
- kVp range: 75–80
- SID: 40 inch (100 cm)

14

17

Radiation Protection

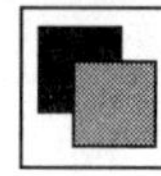

AEC (Phototiming)

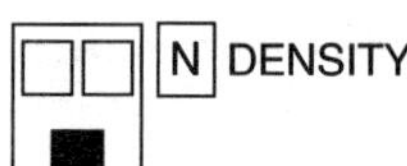

Patient Position

Semi-supine. Arms are placed at the patient's sides or high on the chest.

Part Position Place the spine at a 45° angle to the film; the sagittal plane 1 to 2 inches (3–5 cm) medial to the elevated anterior superior iliac spine is centered to the table.

Central Ray Perpendicular and centered at the level of the iliac crest.

Breathing Instructions Suspend on expiration.

Evaluation Criteria

- Must include all lumbar vertebrae and part of the sacrum.
- In the RPO and LPO positions, the zygapophyseal joints on the side nearer the table should be clearly opened.

Example Exposure Techniques
Measure at CR and Use Chart (p.218)

Room	cm	kVp	mAs	mA	Sec	Beam	Film	Grid	1Ø3Ø
	14								
	18								
	22								
	26								
	30								
	34								
	38								
	42								
	46								

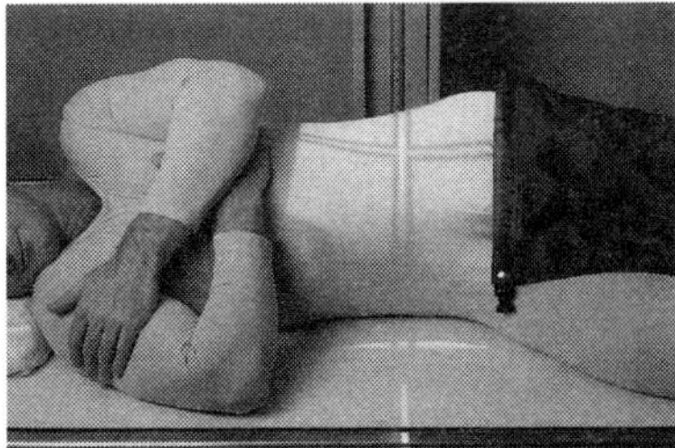

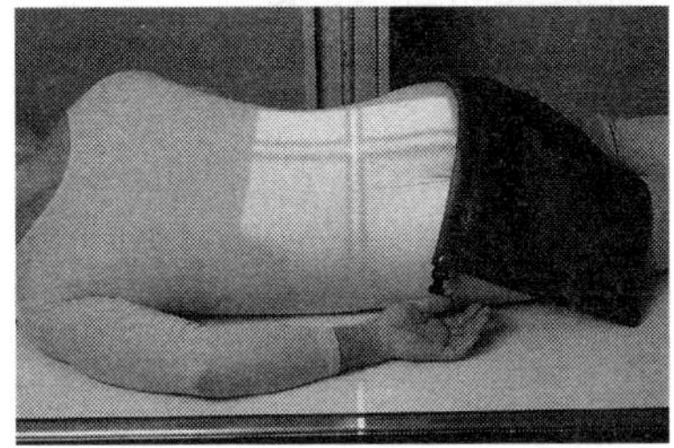

- "Scotty dog" sign should be evident for all five lumbar vertebrae.
- Superior and inferior articulating processes, pedicles, laminae, pars interarticularis, vertebral bodies, and disk spaces should be demonstrated.

Exam Rationale The oblique is a routine position of the lumbar spine that gives a different perspective from the AP, that of a 45° oblique. Both right and left obliques are performed because each demonstrates structures in a slightly different perspective.

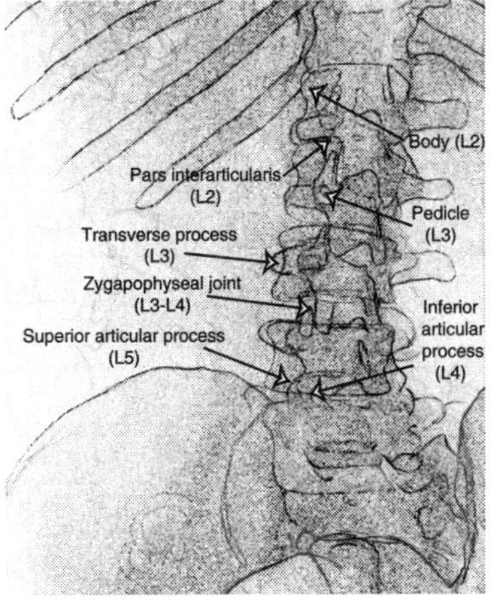

Tips

1. A radiolucent 45° angle sponge may be placed behind the spine to assist the patient in maintaining this position.
2. If the patient cannot be placed supine, oblique PA projections may be performed with the patient semiprone (RAO/LAO). The spine is centered to the midline of the table by placing the central ray 1 inch (3 cm) to the left (for the RAO position) or right (for the LAO position) of the spinous processes. The open zygapophyseal joint is the one farthest from the table (this differs from cervical and thoracic spine obliques).
3. Optimum visualization of the zygapophyseal joint between L5 and S1 may require a 30° patient angle.

Technical Considerations

- Regular screen/film
- Grid
- kVp range: 75–80
- SID: 40 inch (100 cm)

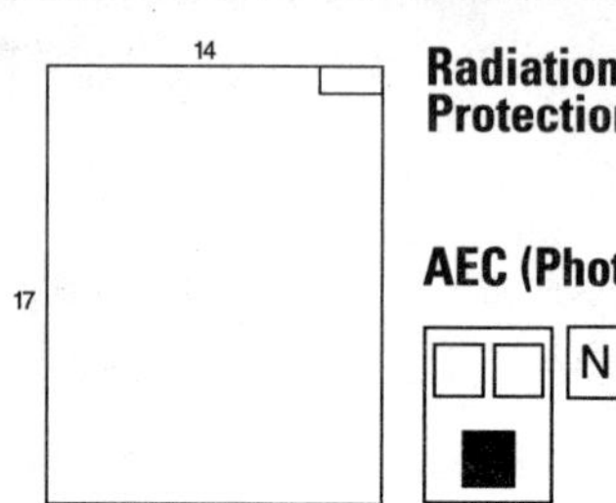

Radiation Protection

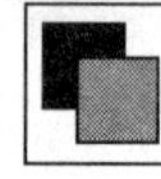

AEC (Phototiming)

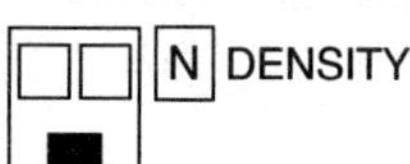

Patient Position

Recumbent left lateral with knees and hips flexed for comfort; arms are placed at right angles to the body with elbows flexed.

Part Position Place the long axis of the spine parallel to the table; the sagittal plane should be parallel and the coronal plane perpendicular to the table; the plane approximately 3 inches (8 cm) anterior to the spinous processes should be centered to the table.

Central Ray Perpendicular and centered at the level of the iliac crest.

Breathing Instructions Suspend on expiration.

Example Exposure Techniques **Measure at CR and Use Chart (p.218)**									
Room	**cm**	**kVp**	**mAs**	**mA**	**Sec**	**Beam**	**Film**	**Grid**	**1Ø3Ø**
	26								
	28								
	30								
	32								
	34								
	36								
	38								
	40								
	42								
	44								

Evaluation Criteria

- Must include all lumbar vertebrae and part of the sacrum.
- Vertebral bodies, intervertebral disk spaces, spinous processes, and intervertebral foramina should be clearly demonstrated.
- The iliac crests and acetabula should be mostly superimposed, indicating minimal rotation.

Exam Rationale The lateral is taken at 90° to the AP. Structures best demonstrated include the vertebral bodies, intervertebral disk spaces, spinous processes, and intervertebral foramina.

Tips

1. If a visible downward sag in the spine is present after placing the patient into a lateral position, a radiolucent sponge should be placed under the thoracolumbar area to make the spine parallel to the table.
2. To better open the intervertebral disk spaces, a 5° caudal angle may be used.
3. If the patient is unable to lie on the left side, a right lateral may be substituted.

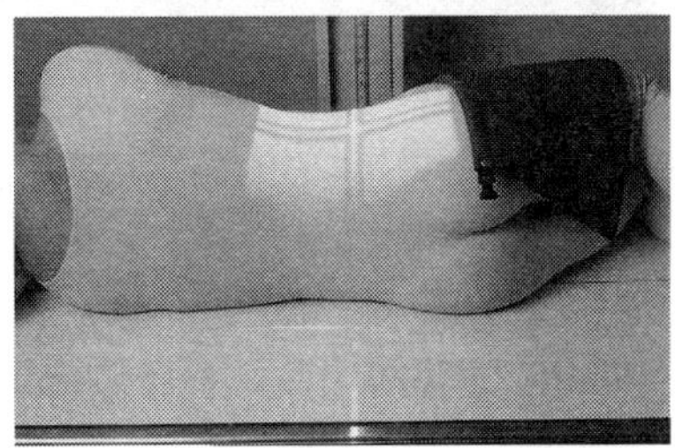

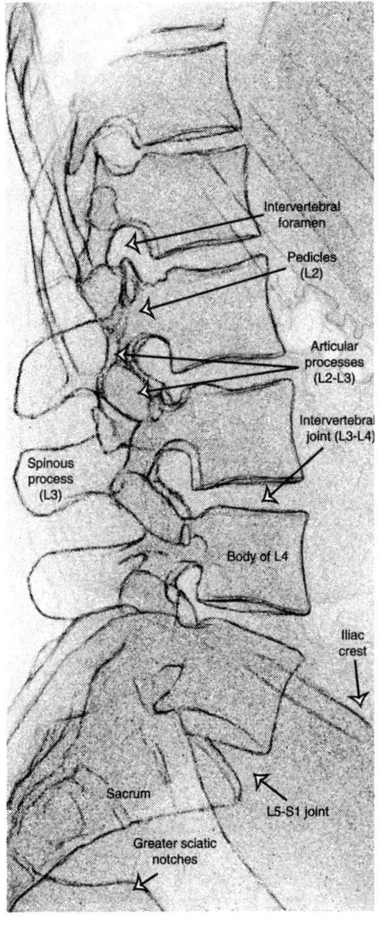

Technical Considerations

- Regular screen/film
- Grid
- kVp range: 90–100
- SID: 40 inch (100 cm)

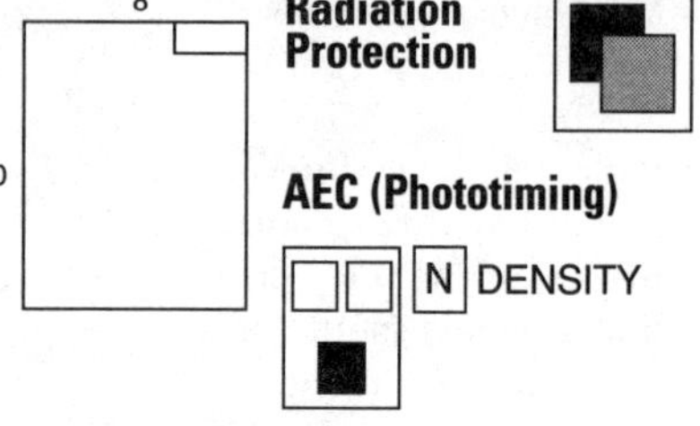

Patient Position

Recumbent left lateral with knees and hips flexed for comfort; arms are placed at right angles to the body with elbows flexed.

Part Position Place the long axis of the spine parallel to the table; the sagittal plane should be parallel and the coronal plane perpendicular to the table; a plane 1 1/2 inches (4 cm) posterior to the midaxillary line should be centered to the table.

Central Ray Directed at a 5° to 10° caudal angle to enter at the L5–S1 joint space; this space is located halfway between the anterior superior iliac spine and the iliac crest and 2 inches (5 cm) anterior to the palpated spinous processes.

Breathing Instructions Suspend on expiration.

Example Exposure Techniques **Measure at CR and Use Chart (p.218)**									
Room	**cm**	**kVp**	**mAs**	**mA**	**Sec**	**Beam**	**Film**	**Grid**	**1Ø3Ø**
	28								
	30								
	32								
	34								
	36								
	38								
	40								
	42								
	44								
	46								

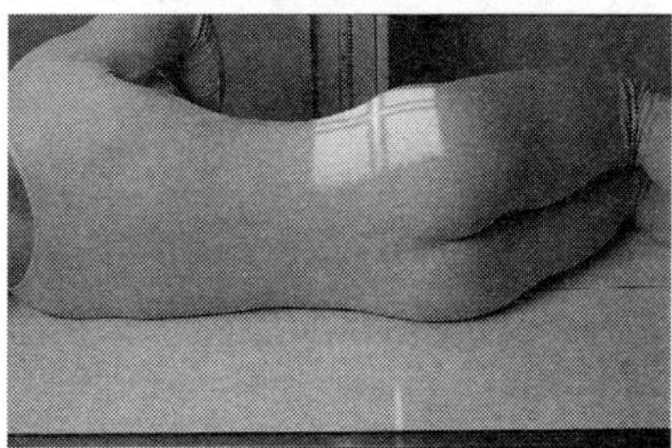

Evaluation Criteria

- L5–S1 joint space should be open.
- The acetabula should be mostly superimposed, indicating minimal rotation.

Exam Rationale The fifth lumbar vertebra and the intervertebral disk between L5 and the sacrum is a common site of pathology. The region is often not well visualized on the lateral lumbar spine because it is much denser than the rest of the lumbar spine and lies at the end of the film, causing the disk space to be closed by the diverging x-ray beam.

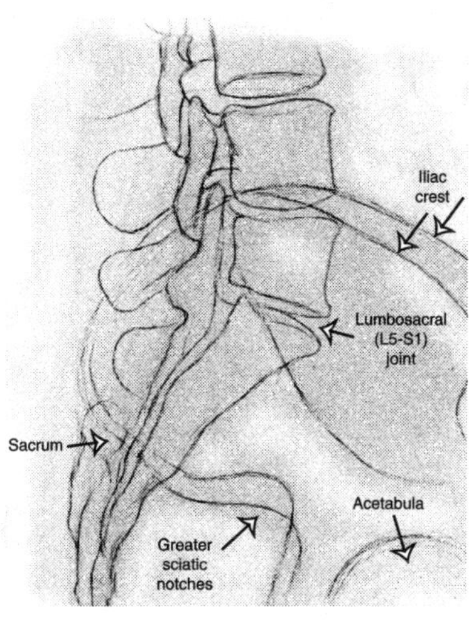

Tips

1. Angulation is not always necessary if the spine is placed parallel to the table.
2. Females may require an increased caudal angle to better open the joint space.
3. To obtain a more uniform density, a lead strip may be placed on the table top behind the patient to limit scatter radiation.

Technical Considerations
- Regular screen/film
- Grid
- kVp range: 80–85
- SID: 40 inch (100 cm)

8

10

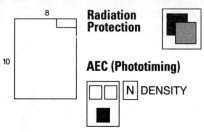

Radiation Protection

AEC (Phototiming)

N DENSITY

Patient Position Supine with the MSP centered to the midline of the table; arms are placed at the patient's sides or high on the chest.

Part Position Flex the knees to place the small of the back in contact with the surface of the table and to help reduce rotation.

Central Ray Directed at a 30° to 35° cephalad angle to enter at the level of the L5–S1 joint space.

Breathing Instructions Suspend on expiration.

Example Exposure Techniques **Measure at CR and Use Chart (p.218)**									
Room	**cm**	**kVp**	**mAs**	**mA**	**Sec**	**Beam**	**Film**	**Grid**	**1Ø3Ø**
	15								
	16								
	17								
	18								
	19								
	20								
	21								
	25								
	23								
	24								

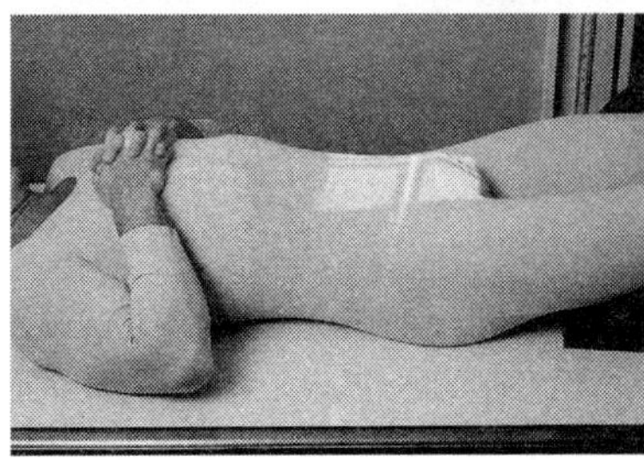

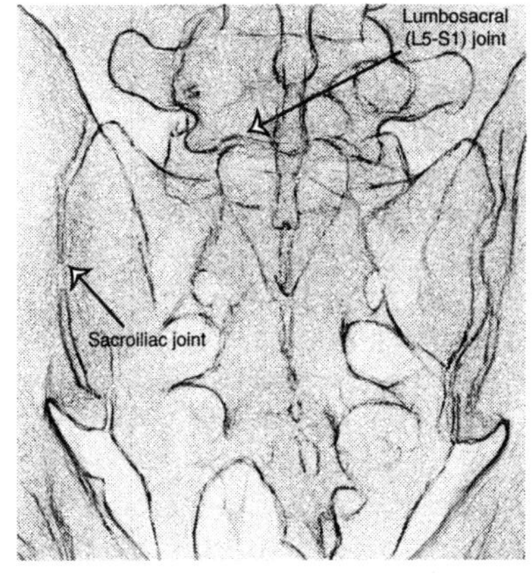

Evaluation Criteria

- L5–S1 joint space should be open.
- Rotation, as evidenced by the asymmetrical appearance of the sacroiliac joints, pedicles, or transverse processes, should not be observed.

Exam Rationale Because the sacrum curves posteriorly, this projection is often necessary to open the intervertebral disk space between L5 and S1.

Tips

1. Females may require an increased cephalad angle to better open the joint space.
2. If the patient cannot be placed supine, a frontal view may be obtained with the patient prone using a 30° to 35° caudal angle. This results in a more magnified view of the L5–S1 disk space.

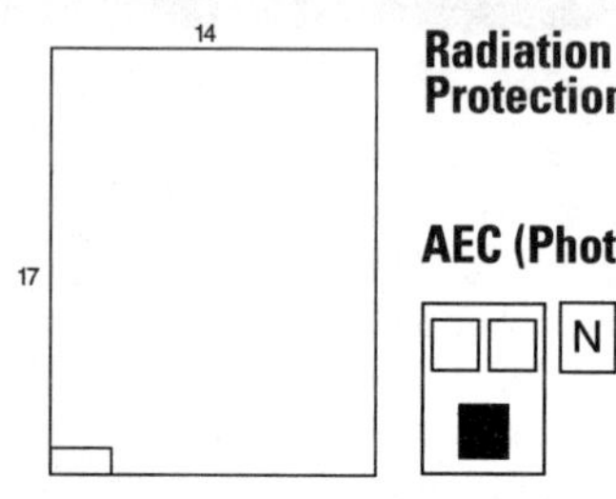

Technical Considerations

- Regular screen/film
- Grid
- kVp range: 80–90
- SID: 40 inch (100 cm)

Patient Position

Standing facing the cassette with arms at the patient's sides; shoes should be removed.

Part Position The MSP is centered to the midline of the film.

Central Ray Perpendicular and centered at a level approximately 4 to 5 inches (10–13 cm) above the iliac crest; the bottom of the film should be placed 2 inches (5 cm) below the level of the iliac crest.

Breathing Instructions Suspend on expiration.

Evaluation Criteria

- All vertebrae affected by the abnormal curvature must be visualized; this normally includes the entire thoracic and lumbar spine.

Example Exposure Techniques **Measure at CR and Use Chart (p.218)**									
Room	**cm**	**kVp**	**mAs**	**mA**	**Sec**	**Beam**	**Film**	**Grid**	**1Ø3Ø**
	10								
	14								
	18								
	22								
	26								
	30								
	34								
	38								
	42								
	46								

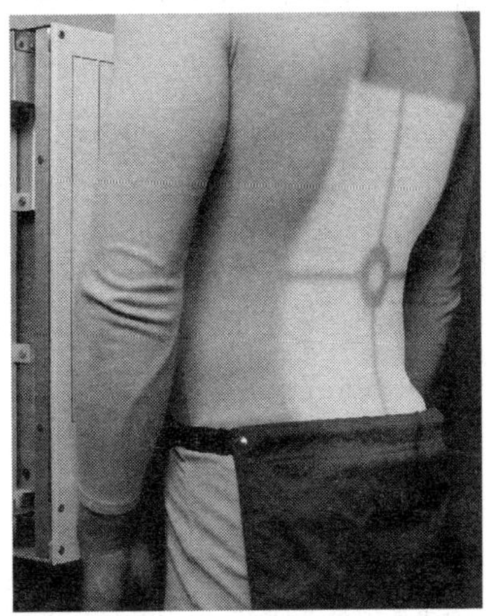

- Excessive rotation, as evidenced by the asymmetrical appearance of the sacroiliac joints, pedicles, or transverse processes, should not be observed; some degree of rotation will likely be present due to the abnormal curvature of the spine.

Exam Rationale Scoliosis, a lateral curvature of the spine, is common. Scoliosis films are taken to periodically monitor the progress of the disease or its treatment. Often a single AP or PA projection is taken to include both the lumbar and thoracic spines because the abnormal curvature usually affects both regions. A lateral film may also be requested.

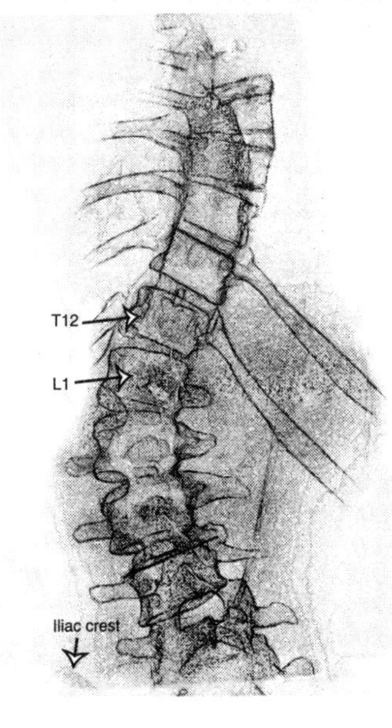

Tips

1. A lateral film may also be requested.
2. Because most patients receive this series over an extended period of time, radiation protection is especially critical. Departments that perform many scoliosis series usually have special shields to cover both the breast and gonadal areas.
3. The PA projection is preferred by most departments because the patient receives less radiation than with an AP.

Technical Considerations

- Regular screen/film
- Grid
- kVp range: 80–90
- SID: 40 inch (100 cm)

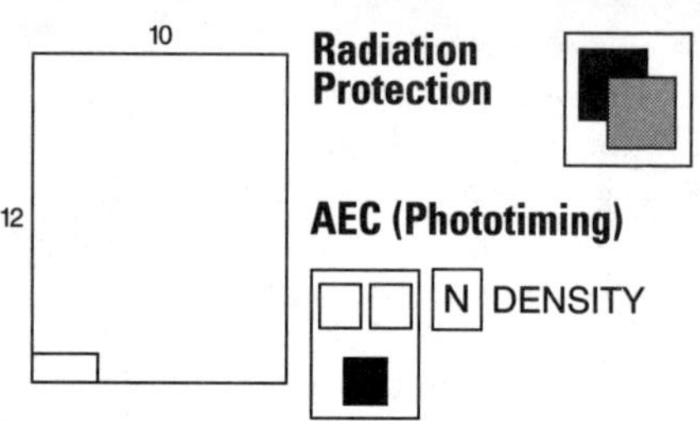

Patient Position

Supine with arms placed at the patient's sides or high on the chest.

Part Position The MSP is centered to the midline of the table; the knees may be flexed to place the small of the back in contact with the surface of the table and to help reduce rotation.

Central Ray Directed at a 15° cephalad angle, entering at a level midway between the symphysis pubis and the anterior superior iliac spine.

Breathing Instructions Suspend on expiration.

Example Exposure Techniques **Measure at CR and Use Chart (p.218)**									
Room	**cm**	**kVp**	**mAs**	**mA**	**Sec**	**Beam**	**Film**	**Grid**	**1Ø3Ø**
	15								
	16								
	17								
	18								
	19								
	20								
	21								
	22								
	23								
	24								

Evaluation Criteria

- Entire sacrum must be included.
- Sacrum should appear more elongated than on an AP lumbar spine projection.
- Rotation, as evidenced by the asymmetrical appearance of the sacroiliac joints and ilia, should not be observed.

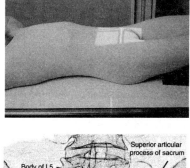

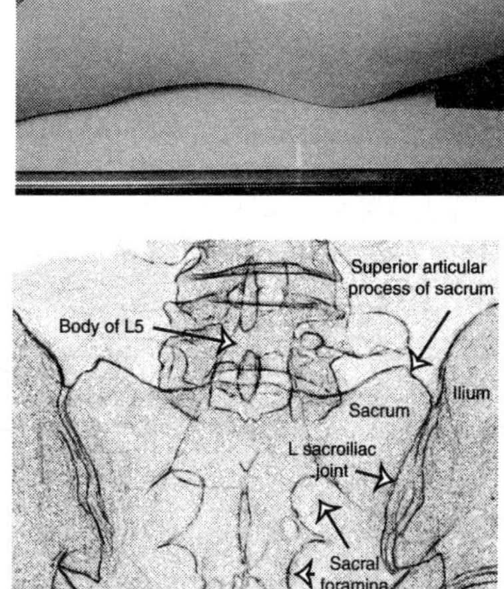

Exam Rationale The most common indication for sacrum examinations is trauma. Structures best demonstrated include the ala, promontory, anterior sacral foramina, and the L5–S1 joint space.

Tips

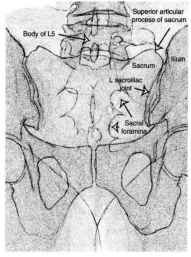

1. Injury to the sacrum may prevent a patient from lying supine. An alternative PA projection can be obtained with the patient lying prone and using a 15° caudal angle, although more radiographic magnification will be evident.
2. Because fecal shadows often overlie the sacrum, the bowel may require cleansing before the radiographic examination to obtain a film of optimum radiographic quality.

Technical Considerations

- Regular screen/film
- Grid
- kVp range: 80–90
- SID: 40 inch (100 cm)

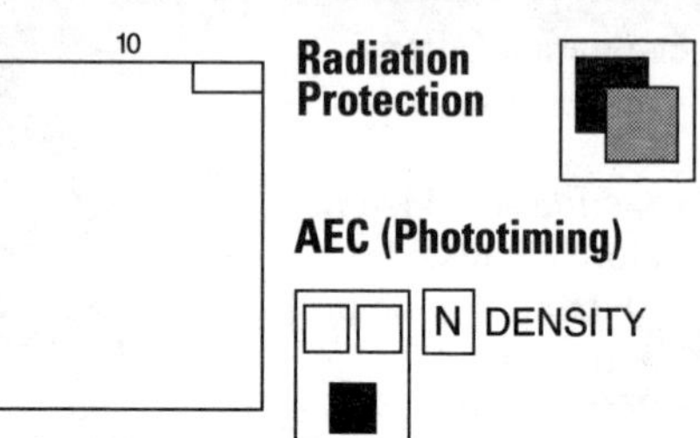

Patient Position

Recumbent left lateral with knees and hips flexed for comfort; arms are placed at right angles to the body with elbows flexed.

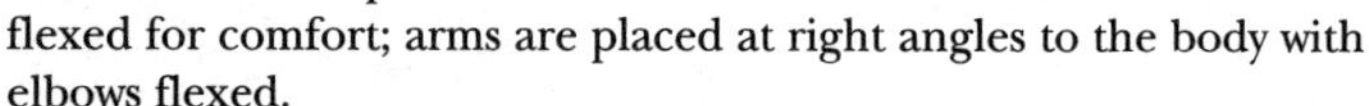

Part Position Place the long axis of the spine parallel to the table; the sagittal plane should be parallel and the coronal plane perpendicular to the table; a plane approximately 3 inches (8 cm) posterior to the midaxillary line should be centered to the table.

Central Ray Perpendicular to the midsacrum, 2 inches (5 cm) anterior to the palpated sacral crest and 1 inch (3 cm) below the ASIS.

Breathing Instructions Suspend on expiration.

Example Exposure Techniques
Measure at CR and Use Chart (p.218)

Room	cm	kVp	mAs	mA	Sec	Beam	Film	Grid	1Ø3Ø
	26								
	28								
	30								
	32								
	34								
	36								
	38								
	40								
	42								
	44								

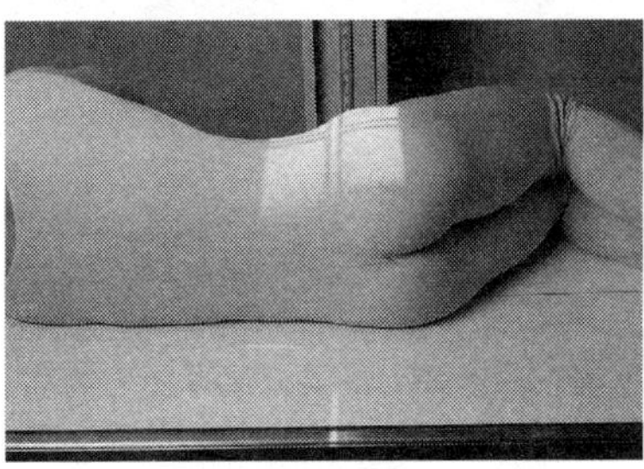

Evaluation Criteria

- The entire sacrum must be included.
- All or part of the L5–S1 joint space must be included.
- The iliac crests and acetabula should be mostly superimposed, indicating minimal rotation.

Exam Rationale The lateral sacrum is taken at 90° to the AP. Structures best demonstrated include the body and median sacral crest.

Tips

1. To obtain a more uniform density, lead blockers may be placed on the table top behind the patient to limit scatter radiation.
2. Close collimation is essential to limit scatter radiation.

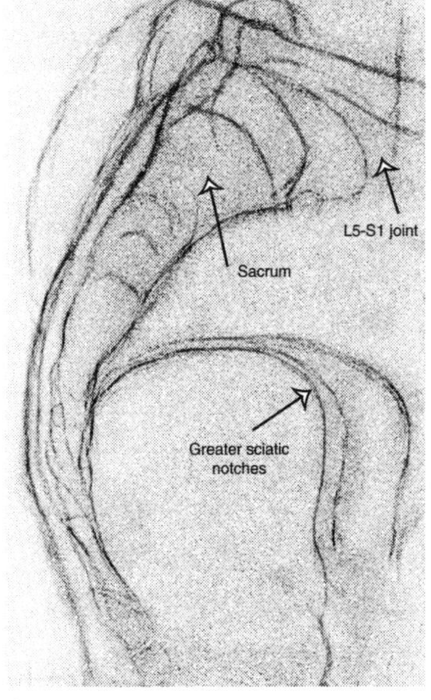

Technical Considerations
- Regular screen/film
- Grid
- kVp range: 75–80
- SID: 40 inch (100 cm)

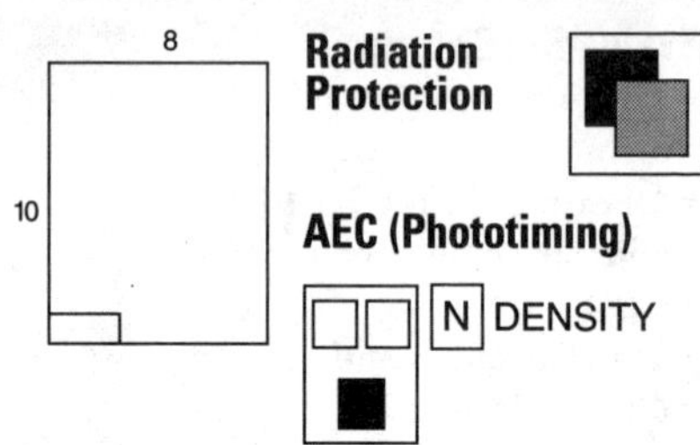

Patient Position Supine with the MSP centered to the midline of the table; arms are placed at the patient's sides or high on the chest.

Part Position The MSP is centered to the midline of the table.

Central Ray Directed at a 10° caudal angle, entering at a level midway between the symphysis pubis and the anterior superior iliac spine.

Patient Instruction Suspend on expiration.

Evaluation Criteria
- Entire coccyx must be included.
- Coccyx should appear more elongated than on an AP lumbar spine examination.

Example Exposure Techniques **Measure at CR and Use Chart (p.218)**									
Room	**cm**	**kVp**	**mAs**	**mA**	**Sec**	**Beam**	**Film**	**Grid**	**1Ø3Ø**
	15								
	16								
	17								
	18								
	19								
	20								
	21								
	22								
	23								
	24								

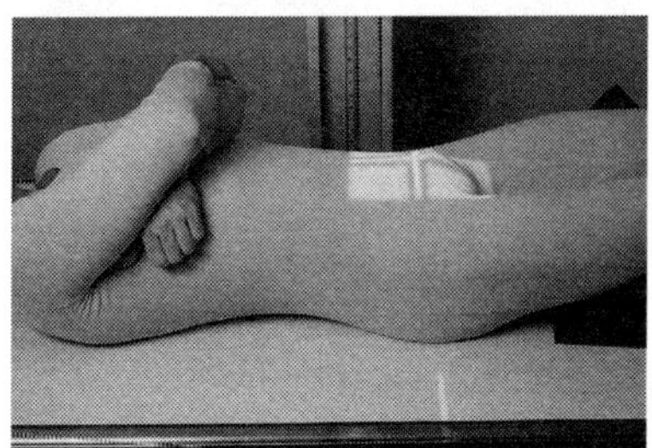

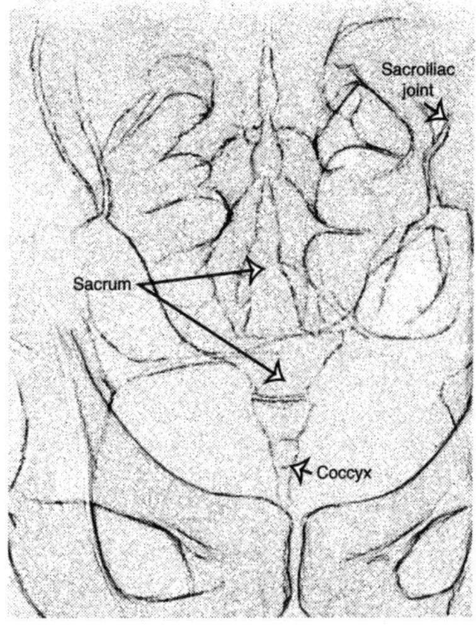

- Rotation, as evidenced by the asymmetrical appearance of the ischial or pubic rami and the obturator foramina, should not be observed.

Exam Rationale The most common indication for radiographic examination of the coccyx is trauma. The AP is one of two routine positions.

Tips

1. Injury to the coccyx may prevent a patient from lying supine. An alternative PA projection can be obtained with the patient lying prone and using a 10° cephalad angle, although more radiographic magnification will be evident.
2. Because the rectal and bladder shadows overlie the coccyx, it is often desirable to have the patient void and defecate before the radiographic examination.

Technical Considerations

- Regular screen/film
- Grid
- kVp range: 75–80
- SID: 40 inch (100 cm)

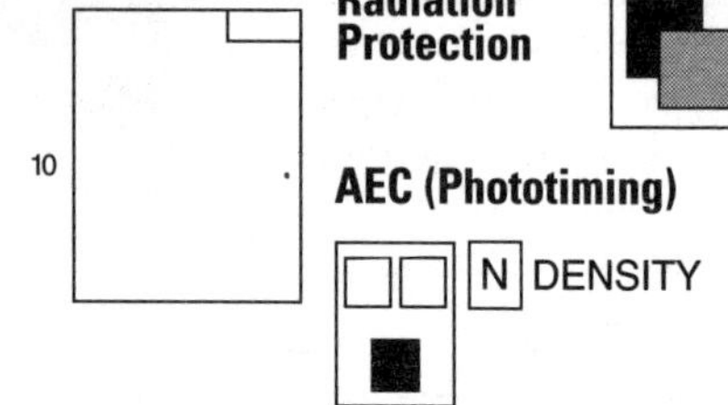

Patient Position

Recumbent left lateral with knees and hips are flexed for comfort; arms are placed at right angles to the body with elbows flexed.

Part Position Place the long axis of the spine parallel to the table; the sagittal plane should be parallel and the coronal plane perpendicular to the table; a plane approximately 5 inches (13 cm) posterior to the midaxillary line should be centered to the table.

Central Ray Perpendicular, 1 inch (3 cm) anterior to the palpated posterior coccyx.

Breathing Instructions Suspend on expiration.

Example Exposure Techniques **Measure at CR and Use Chart (p.218)**									
Room	**cm**	**kVp**	**mAs**	**mA**	**Sec**	**Beam**	**Film**	**Grid**	**1Ø3Ø**
	22								
	24								
	26								
	28								
	30								
	32								
	34								
	36								
	38								
	40								

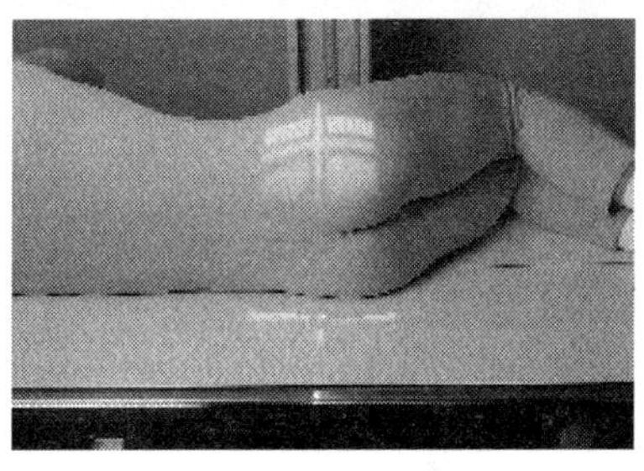

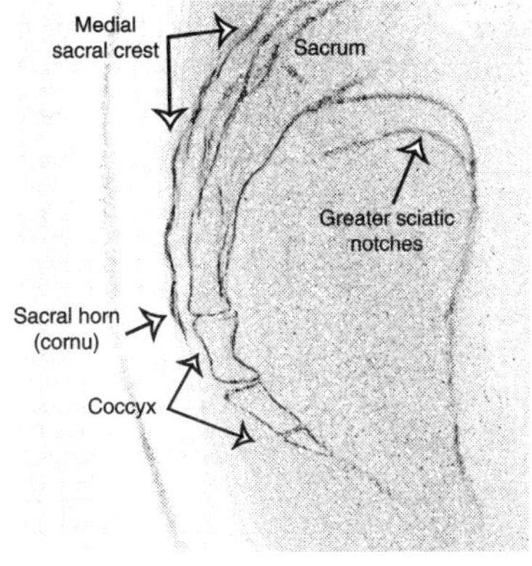

Evaluation Criteria

- The entire coccyx and a portion of the distal sacrum must be included.
- The acetabula should be mostly superimposed, indicating minimal rotation.

Exam Rationale The lateral coccyx is taken at 90° to the AP. The most common indication for radiographic examination of the coccyx is trauma.

Tips

1. To obtain a more uniform density, lead blockers may be placed on the table top behind the patient to limit scatter radiation.
2. Close collimation is essential to limit scatter radiation.

Trauma Considerations Spinal trauma is common and the radiographer must give special attention to such patients. Patients with acute spinal trauma should be moved as little as possible. In general the AP and cross-table lateral are taken and reviewed by a physician before continuing with obliques or special projections.

Pediatric Considerations Motion is always a consideration in pediatric radiography and exposure times must be kept as low as diagnostically possible.

Geriatric Considerations Several major degenerative diseases affect the spine of geriatric patients. These diseases will give the patient less flexibility and mobility. The radiographer will need to adapt to this loss of vertebral motion.

ALTERNATIVE POSITIONS/PROJECTIONS

Part	Alternative	Page
Cervical spine (trauma)	Cross-table Lateral	266
	Oblique	268
Thoracic spine (trauma)	Cross-table Lateral	270
	Cross-table Swimmer's Lateral	272
Lumbar spine (trauma)	Cross-table Lateral	274

Fundamental Principles The basic views for trauma patients are two projections taken at right angles to each other. For trauma spine this would include an AP and a cross-table lateral projection. This is generally sufficient for patients who have a neurologic deficit.

All trauma patients are brought into the emergency room with a cervical collar. This prevents the patient from moving the neck and limits further injury to the spinal cord. A cross-table lateral projection of the cervical spine must be taken with the cervical collar in place. Specific instructions from a physician to either leave the collar on the patient or remove it should be obtained before proceeding.

It is especially important for radiographers to be accurate in positioning and technique when radiographing trauma patients. They should be familiar with the mobile equipment, emergency room personnel, and specific hospital policies regarding trauma patients. This will enable them to work efficiently. It is critical to get a diagnostic film on the first attempt to ensure a quick diagnosis.

In radiographing trauma patients, a common error is failure to remove artifacts from the area of interest. Even though the cervical collar must stay in place, necklaces and earrings can be carefully removed without moving the patient's neck.

Technical Considerations

- Regular screen/film
- Grid or non-grid
- kVp range: 75–85
- SID: 72 inch (180 cm)

12

10

Radiation Protection

Patient Position Remains recumbent on the spine board or stretcher; all potential artifacts are removed if possible, but the cervical collar is left on; the cassette/grid is placed in the vertical position with its bottom portion touching the shoulder.

Part Position The neck remains in the cervical collar and the cervical spine is not adjusted.

Central Ray Perpendicular to the upper margin of the thyroid cartilage; align the coronal plane, which passes through the mastoid processes, to the midline of the film.

Breathing Instructions Suspend on expiration. Relax shoulders.

Example Exposure Techniques
Measure at CR and Use Chart (p.218)

Room	cm	kVp	mAs	mA	Sec	Beam	Film	Grid	1Ø3Ø
	9								
	10								
	11								
	12								
	13								
	14								
	15								
	16								
	17								
	18								

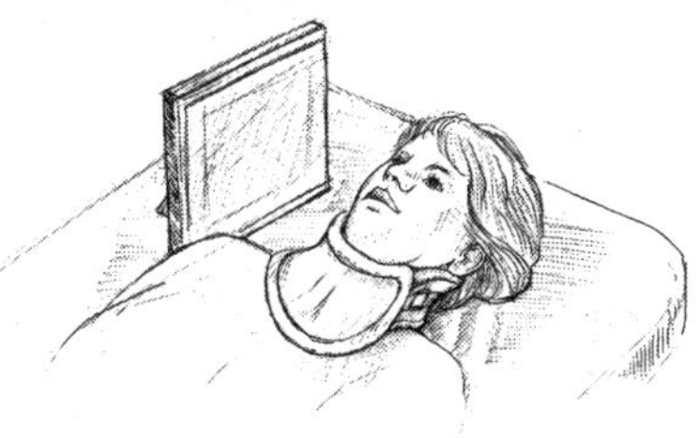

Evaluation Criteria

- All seven cervical vertebrae should be demonstrated.
- The rami of the mandible should not be superimposed on the upper cervical vertebrae.
- The technique used should adequately show the bony structures and soft tissues.

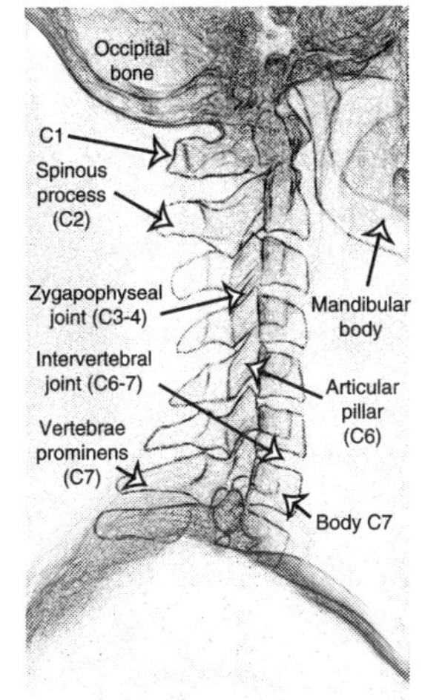

Exam Rationale A cross-table lateral of the cervical spine is performed on all patients who have sustained a traumatic injury to rule out the possibility of fracture or dislocation. Structures demonstrated include the bodies of all seven cervical vertebrae, the intervertebral joint spaces, articular pillars, superior and inferior articulating facets, zygapophyseal joints, and spinous processes.

Tips

1. The patient may need help depressing the shoulders. This can be done by:
   —Having someone pull down on the patient's arms.
   —Having the patient pull on a strap that is wrapped around the feet.
   —These procedures should be done only with the consent of the physician and patient.
2. The divergence of the x-ray beam can project C7 into the shoulder; therefore, it may be necessary to center at C7.
3. If all seven vertebrae are not demonstrated, it may be necessary to perform a swimmer's position.
4. It is best to use the correct film size and collimate to the part to reduce scatter radiation.

Technical Considerations

- Regular screen/film
- Grid
- kVp range: 70–80
- SID: 40 inch (100 cm)

Patient Position

Recumbent

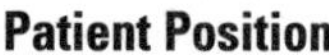

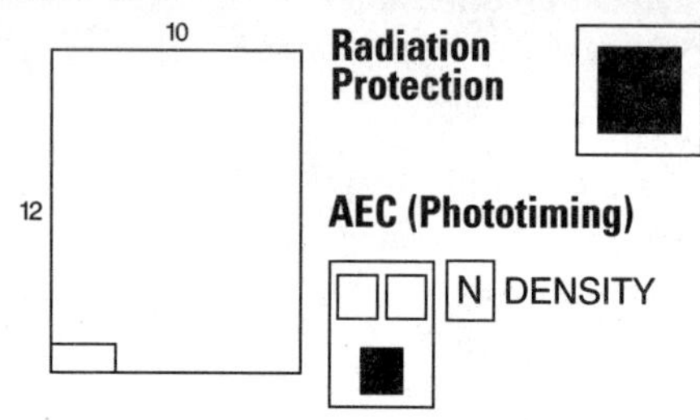

Part Position Adjust the entire body to form an angle of 45° with the plane of the film; the head should look straight ahead; chin should be extended slightly.

Central Ray Angle 15° to 20° cephalic to upper margin of thyroid cartilage.

Breathing Instructions Normal respiration.

Evaluation Criteria

- Intervertebral foramina and disk spaces should be open.
- Vertebrae demonstrated are C1–C7.
- Chin should be sufficiently elevated so the mandibular rami do not overlap C1 and C2.

Example Exposure Techniques **Measure at CR and Use Chart (p.218)**									
Room	**cm**	**kVp**	**mAs**	**mA**	**Sec**	**Beam**	**Film**	**Grid**	**1Ø3Ø**
	9								
	10								
	11								
	12								
	13								
	14								
	15								
	16								
	17								
	18								

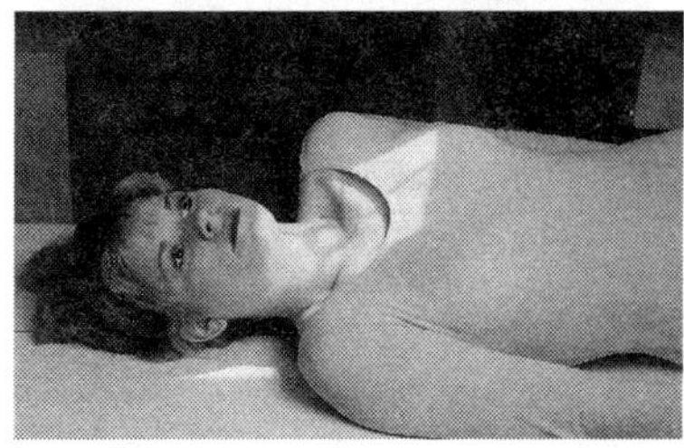

Exam Rationale The oblique projections are typically not performed as part of an initial examination of the trauma spine but may be used with patients who have injuries to areas of the body other than their spine, precluding filming in the erect position. Structures demonstrated on the oblique projections include the intervertebral foramina and pedicles farthest from the film (the up side). Both sides are examined for comparison.

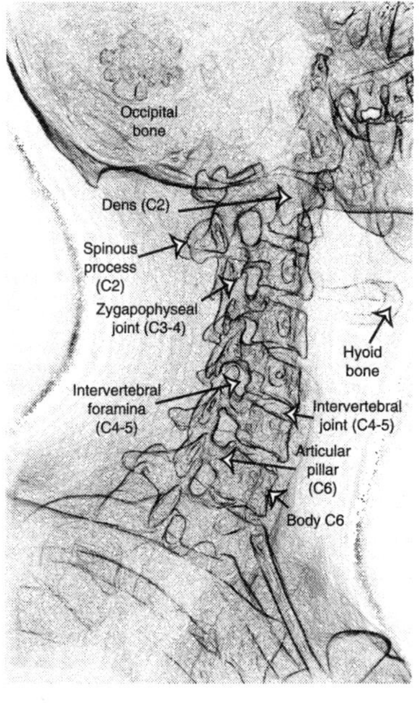

Tips

1. The patient can remain on the spine board. The patient can be positioned on either the trauma cart or on the radiographic table.
2. When it is not possible to rotate the patient, the x-ray tube can be angled 45° into the neck and 15° to 20° cephalic. Because there is a double angle on the tube, it is not possible to use a grid.

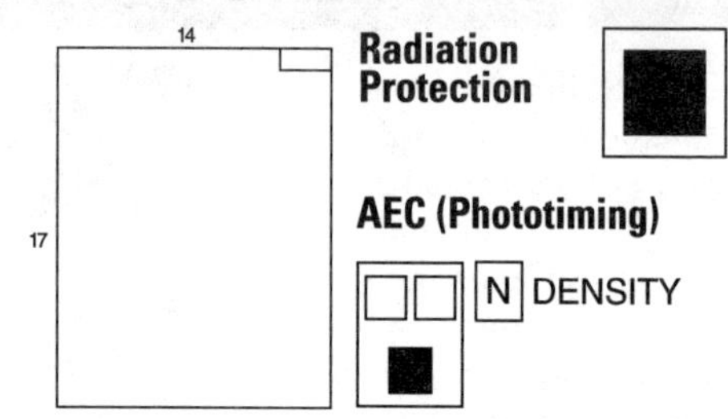

Technical Considerations

- Regular screen/film
- Grid
- kVp range: 70–80
- SID: 40 inch (100 cm)

Patient Position

Recumbent on the spine board or stretcher with the midcoronal plane centered to the cassette.

Part Position Raise the patient's arms over the head.

Central Ray Perpendicular to T8.

Breathing Instructions Normal respiration.

Evaluation Criteria

- The vertebrae from T3 to L2 should be visualized.
- Disk spaces and intervertebral foramina should be clearly demonstrated.

Example Exposure Techniques
Measure at CR and Use Chart (p.218)

Room	cm	kVp	mAs	mA	Sec	Beam	Film	Grid	1Ø3Ø
	20								
	22								
	24								
	26								
	28								
	30								
	32								
	34								
	36								
	38								

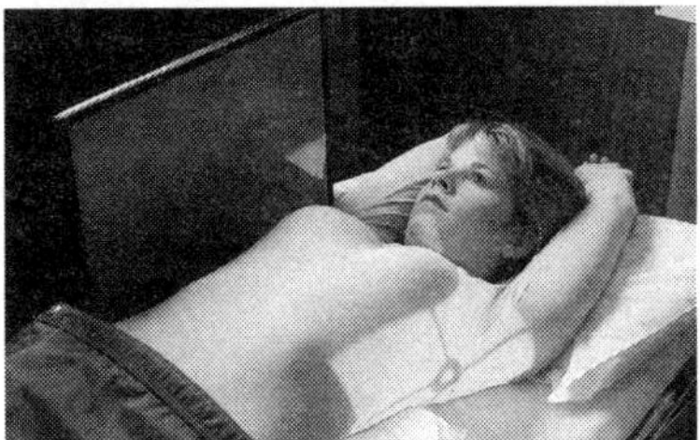

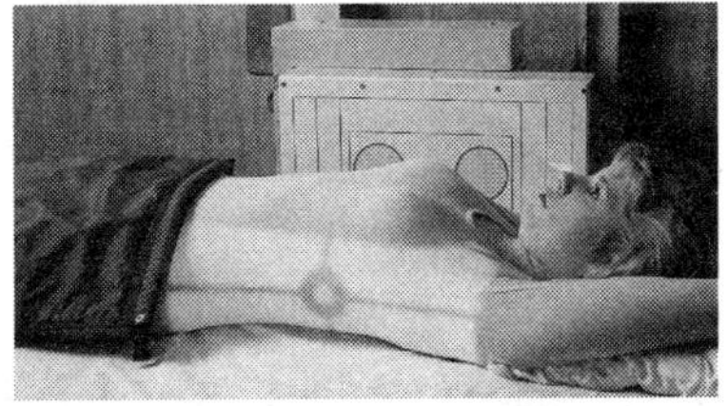

Exam Rationale A cross-table lateral of the thoracic spine is performed on all patients who have sustained a traumatic injury to the thoracic spine to rule out the possibility of fracture or dislocation. Structures demonstrated include the thoracic bodies, intervertebral disk spaces, intervertebral foramina of T3–L2, and the spinous processes of the lower thoracic and upper lumbar regions.

Tips

1. The lower margin of the film should be 1 inch (3 cm) above the lower margin of the ribs; this will place L2 at the bottom of the film.
2. Use of an upright Bucky versus a grid/cassette will produce a significantly better image.
3. Use AEC only with upright Bucky device.

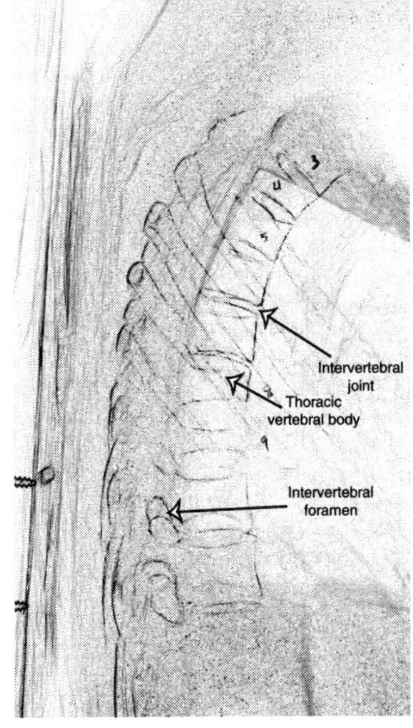

Technical Considerations
- Regular screen/film
- Grid
- kVp range: 75–85
- SID: 40 inch (100 cm)

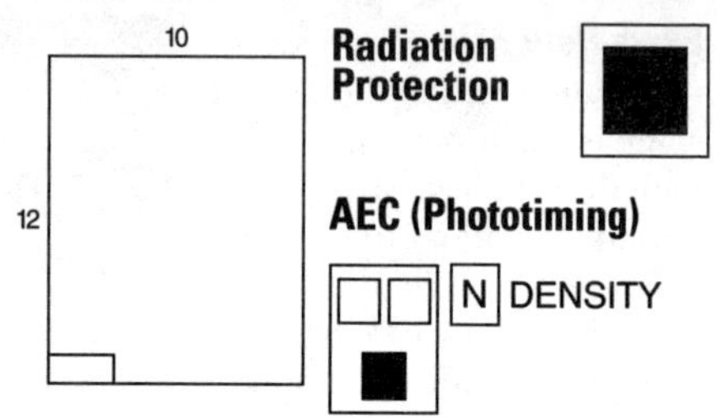

Patient Position Recumbent on the spine board with the midaxillary line centered to the cassette .

Part Position Raise the arm that is closest to the film and lower the arm that is farthest from the film.

Central Ray Perpendicular to T2.

Breathing Instructions Suspend on expiration.

Evaluation Criteria
- The humeral heads should not be superimposed on the vertebral bodies.
- The disk spaces between Cl and Tl and the first three to four thoracic vertebrae should be visualized.

Example Exposure Techniques
Measure at CR and Use Chart (p.218)

Room	cm	kVp	mAs	mA	Sec	Beam	Film	Grid	1Ø3Ø
	9								
	10								
	11								
	12								
	13								
	14								
	15								
	16								
	17								
	18								

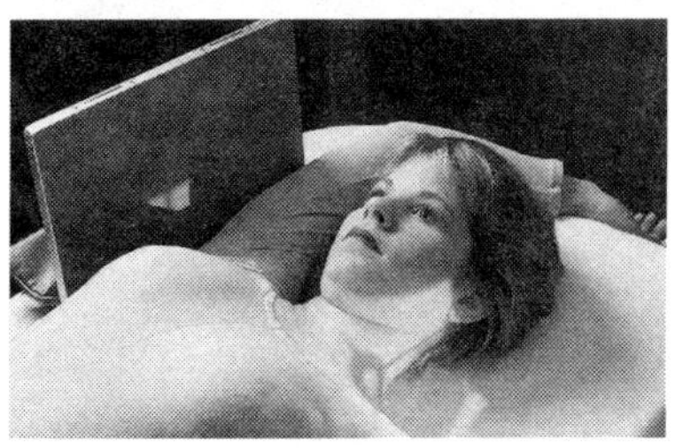

Exam Rationale Structures demonstrated on the swimmer's lateral position include the bodies, intervertebral disk spaces, spinous processes, and zygapophyseal joints of upper thoracic and/or lower cervical vertebrae.

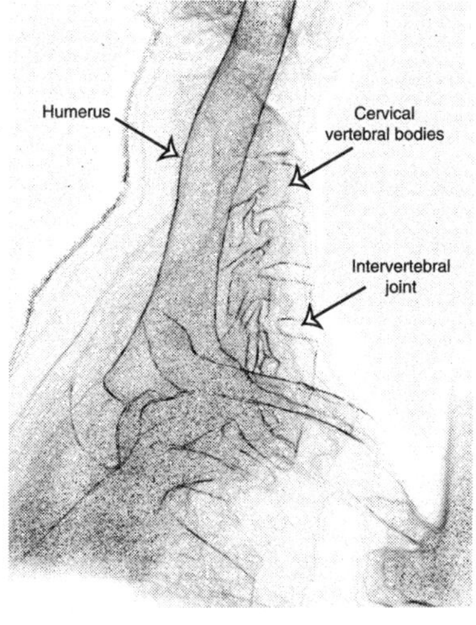

Tips

1. If the patient cannot separate the shoulders enough, a 5° caudal angle may be used.
2. If the patient cannot raise the arm closest to the film, the other arm may be raised while depressing the arm closest to the film.
3. If the lower cervical vertebrae are of interest, the central ray should be directed to C7.

Technical Considerations

- Regular screen/film
- Grid
- kVp range: 75–85
- SID: 40 inch (100 cm)

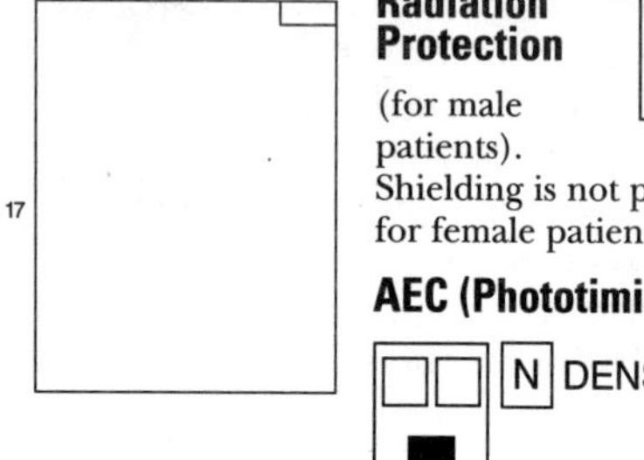

Radiation Protection

(for male patients). Shielding is not possible for female patients.

AEC (Phototiming)

N DENSITY

Patient Position The patient remains recumbent on the spine board or stretcher with the midcoronal plane centered to the cassette.

Part Position Raise the patient's arms over the head.

Central Ray Perpendicular to L4.

Breathing Instructions Suspend respiration.

Evaluation Criteria

- The vertebra from T12 to S1 should be visualized.

Example Exposure Techniques **Measure at CR and Use Chart (p.218)**									
Room	**cm**	**kVp**	**mAs**	**mA**	**Sec**	**Beam**	**Film**	**Grid**	**1Ø3Ø**
	26								
	28								
	30								
	32								
	34								
	36								
	38								
	40								
	42								
	44								

Exam Rationale A cross-table lateral of the lumbar spine is performed on patients who have sustained a traumatic injury to the lower back to rule out the possibility of a fracture or dislocation. Structures demonstrated include the lumbar bodies, intervertebral disk spaces, intervertebral foramina, and the spinous processes of T12–S1.

Tip Use of an upright Bucky versus a grid/cassette will produce a significantly better image.

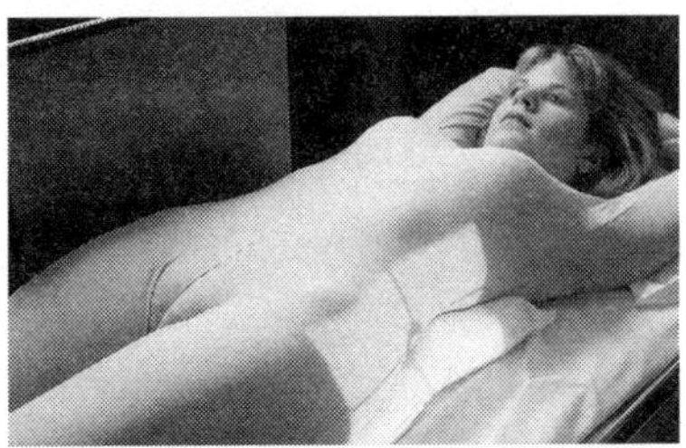

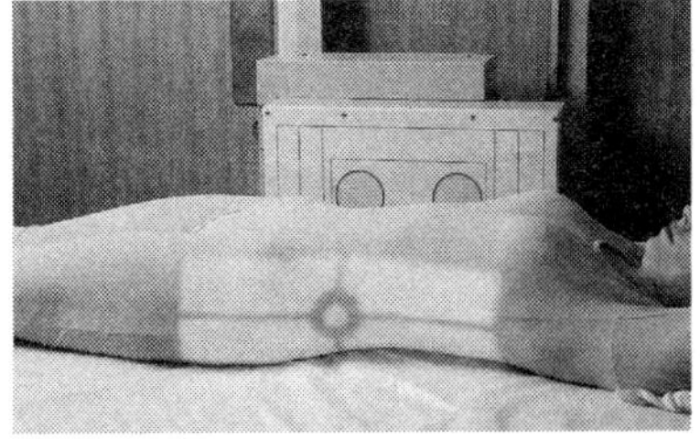

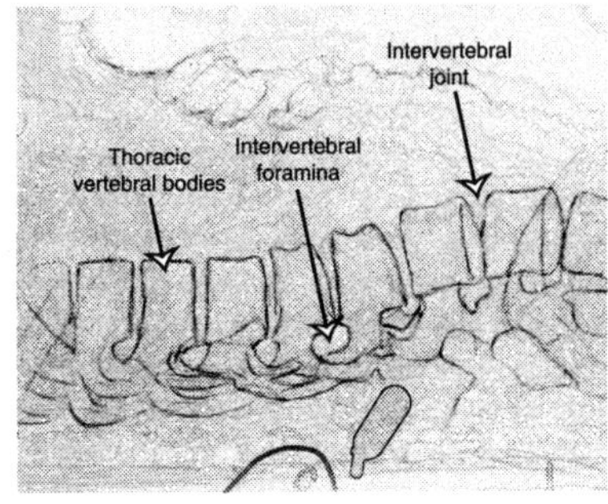

SKULL AND FACIAL BONES

ROUTINE AND ALTERNATIVE POSITIONS/PROJECTIONS

Part	Routine	Page	Alternative	Page
Skull	Axial AP	278		
	PA	280		
	Lateral	282		
	Submentovertical	284		
Facial bones	PA Caldwell	286		
	Parietoacanthial (Waters)	288		
	Lateral	290		
Nasal bones	PA Caldwell	292		
	Parietoacanthial (Waters)	294		
	Lateral	296		
	Superoinferior (axial)	298		
Orbits	PA	300		
	Modified parietoacanthial (modified Waters)	302		
	Lateral	304		
	Parieto-orbital oblique (Rhese)	306		
Zygomatic arches	Axial AP (Towne/Grashey)	308		
	Submentovertical	310	Oblique axial (May)	312
Mandible	Axial AP (Towne/Grashey)	314		
	PA	316		
	Axiolateral	318		
Temporomandibular joints	Axiolateral transcranial (Schuller)	320		
	Transcranial lateral	322		
Sinuses	PA Caldwell	324		
	Parietoacanthial (Waters)	326		
	Lateral	328		
	Submentovertical	330		
	Axial transoral (Pirie)	332		
Temporal bones	Axial AP (Towne/Grashey)	334		
	Axiolateral oblique (Law)	336		
	Posterior profile (Stenvers/Arcelin)	338		
	Axioposterior oblique (Mayer)	340		
	Submentovertical	342		
Sella turcica	Axial AP (Towne/Grashey)	344	Axial PA (Haas)	346
	Lateral	348		

Technical Considerations

- Regular screen/film
- Grid
- kVp range: 70–80
- SID: 40 inch (100 cm)

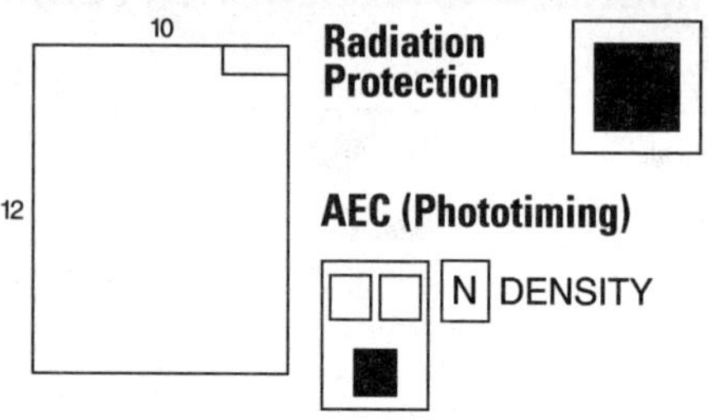

Patient Position
Facing the tube; all potential artifacts removed.

Part Position MSP is perpendicular to the midplane of the cassette; film is centered to the foramen magnum with the top of the cassette at the top of the patient's head; chin is depressed to place OML perpendicular to the film.

Central Ray 30° caudal to OML.

Breathing Instructions Suspend respiration.

Example Exposure Techniques **Measure at CR and Use this Chart**									
Room	**cm**	**kVp**	**mAs**	**mA**	**Sec**	**Beam**	**Film**	**Grid**	**1Ø3Ø**
	16								
	17								
	18								
	19								
	20								
	21								
	22								
	23								
	24								
	25								

Evaluation Criteria

- Entire skull is demonstrated.
- The dorsum sella and posterior clinoids should be seen within the foramen magnum.
- The petrous pyramids should be symmetrical to evidence no rotation.
- The distance from the lateral border of the skull to the foramen magnum should be equal on each side to evidence no rotation.

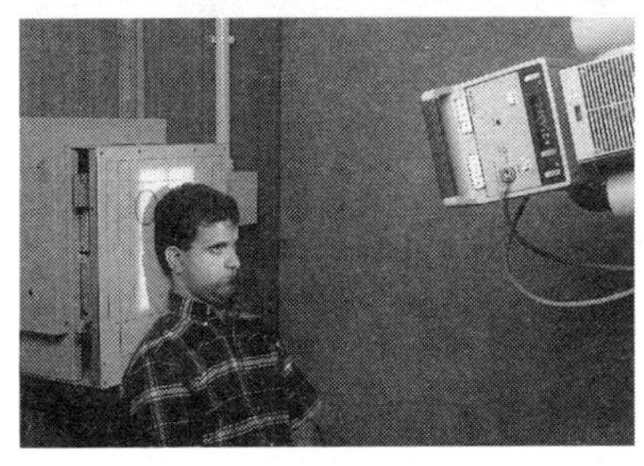

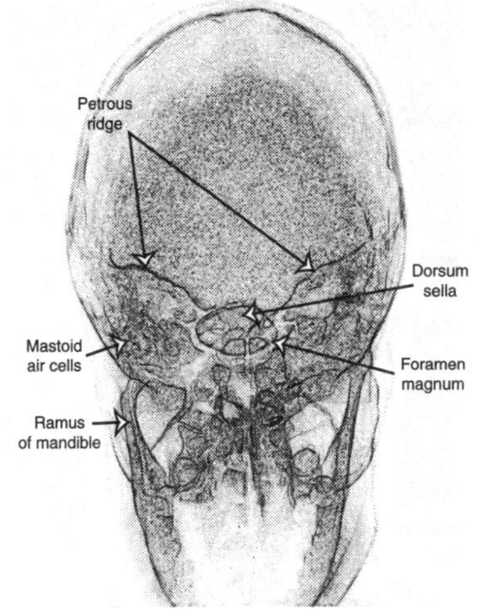

Exam Rationale This projection demonstrates the occipital bone, the petrous ridges, the mastoid air cells, and the foramen magnum with the dorsum sella and posterior clinoid processes projected within its shadow. It is used to rule out fractures and disease processes.

Tip If the patient is unable to depress the chin enough to place OML perpendicular to the film, place the IOML perpendicular to the film and increase the central ray to 37° caudal.

Technical Considerations

- Regular screen/film
- Grid
- kVp range: 70–80
- SID: 40 inch (100 cm)

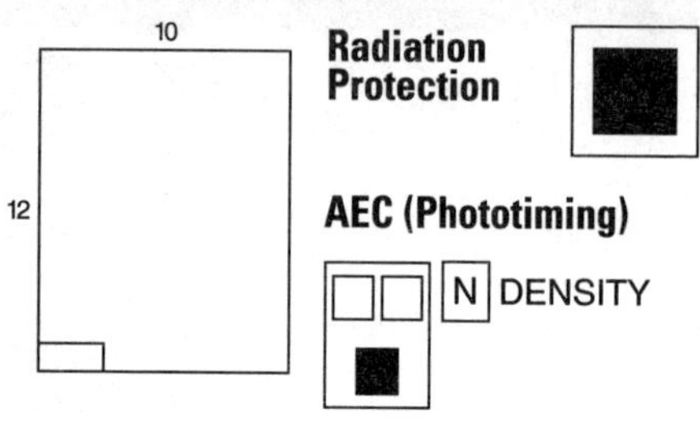

Patient Position

Facing the film; all potential artifacts removed.

Part Position Cassette is centered to the nasion with the top of the film approximately 1 1/2 inches (4 cm) above the vertex of the skull; MSP is perpendicular to the midline of the cassette; OML is perpendicular to the film.

Central Ray Perpendicular to the film exiting at the nasion.

Breathing Instructions Suspend respiration.

Example Exposure Techniques

Measure at CR and Use Chart (p.278)

Room	cm	kVp	mAs	mA	Sec	Beam	Film	Grid	1Ø3Ø
	16								
	17								
	18								
	19								
	20								
	21								
	22								
	23								
	24								
	25								

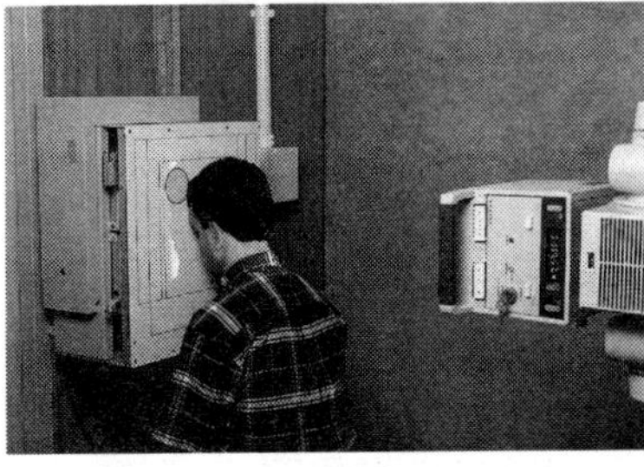

Evaluation Criteria

- Entire skull is demonstrated.
- The distance from the lateral border of the skull to the lateral border of the orbit should be equal on each side to evidence no rotation.
- The petrous pyramids will fill the entire orbit.

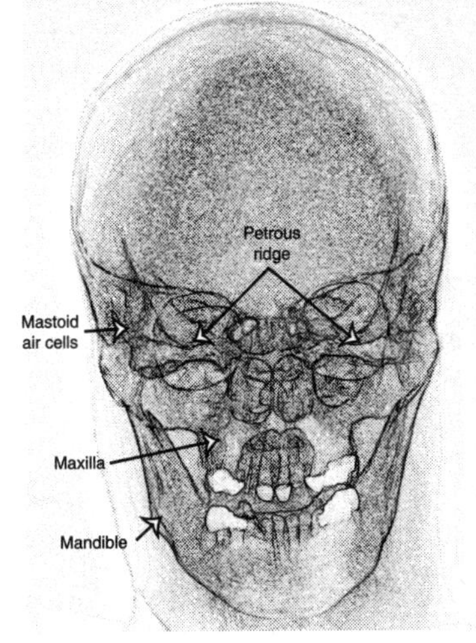

Exam Rationale This projection is used to demonstrate the frontal bone, the frontal and ethmoid air cells, facial bones, orbital margin, and the mandibular condyles and rami. It is frequently used in conjunction with other modalities to confirm disease processes as well as in trauma situations.

Tip Some department protocols use a PA Caldwell in which case the central ray is directed 15° caudally. This would project the petrous pyramids into the lower third of the orbits.

Technical Considerations

- Regular screen/film
- Grid
- kVp range: 70–80
- SID: 40 inch (100 cm)

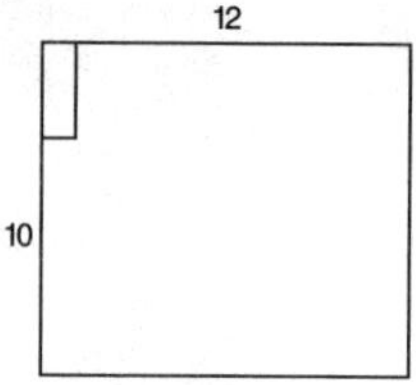

12

10

Radiation Protection

AEC (Phototiming)

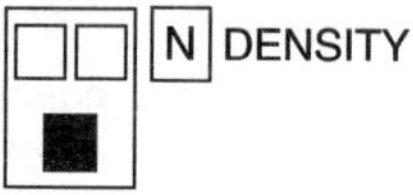

N DENSITY

Patient Position

In lateral position; all potential artifacts removed.

Part Position EAM is centered to the midline of the cassette with the top of the film approximately 2 inches (5 cm) above the vertex of the skull; MSP is parallel to the cassette, inter-pupillary line is perpendicular to the cassette; IOML is parallel to the transverse axis of the cassette.

Central Ray Perpendicular to the film entering 2 inches (5 cm) superior to the EAM.

Breathing Instructions Suspend respiration.

Example Exposure Techniques
Measure at CR and Use Chart (p.278)

Room	cm	kVp	mAs	mA	Sec	Beam	Film	Grid	1Ø3Ø
	11								
	12								
	13								
	14								
	15								
	16								
	17								
	18								
	19								
	20								

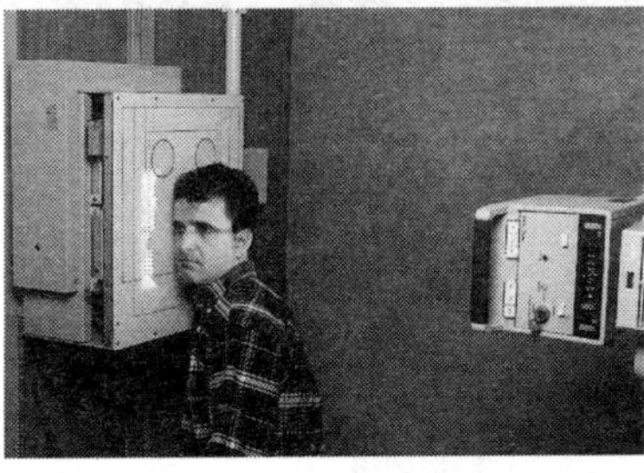

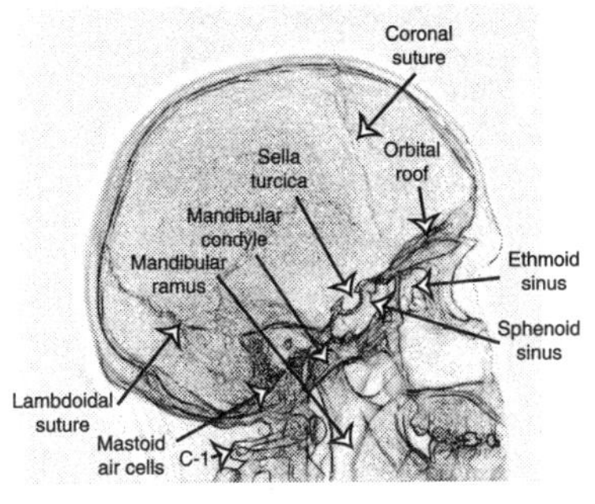

Evaluation Criteria

- The entire skull should be demonstrated.
- Superimposition of the mandibular rami, the orbital roofs, and the external auditory canals indicates no rotation or tilt.
- The sella turcica should be seen in profile (indicates no rotation or tilt).

Exam Rationale This position demonstrates the lateral cranium closest to the film with the other side superimposed, the sella turcica, and the anterior and posterior clinoid processes. To determine fracture localization, both right and left laterals should be obtained. It will also demonstrate upper cervical spine alignment.

Tips

1. If recumbent, place the patient in the RAO position for the right lateral and the LAO position for the left lateral.
2. A cross-table lateral should be used for patients with trauma or cervical spine injury. This would demonstrate fluid levels that would indicate a basal fracture.

Technical Considerations

- Regular screen/film
- Grid
- kVp range: 70–80
- SID: 40 inch (100 cm)

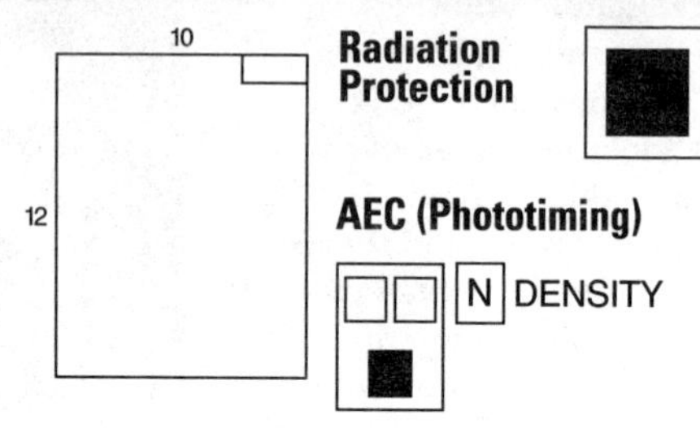

Patient Position

Facing the tube; all potential artifacts removed.

Part Position Patient's neck is extended until the head is resting on the vertex; cassette is centered to the level of the sella turcica; MSP is perpendicular to the midplane of the cassette; IOML parallel to the cassette.

Central Ray Perpendicular to the IOML entering between the angles of the mandible.

Breathing Instructions Suspend respiration.

Example Exposure Techniques **Measure at CR and Use Chart (p.278)**									
Room	**cm**	**kVp**	**mAs**	**mA**	**Sec**	**Beam**	**Film**	**Grid**	**1Ø3Ø**
	18								
	19								
	20								
	21								
	22								
	23								
	24								
	25								
	26								
	27								

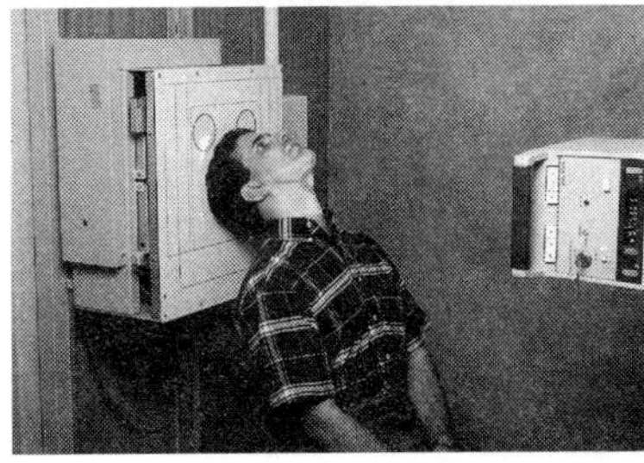

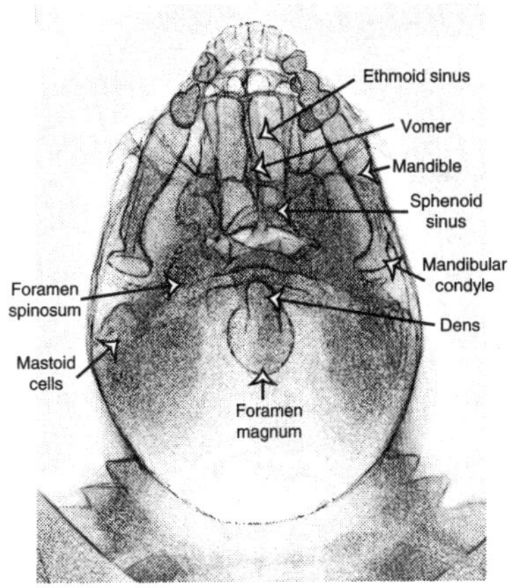

Evaluation Criteria

- Entire skull is demonstrated.
- The mandibular symphysis should superimpose the anterior frontal bone (indicates adequate extension or tube angle).
- The mandibular condyles should be demonstrated anterior to the petrous pyramids (indicates adequate extension or tube angle).
- The distance from the lateral border of the skull to the mandibular condyles should be equal on each side (indicates no rotation).
- The petrous ridges should be symmetrical (indicates no rotation).

Exam Rationale This projection is used to demonstrate the petrous pyramids, the mastoid processes, the foramina ovale and spinosum, the mandible, the sphenoid and ethmoid sinuses, the foramen magnum, the zygomatic arches, the nasal passages, and the occipital bone.

Tips

1. Work quickly because this position is uncomfortable for the patient.
2. The preferred position is erect; if recumbent, place pillows or sponges under the shoulders.
3. If unable to place the IOML parallel to the film, the central ray should be perpendicular to the IOML.

Technical Considerations

- Regular screen/film
- Grid
- kVp range: 70–80
- SID: 40 inch (100 cm)

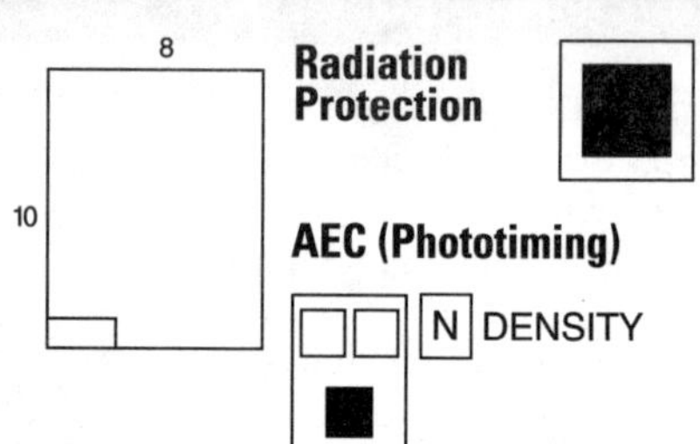

Patient Position Facing the film; all potential artifacts removed.

Part Position Cassette is centered to the nasion; MSP is perpendicular to the midline of the cassette; OML is perpendicular to the film.

Central Ray 15° caudal to nasion.

Breathing Instructions Suspend respiration.

Evaluation Criteria

- No rotation.
- The petrous pyramids will fill the lower one-third of the orbit.

Example Exposure Techniques **Measure at CR and Use Chart (p.278)**									
Room	**cm**	**kVp**	**mAs**	**mA**	**Sec**	**Beam**	**Film**	**Grid**	**1Ø3Ø**
	16								
	17								
	18								
	19								
	20								
	21								
	22								
	23								
	24								
	25								

Exam Rationale This projection is performed to demonstrate fractures of the facial bones and is especially helpful to determine alveolar ridge fractures. It demonstrates the orbital rim, the nasal septum, and the mandibular condyles.

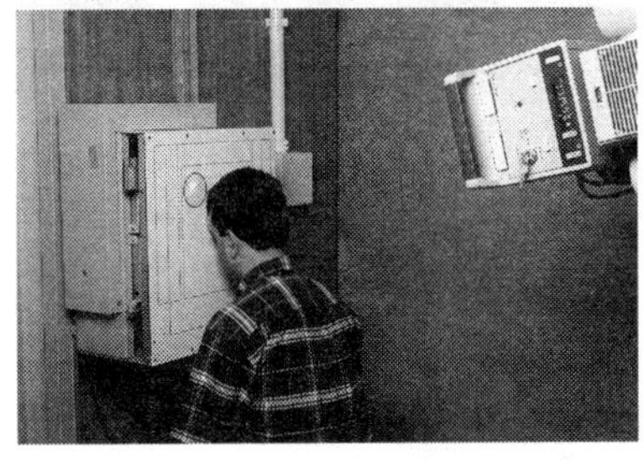

Tip Some department protocols call for a perpendicular central ray in which case the petrous pyramids would fill the orbits.

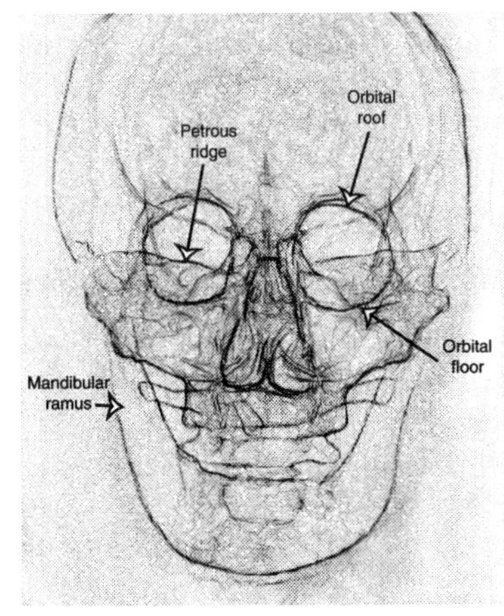

Technical Considerations

- Regular screen/film
- Grid
- kVp range: 70–80
- SID: 40 inch (100 cm)

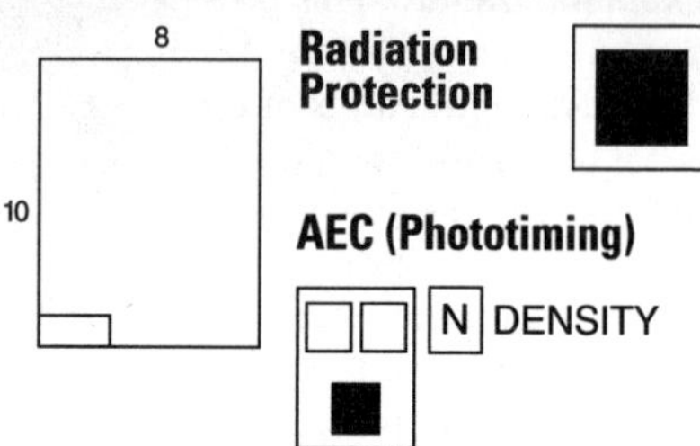

Patient Position Facing the film; all potential artifacts removed.

Part Position The neck is extended and the chin placed on the Bucky; the cassette is centered to the acanthion; MSP is perpendicular to the midline of the cassette; OML forms a 37° angle to the film.

Central Ray Perpendicular to the film exiting at the acanthion.

Breathing Instructions Suspend respiration.

Evaluation Criteria

- No rotation as evidenced by an equal distance from the orbit to the lateral border of the skull on both sides.
- Petrous ridges should be projected immediately below the maxillary sinuses.

Example Exposure Techniques
Measure at CR and Use Chart (p.278)

Room	cm	kVp	mAs	mA	Sec	Beam	Film	Grid	1Ø3Ø
	16								
	17								
	18								
	19								
	20								
	21								
	22								
	23								
	24								
	25								

Exam Rationale This projection is especially good for demonstrating fractures of the orbit and depressed fractures of the nasal wings.

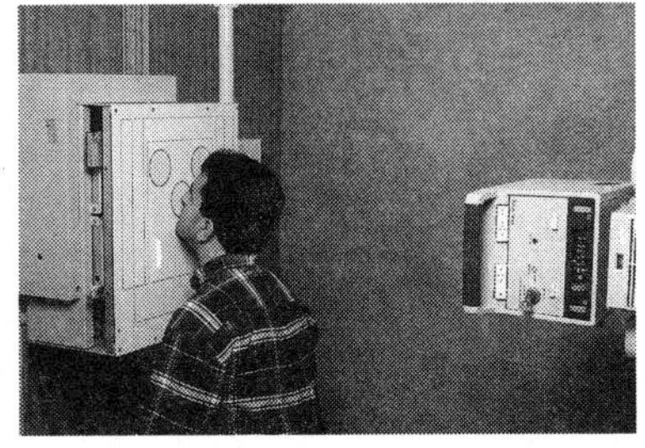

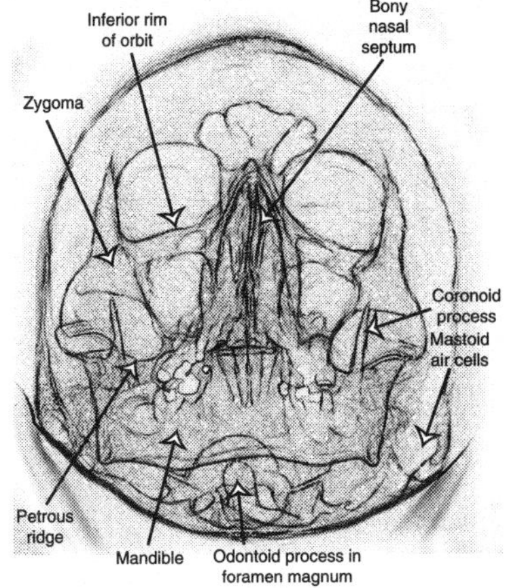

Tips

1. To better demonstrate the orbital floor, the modified parietoacanthial may be used. Extend the neck and place the chin on the cassette holder; center the film to the acanthion; adjust the flexion of the neck to place OML at a 55° angle to the plane of the film. The petrous ridges would be demonstrated immediately below the inferior border of the orbits.
2. Use of stereoscopy in this projection is especially helpful to demonstrate subtle fractures of the zygoma.

Technical Considerations

- Regular screen/film
- Grid
- kVp range: 70–80
- SID: 40 inch (100 cm)

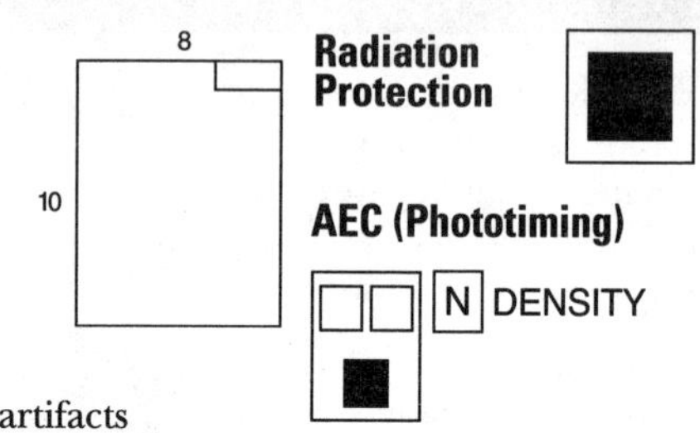

Patient Position In lateral position; all potential artifacts removed.

Part Position Cassette is centered to the zygoma; MSP is parallel to the film; interpupillary line is perpendicular to the film; IOML is parallel to the transverse axis of the cassette.

Central Ray Perpendicular to the film entering at the zygoma.

Breathing Instructions Suspend respiration.

Example Exposure Techniques **Measure at CR and Use Chart (p.278)**									
Room	cm	kVp	mAs	mA	Sec	Beam	Film	Grid	1Ø3Ø
	11								
	12								
	13								
	14								
	15								
	16								
	17								
	18								
	19								
	20								

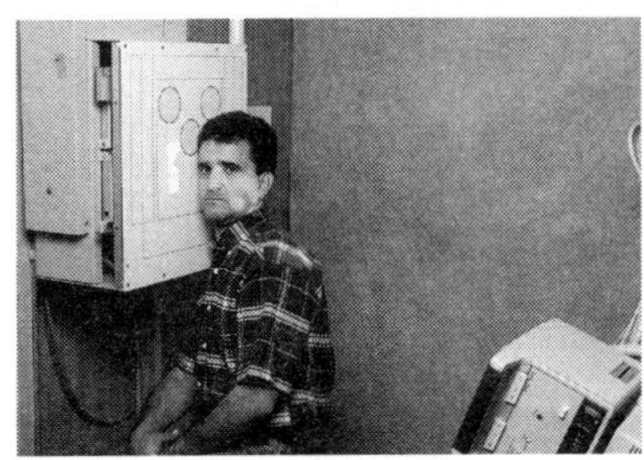

Evaluation Criteria

- Includes all facial bones.
- True lateral as evidenced by:
  - —Superimposition of the mandibular rami.
  - —Superimposition of the orbital roofs.
  - —No rotation seen in the sella turcica.

Exam Rationale This position is used to demonstrate the facial bones of the side closest to the film with the opposite side superimposed. It is useful for demonstrating depressed fractures of the frontal sinus. It also demonstrates the orbital roof, sella turcica, and mandible.

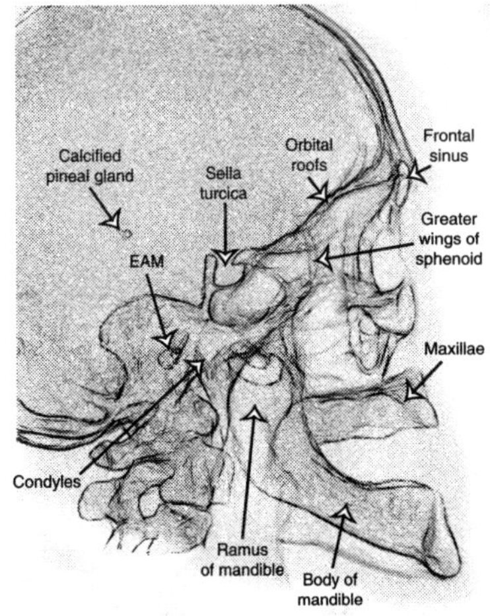

Technical Considerations

- Regular screen/film
- Grid
- kVp range: 70–80
- SID: 40 inch (100 cm)

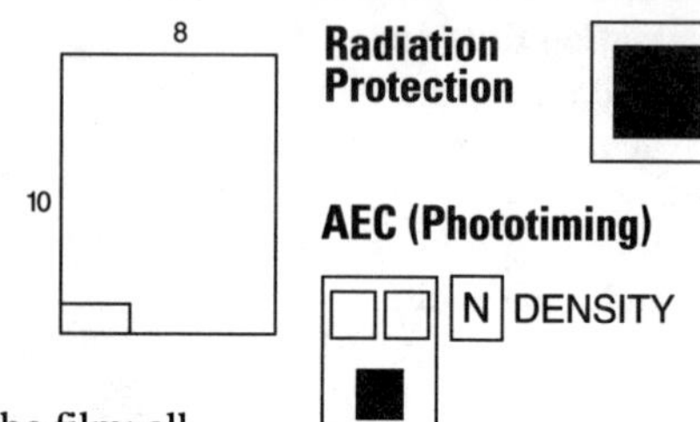

Patient Position Facing the film; all potential artifacts removed.

Part Position Cassette is centered to the nasion; OML is perpendicular to the film; MSP is perpendicular to the midline of the cassette.

Central Ray 15° caudal to nasion.

Breathing Instructions Suspend respiration.

Example Exposure Techniques **Measure at CR and Use Chart (p.278)**									
Room	**cm**	**kVp**	**mAs**	**mA**	**Sec**	**Beam**	**Film**	**Grid**	**1Ø3Ø**
	16								
	17								
	18								
	19								
	20								
	21								
	22								
	23								
	24								
	25								

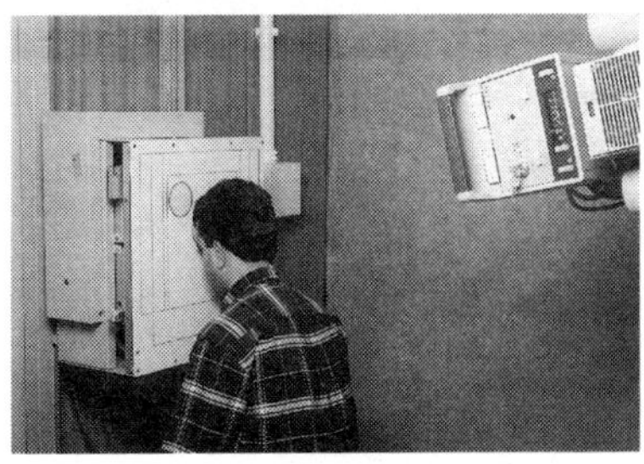

Evaluation Criteria

- The petrous ridges are projected in the lower one-third of the orbit.
- No rotation as evidenced by an equal distance from the crista galli to the lateral border of the orbit on each side.

Exam Rationale This projection best demonstrates the bony nasal septum.

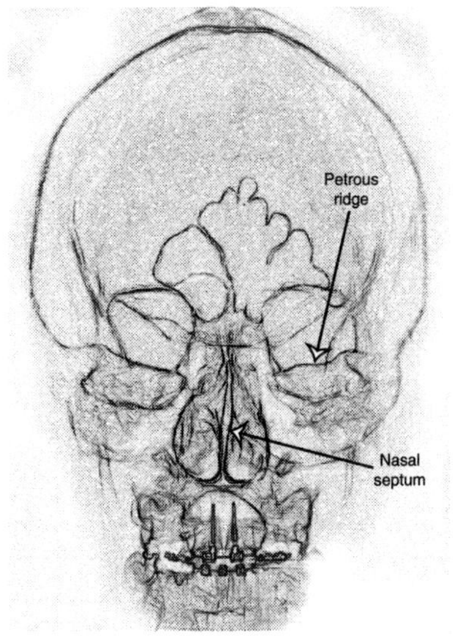

Technical Considerations
- Regular screen/film
- Grid
- kVp range: 70–80
- SID: 40 inch (100 cm)

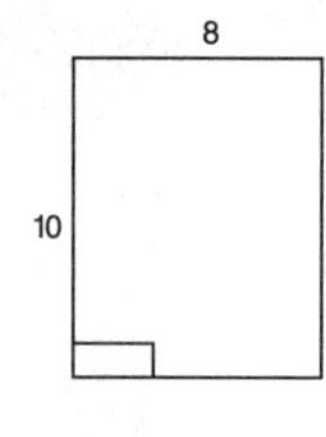

Radiation Protection

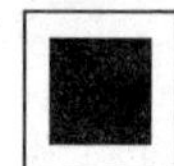

AEC (Phototiming)

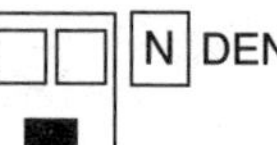

Patient Position Facing the film; all potential artifacts removed.

Part Position The neck is extended and the chin placed on the Bucky; the cassette is centered to the acanthion; MSP is perpendicular to midline of cassette; OML forms a 37° angle to the film.

Central Ray Perpendicular to the film exiting at the acanthion.

Breathing Instructions Suspend respiration.

Example Exposure Techniques **Measure at CR and Use Chart (p.278)**									
Room	**cm**	**kVp**	**mAs**	**mA**	**Sec**	**Beam**	**Film**	**Grid**	**1Ø3Ø**
	16								
	17								
	18								
	19								
	20								
	21								
	22								
	23								
	24								
	25								

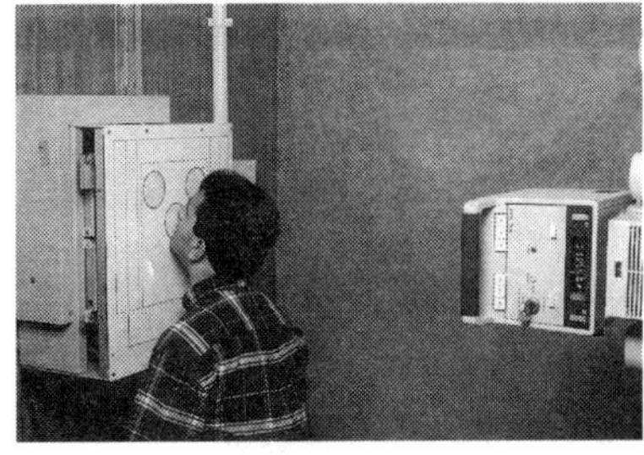

Evaluation Criteria

- The petrous ridges are projected immediately below the maxillary sinuses.
- No rotation as evidenced by equal distance from the orbit to the lateral border of the skull on each side.

Exam Rationale This projection is used to demonstrate displacement of the bony nasal septum and depressed fractures of the nasal wings.

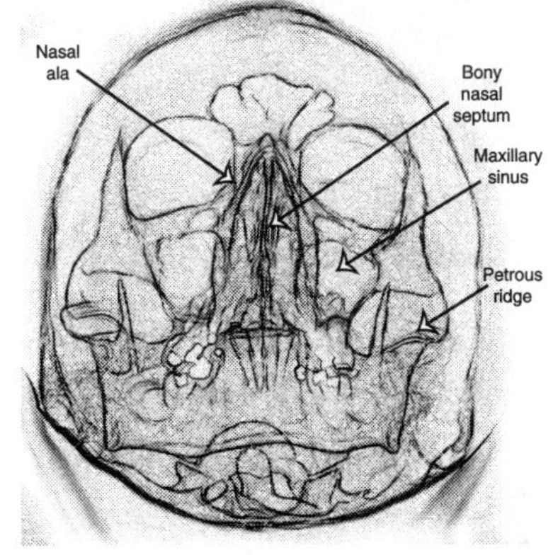

Technical Considerations

- Detail screen/film
- Non-grid
- kVp range: 60–65
- SID: 40 inch (100 cm)

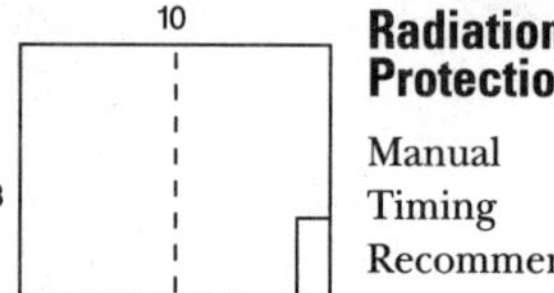

Radiation Protection

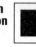

Manual
Timing
Recommended

Patient Position In lateral position; all potential artifacts removed.

Part Position Side of the head against the film; centered to the nasal bones; MSP is parallel and interpupillary line perpendicular to the film; IOML is parallel to the transverse axis of the cassette.

Central Ray Perpendicular to the film at a point 1/2 inch (1 cm) inferior and posterior to the nasion.

Breathing Instructions Suspend respiration.

Evaluation Criteria

- The frontonasal suture, the nasal bones, the anterior nasal spine, and the soft tissue should be included.
- There should be no rotation.

Example Exposure Techniques **Measure at CR and Use Chart (p.278)**									
Room	**cm**	**kVp**	**mAs**	**mA**	**Sec**	**Beam**	**Film**	**Grid**	**1Ø3Ø**
	1								
	2								
	3								
	4								
	5								

Exam Rationale This position is used to demonstrate the nasal bones and soft tissue structures of the nose. It is the best position to demonstrate nondisplaced, linear fractures of the nasal bones. Both laterals are normally done for comparison.

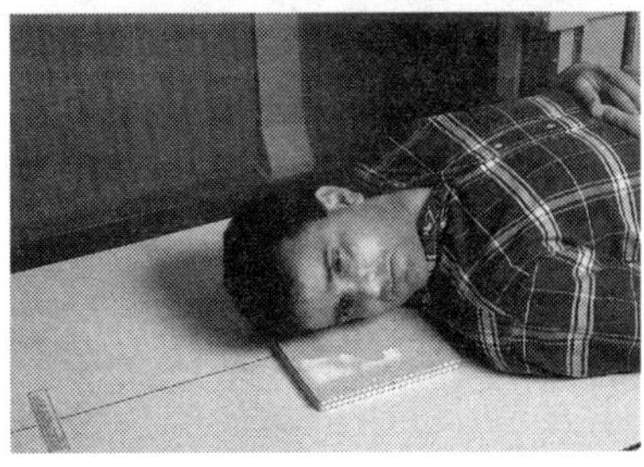

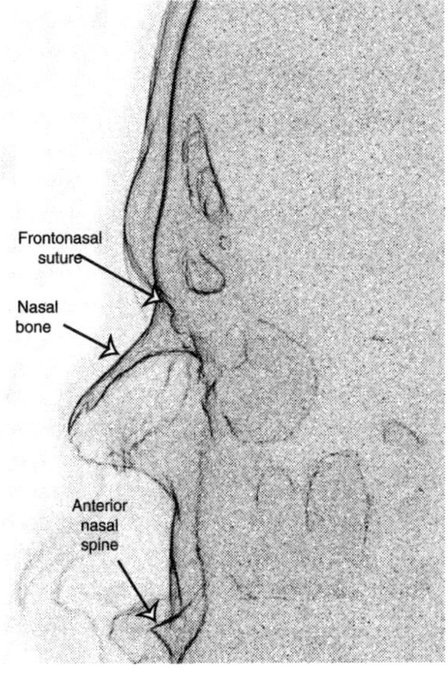

Technical Considerations
- Detail screen/film
- Non-grid
- kVp range: 58–60
- SID: 40 inch (100 cm)

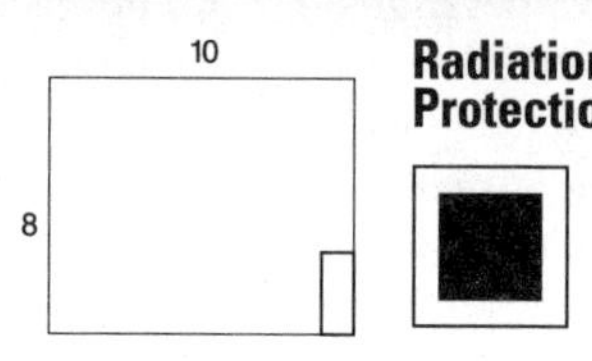

Patient Position Seated in a chair.

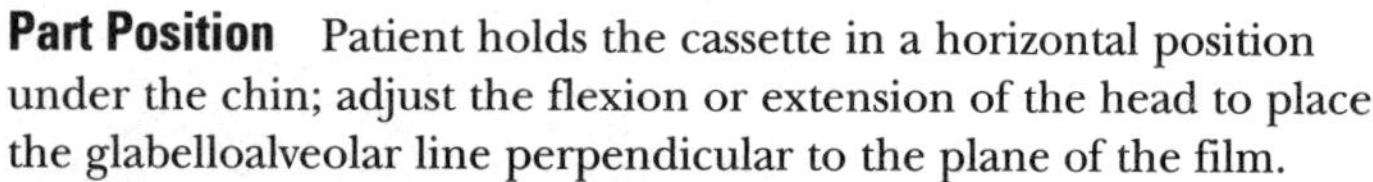

Part Position Patient holds the cassette in a horizontal position under the chin; adjust the flexion or extension of the head to place the glabelloalveolar line perpendicular to the plane of the film.

Central Ray Perpendicular to the film along the glabelloalveolar line.

Breathing Instructions Suspend respiration.

Evaluation Criteria
- Demonstrates the nasal bones.
- Soft tissue should also be demonstrated.

Exam Rationale This projection demonstrates medial or lateral displacement of nasal bone fractures.

Example Exposure Techniques
Measure at CR and Use Chart (p.278)

Room	cm	kVp	mAs	mA	Sec	Beam	Film	Grid	1Ø3Ø
	2								
	3								
	4								
	5								
	6								

Tip With the patient in the supine position, place the cassette under the chin in a vertical position; adjust the flexion or extension of the head to place the glabelloalveolar line perpendicular to the plane of the film. This position will not adequately demonstrate the nasal bones on individuals with a prominent forehead or chin or protruding front teeth. If intraoral film is available, place it in the mouth and position the patient and central ray as described above.

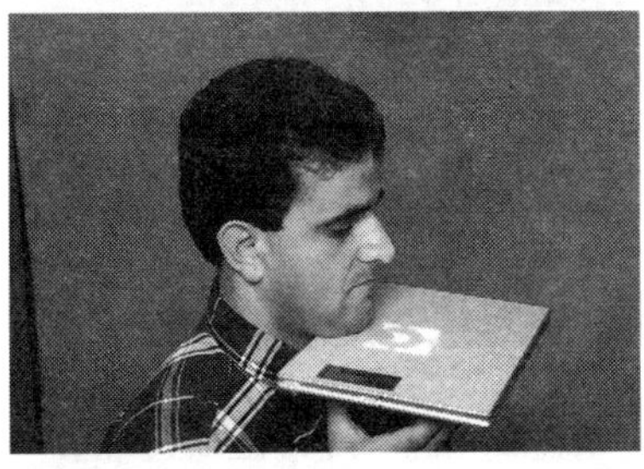

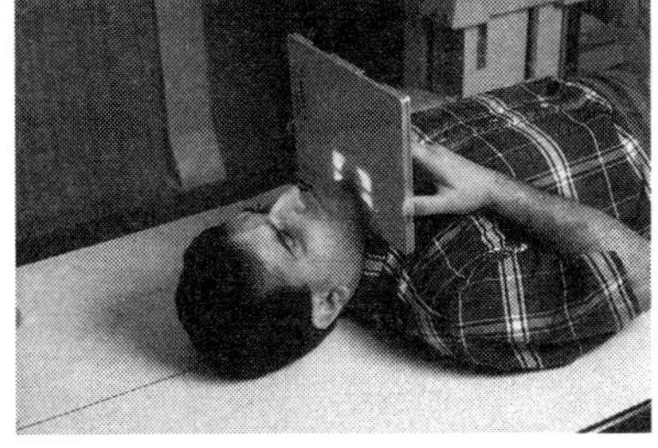

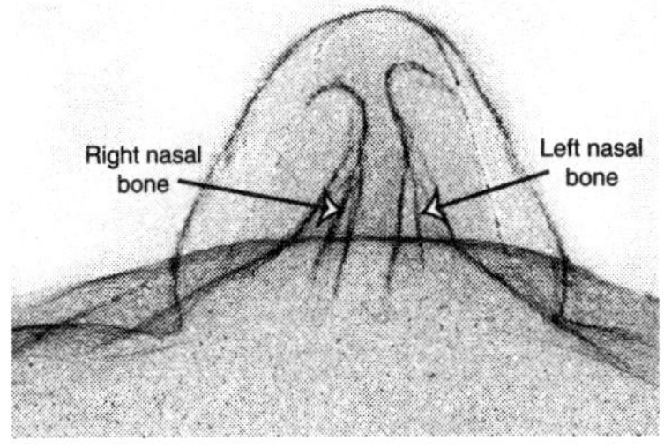

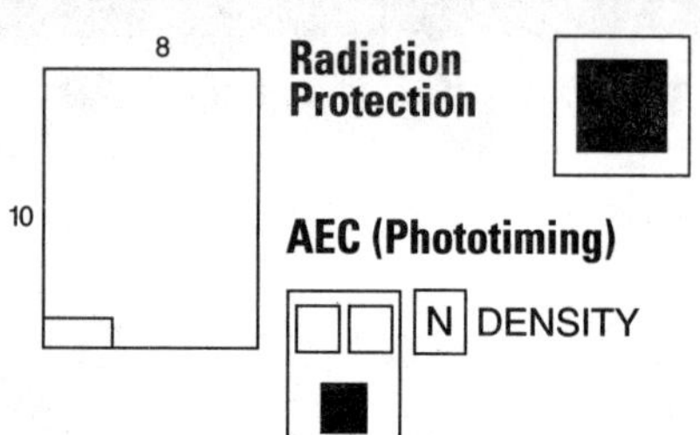

Technical Considerations
- Regular screen/film
- Grid
- kVp range: 70–80
- SID: 40 inch (100 cm)

Patient Position Facing the film; all potential artifacts removed.

Part Position Cassette is centered to the orbits; MSP is perpendicular to the midpoint of the cassette; OML is perpendicular to the film.

Central Ray Perpendicular to the film.

Breathing Instructions Suspend respiration.

Example Exposure Techniques **Measure at CR and Use Chart (p.278)**									
Room	**cm**	**kVp**	**mAs**	**mA**	**Sec**	**Beam**	**Film**	**Grid**	**1Ø3Ø**
	16								
	17								
	18								
	19								
	20								
	21								
	22								
	23								
	24								
	25								

Evaluation Criteria

- No rotation as evidenced by equal distance from the lateral border of the orbit to the lateral border of the skull on each side.
- Petrous ridges fill the orbit.

Exam Rationale This projection demonstrates the upper two-thirds of the orbit.

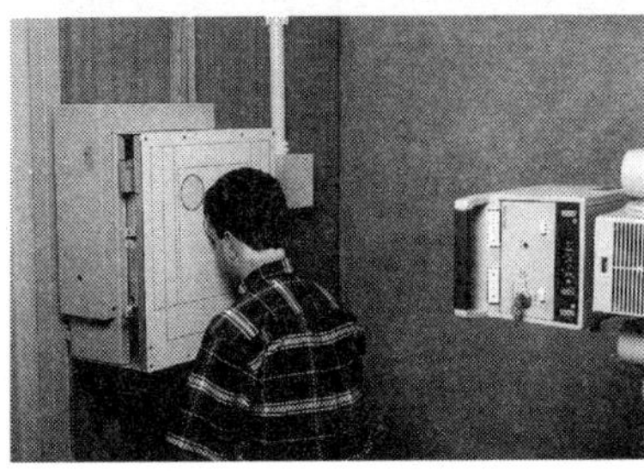

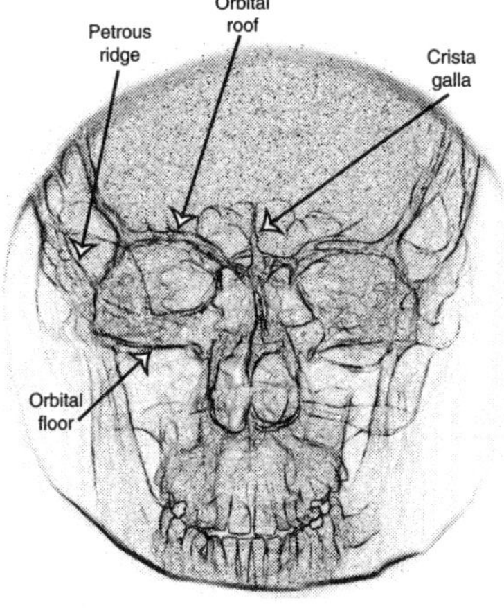

Technical Considerations

- Regular screen/film
- Grid
- kVp range: 70–80
- SID: 40 inch (100 cm)

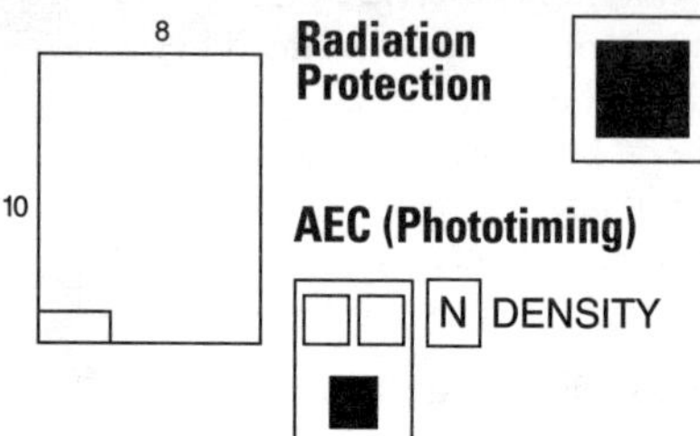

Patient Position Facing the film; all potential artifacts removed.

Part Position Extend the neck and place the chin on the Bucky; cassette is centered to the level of the acanthion; MSP is centered to the film; OML forms a 55° angle with the plane of the film.

Central Ray Perpendicular to the film exiting at the acanthion.

Breathing Instructions Suspend respiration.

Evaluation Criteria

- The entire orbital rim and the maxillae should be demonstrated.
- No rotation as evidenced by an equal distance from the lateral orbital border to the lateral border of the skull on each side.
- The petrous ridges are projected into the maxillary sinuses.

Example Exposure Techniques
Measure at CR and Use Chart (p.278)

Room	cm	kVp	mAs	mA	Sec	Beam	Film	Grid	1Ø3Ø
	16								
	17								
	18								
	19								
	20								
	21								
	22								
	23								
	24								
	25								

Exam Rationale This projection demonstrates the floor of the orbits and is especially helpful in demonstrating "blowout" fractures.

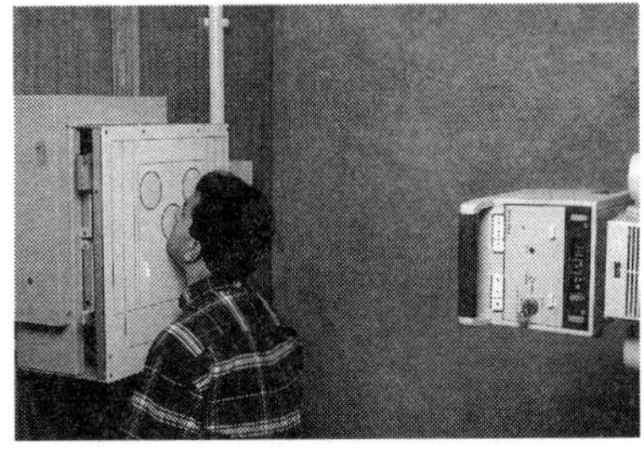

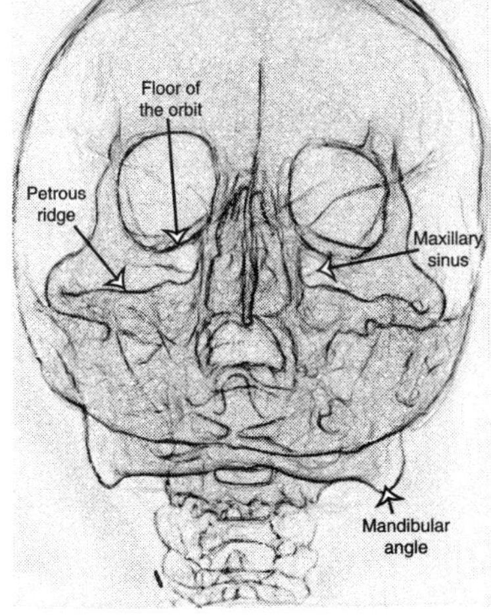

Technical Considerations

- Regular screen/film
- Grid
- kVp range: 70–80
- SID: 40 inch (100 cm)

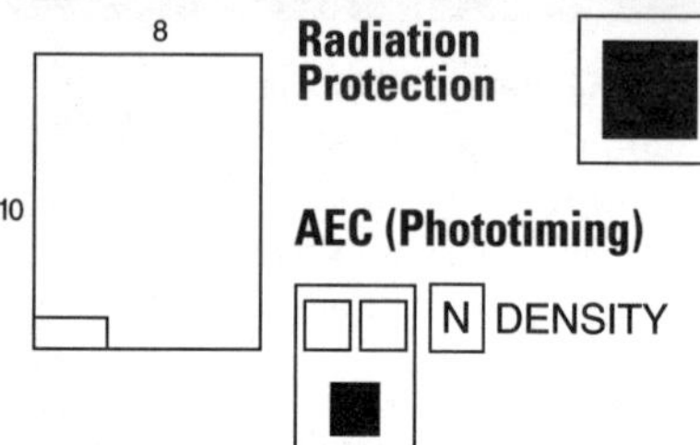

Patient Position In lateral position; all potential artifacts removed.

Part Position Cassette is centered to the orbit; MSP is parallel and interpupillary line is perpendicular to the film.

Central Ray Perpendicular to the film.

Breathing Instructions Suspend respiration.

Example Exposure Techniques **Measure at CR and Use Chart (p.278)**									
Room	**cm**	**kVp**	**mAs**	**mA**	**Sec**	**Beam**	**Film**	**Grid**	**1Ø3Ø**
	11								
	12								
	13								
	14								
	15								
	16								
	17								
	18								
	19								
	20								

Evaluation Criteria

- Superimposition of both orbits.

Exam Rationale This position is used to demonstrate foreign bodies.

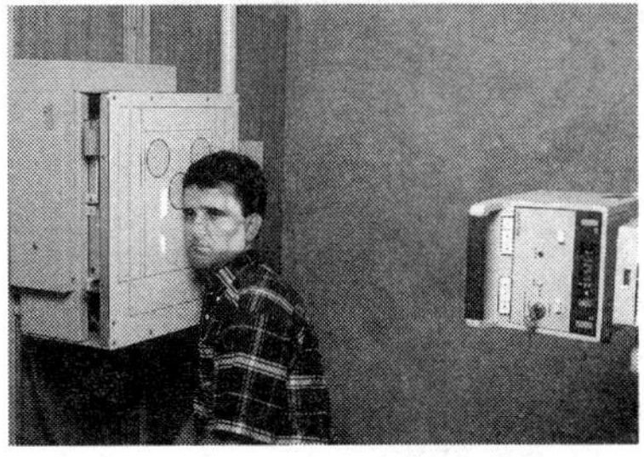

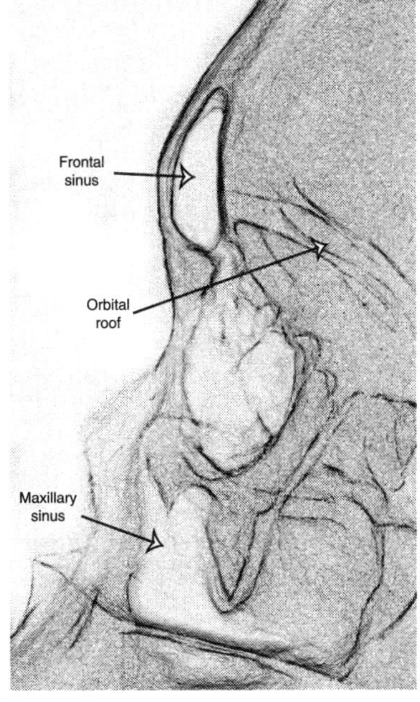

Technical Considerations
- Regular screen/film
- Grid
- kVp range: 70–80
- SID: 40 inch (100 cm)

Radiation Protection

AEC (Phototiming)

Patient Position Facing the film; all potential artifacts removed.

Part Position Center affected orbit to midline of the grid and center the film to the orbit; patient's zygoma, nose, and chin rest on the table; MSP forms a 53° angle to the film; acanthiomeatal line is perpendicular to the plane of the film.

Central Ray Perpendicular to the film exiting through the affected orbit.

Breathing Instructions Suspend respiration.

Evaluation Criteria
- The entire orbit should be included.
- The optic foramen should be projected in the lower, outer quadrant of the orbit.

Example Exposure Techniques
Measure at CR and Use Chart (p.278)

Room	cm	kVp	mAs	mA	Sec	Beam	Film	Grid	1Ø3Ø
	16								
	17								
	18								
	19								
	20								
	21								
	22								
	23								
	24								
	25								

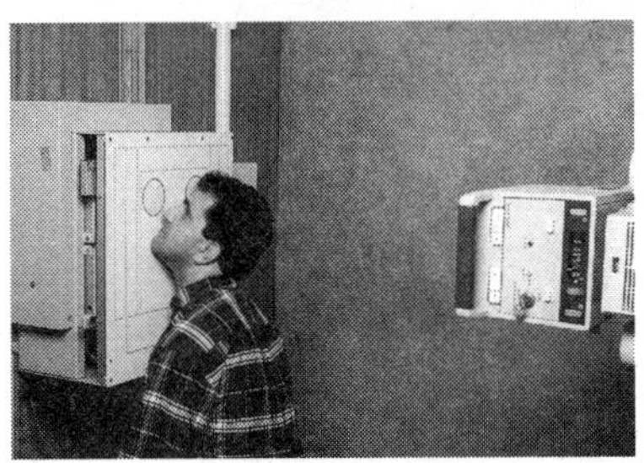

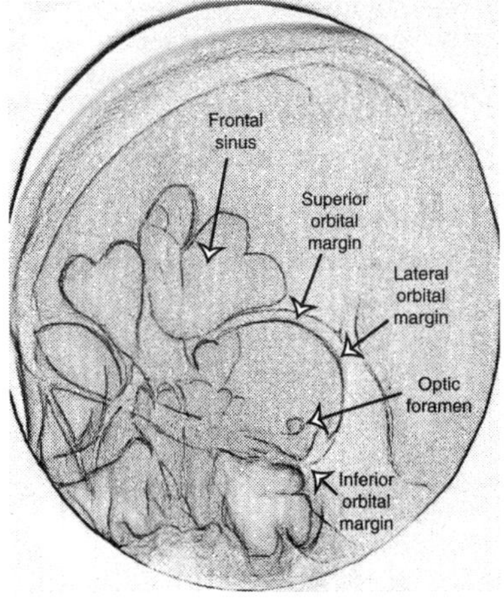

- The optic foramen should be found at the end of the sphenoid ridge.

Exam Rationale This projection demonstrates the optic foramen. Enlargement or erosion is usually associated with tumor; narrowing could indicate abnormal bone growth. Normally both sides are taken for comparison.

Tips

1. It is important to collimate to the orbit to maximize detail.
2. If the optic foramen does not lie in the lower quadrant, the acanthiomeatal line is not perpendicular to the film; if it does not lie in the outer quadrant, the MSP is not at a 53° angle to the film.

Technical Considerations
- Regular screen/film
- Grid
- kVp range: 60–70
- SID: 40 inch (100 cm)

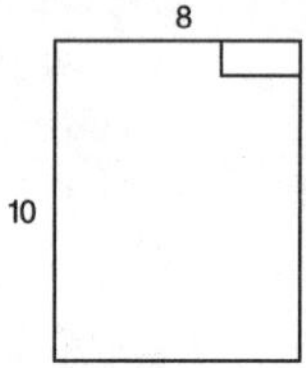

8

10

Radiation Protection

AEC (Phototiming)

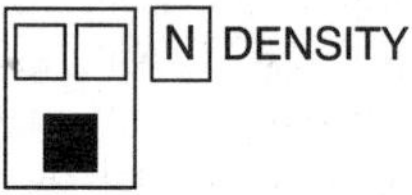

N DENSITY

Patient Position Facing the tube; all potential artifacts removed.

Part Position Cassette is centered to the level of the mandibular angles; MSP is perpendicular to the center of the grid; OML is perpendicular to the plane of the film.

Central Ray 30° caudal entering the glabella.

Breathing Instructions Suspend respiration.

Evaluation Criteria
- Zygomatic arches projected free of the mandible.
- No rotation demonstrated as evidenced by the symmetrical demonstration of the zygomatic arches.

Example Exposure Techniques
Measure at CR and Use Chart (p.278)

Room	cm	kVp	mAs	mA	Sec	Beam	Film	Grid	1Ø3Ø
	16								
	17								
	18								
	19								
	20								
	21								
	22								
	23								
	24								
	25								

Exam Rationale This projection is used to demonstrate the zygomatic arches free of superimposition. It is normally used to demonstrate fracture.

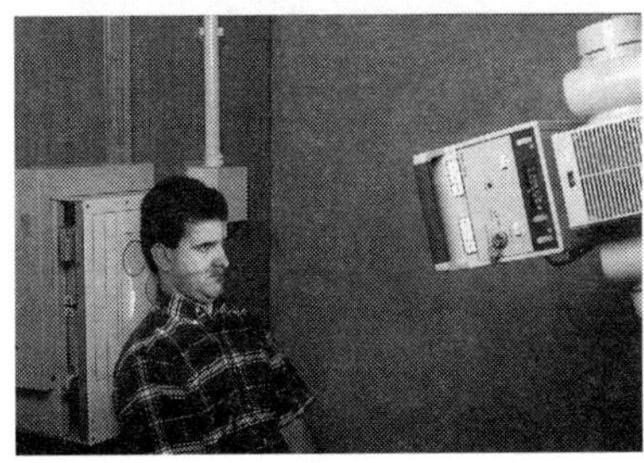

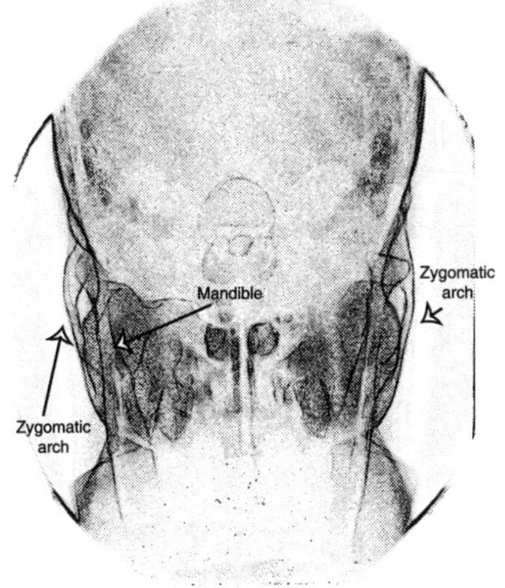

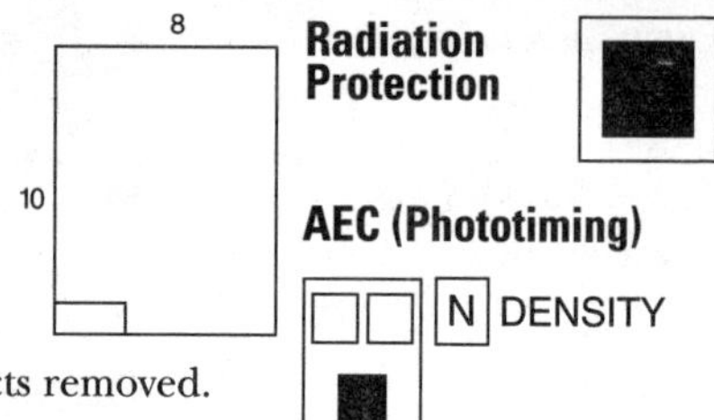

Technical Considerations
- Regular screen/film
- Grid
- kVp range: 60–70
- SID: 40 inch (100 cm)

Patient Position Facing the tube; all potential artifacts removed.

Part Position Patient's neck is extended until head is resting on the vertex; cassette is centered to a level 1 inch (3 cm) posterior to the outer canthus; MSP is perpendicular to the plane of the film; IOML is parallel to the cassette.

Central Ray Perpendicular to IOML entering midway between the zygomatic arches.

Breathing Instructions Suspend respiration.

Evaluation Criteria
- The zygomatic arches should be projected free of superimposition.
- No rotation is demonstrated.

Example Exposure Techniques **Measure at CR and Use Chart (p.278)**									
Room	**cm**	**kVp**	**mAs**	**mA**	**Sec**	**Beam**	**Film**	**Grid**	**1Ø3Ø**
	16								
	17								
	18								
	19								
	20								
	21								
	22								
	23								
	24								
	25								

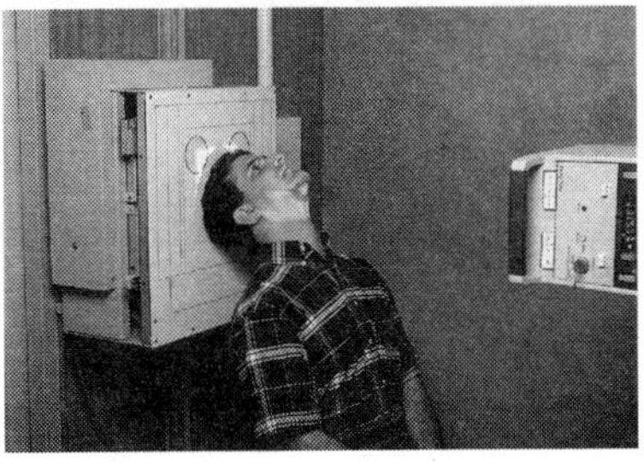

Exam Rationale This projection can be used to demonstrate the lateral margins of the zygomatic arches free of superimposition. It is usually performed to identify fractures.

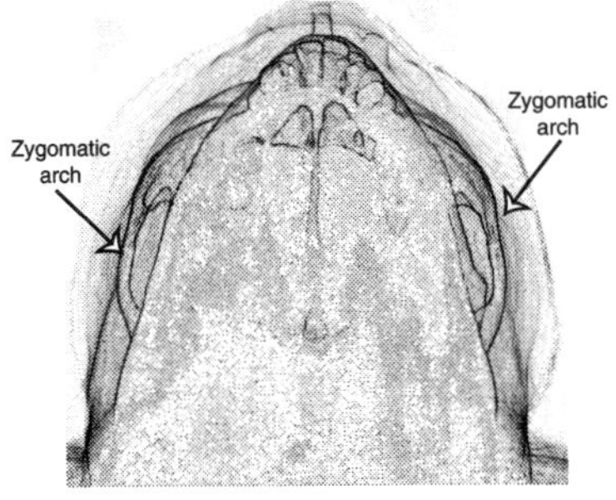

Tips

1. Due to the difficulty of maintaining this position, do this projection as quickly as possible.
2. Decreasing the mAs approximately 50% from the SMV to demonstrate the base of the cranium should demonstrate the arches with the proper density.

Technical Considerations
- Regular screen/film
- Grid
- kVp range: 60–70
- SID: 40 inch (100 cm)

8

10

Radiation Protection

AEC (Phototiming)

N DENSITY

Patient Position Facing the film; all potential artifacts removed.

Part Position Extend the neck and place the vertex of the head on the cassette holder; center the affected zygomatic arch to the center of the grid; center the film to a point approximately 3 inches (8 cm) inferior to the zygomatic bone; IOML as close to parallel to the film as possible; tilt the head 15° away from the affected side.

Central Ray Angle the tube caudally to place the central ray perpendicular to the IOML; center the central ray to the affected zygomatic arch (approximately 1 inch [3 cm] posterior to the outer canthus); center the cassette to the central ray.

Breathing Instructions Suspend respiration.

Example Exposure Techniques
Measure at CR and Use Chart (p.278)

Room	cm	kVp	mAs	mA	Sec	Beam	Film	Grid	1Ø3Ø
	5								
	6								
	7								
	8								
	9								
	10								
	11								
	12								

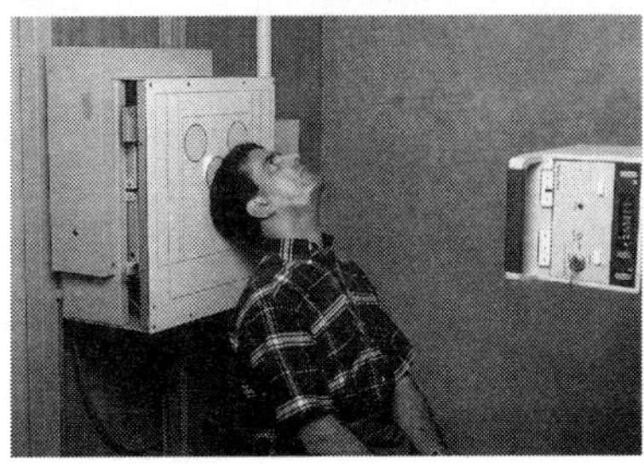

Evaluation Criteria

- Affected zygomatic arch projected free of superimposition.

Exam Rationale This position is used to demonstrate a unilateral zygomatic arch projected free from superimposition. It is particularly helpful with patients who have flat cheekbones or a depressed fracture of the zygomatic arch. Both sides are usually done for comparison.

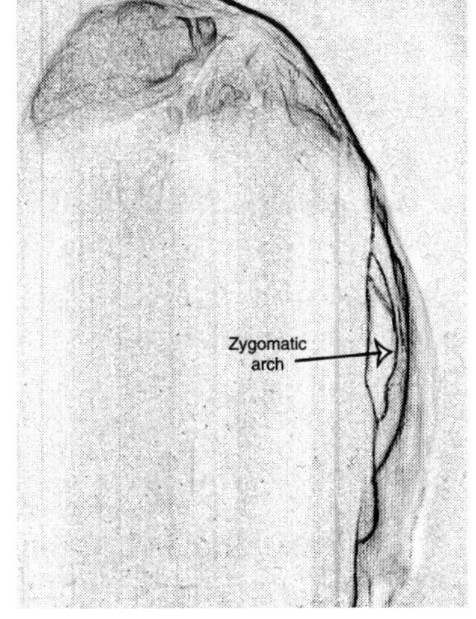

Technical Considerations
- Regular screen/film
- Grid
- kVp range: 70–80
- SID: 40 inch (100 cm)

8

10

Radiation Protection

AEC (Phototiming)

N DENSITY

Patient Position Facing the tube; all potential artifacts removed.

Part Position OML and MSP are perpendicular to the film.

Central Ray 35° caudally entering the glabella.

Breathing Instructions Suspend respiration.

Evaluation Criteria
- The condyloid processes and mandibular rami are demonstrated without rotation as evidenced by symmetrical views of the rami.

Exam Rationale This projection demonstrates the mandibular rami, the mandibular condyles, and the temporomandibular fossae.

Example Exposure Techniques
Measure at CR and Use Chart (p.278)

Room	cm	kVp	mAs	mA	Sec	Beam	Film	Grid	1Ø3Ø
	16								
	17								
	18								
	19								
	20								
	21								
	22								
	23								
	24								
	25								

Tip If unable to place the OML perpendicular to the film, place the IOML perpendicular to the film and increase the central ray angle by 7°.

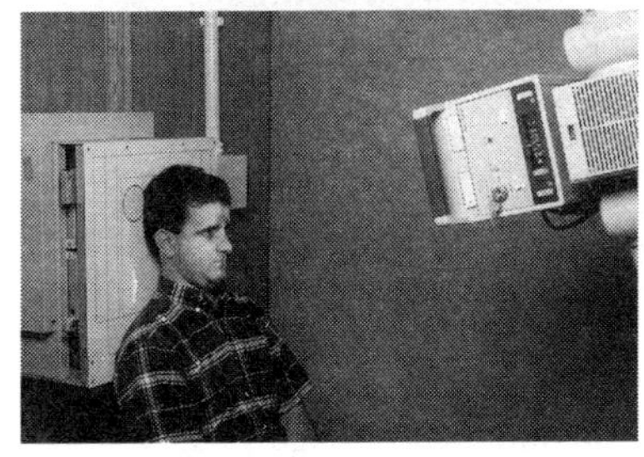

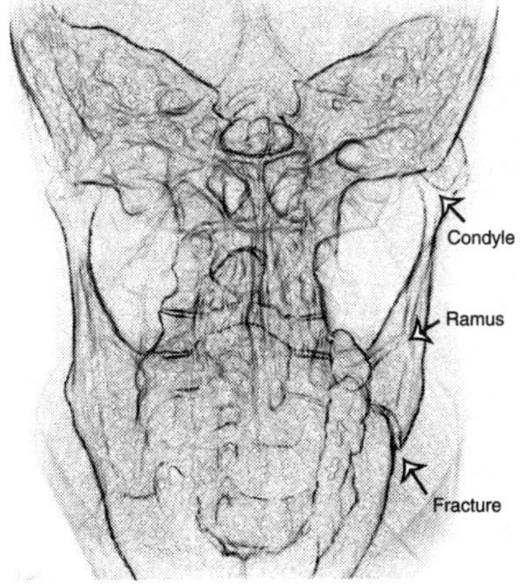

Technical Considerations

- Regular screen/film
- Grid
- kVp range: 70–80
- SID: 40 inch (100 cm)

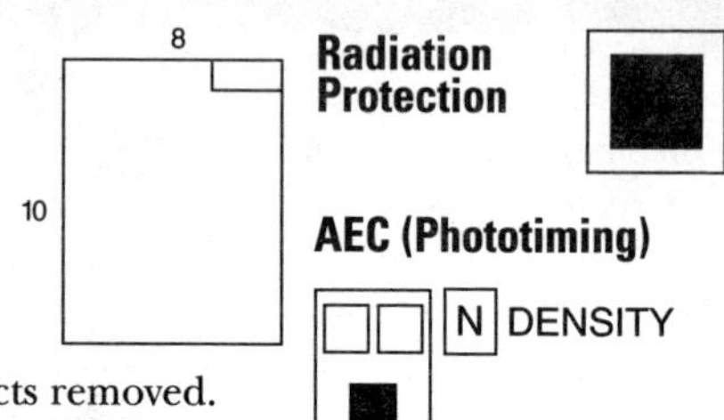

Patient Position Facing the film; all potential artifacts removed.

Part Position MSP is perpendicular to the midline of the grid; OML is perpendicular to film; cassette is centered to the level of the lips.

Central Ray Perpendicular to the film exiting at the lips.

Breathing Instructions Suspend respiration.

Evaluation Criteria

- The entire mandible should be included.
- No rotation as evidenced by symmetrical visualization of the rami.

Exam Rationale This projection is used to demonstrate the mandibular rami and body.

Example Exposure Techniques **Measure at CR and Use Chart (p.278)**									
Room	**cm**	**kVp**	**mAs**	**mA**	**Sec**	**Beam**	**Film**	**Grid**	**1Ø3Ø**
	16								
	17								
	18								
	19								
	20								
	21								
	22								
	23								
	24								
	25								

Tip To demonstrate the mentum, place the nose and chin on the table top with the MSP perpendicular to the midline of the grid.

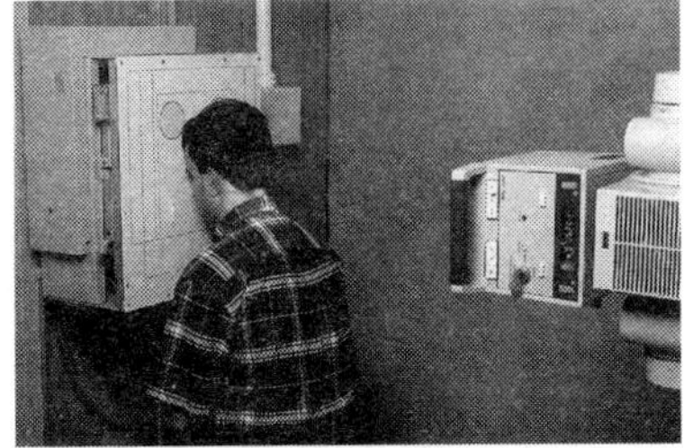

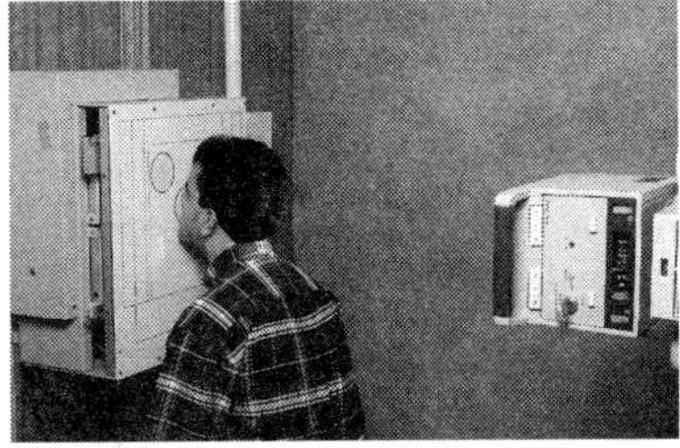

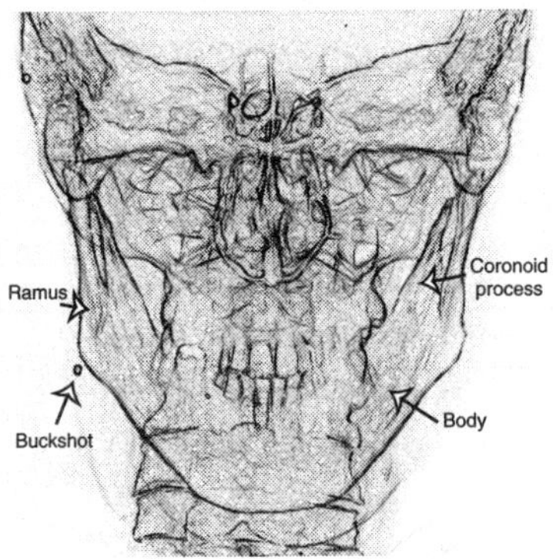

Technical Considerations
- Regular screen/film
- Grid
- kVp range: 70–80
- SID: 40 inch (100 cm)

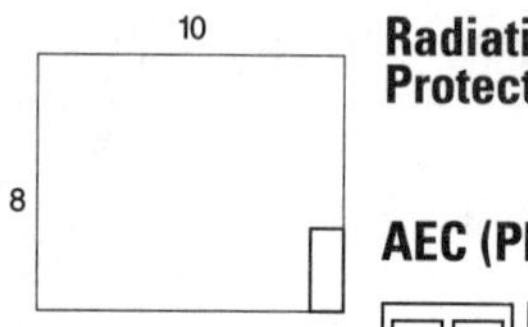

Radiation Protection

AEC (Phototiming)

N DENSITY

Patient Position In lateral position; all potential artifacts removed.

Part Position Head in a lateral position with side of interest closest to the film; extend the chin to prevent superimposition on the cervical spine; to demonstrate the ramus, the head should be in a true lateral position; to demonstrate the body, rotate the head approximately 30° toward the film; to demonstrate the mentum, rotate the head approximately 45° toward the film.

Central Ray 25° to 35° cephalic to the area of interest.

Breathing Instructions Suspend respiration.

Example Exposure Techniques
Measure at CR and Use Chart (p.278)

Room	cm	kVp	mAs	mA	Sec	Beam	Film	Grid	1Ø3Ø
	8								
	9								
	10								
	11								
	12								
	13								
	14								
	15								
	16								
	17								

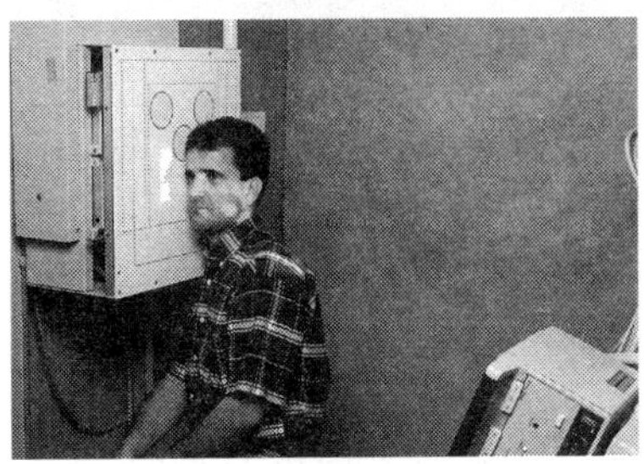

Evaluation Criteria

- Area of interest is well demonstrated.
- No superimposition of the opposite side of the mandible.

Exam Rationale This position demonstrates the temporomandibular joint (TMJ), condyle, coronoid process, ramus, body, and mentum of the side of the mandible closest to the film. Both sides are taken for comparison.

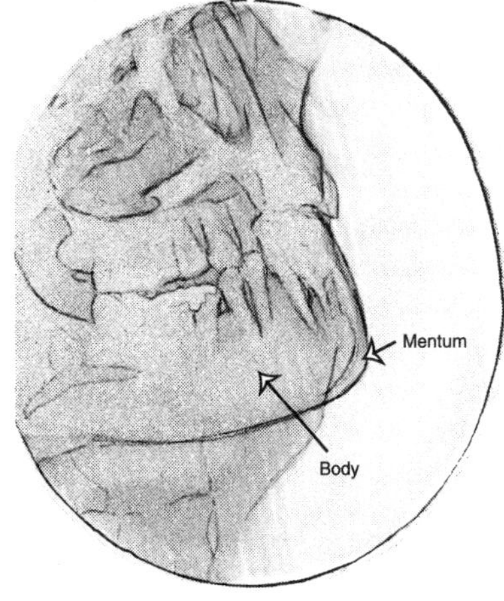

Technical Considerations
- Regular screen/film
- Grid
- kVp range: 70–80
- SID: 40 inch (100 cm)

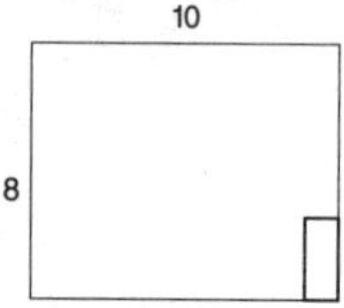

10

8

Radiation Protection

AEC (Phototiming)

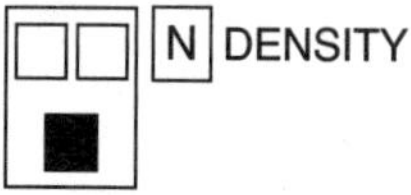

N DENSITY

Patient Position In the lateral position; all potential artifacts removed.

Part Position Cassette is centered to the TMJ; MSP is parallel to the film; interpupillary line is perpendicular to the film; IOML is parallel to the transverse axis of the film.

Central Ray 25° to 30° caudal centered to the center of the film.

Breathing Instructions
- Closed mouth: suspend respiration. Keep mouth closed.
- Open mouth: suspend respiration. Keep mouth open.

Example Exposure Techniques
Measure at CR and Use Chart (p.278)

Room	cm	kVp	mAs	mA	Sec	Beam	Film	Grid	1Ø3Ø
	11								
	12								
	13								
	14								
	15								
	16								
	17								
	18								
	19								
	20								

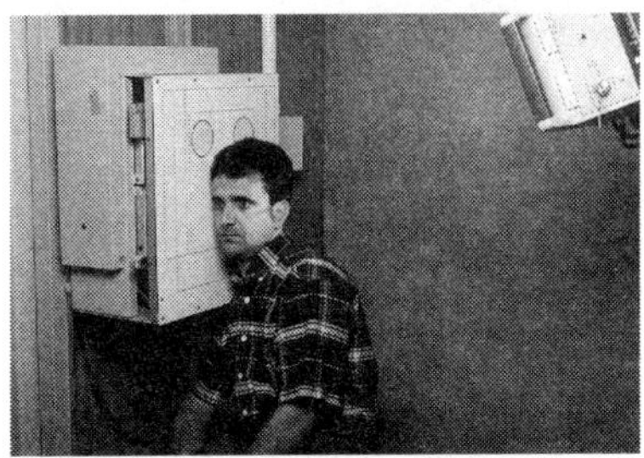

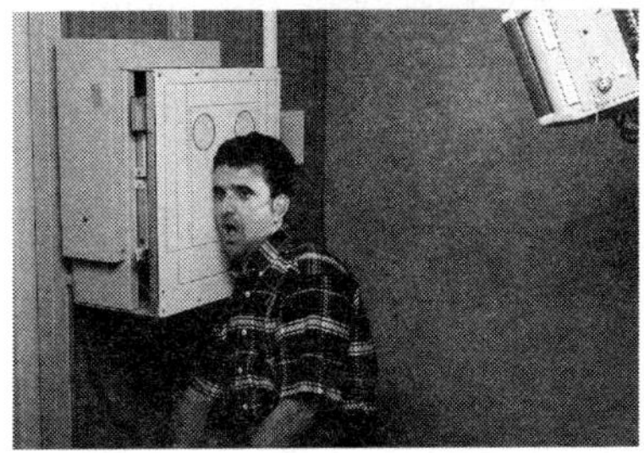

Evaluation Criteria

- With the mouth closed, the mandibular condyle will be visualized within the mandibular fossa.
- With the mouth open, the mandibular condyle will move inferior and anterior and will be demonstrated inferior to the articular tubercle.

Exam Rationale This projection better demonstrates the TMJ closest to the film. The configuration of the condyle and mandibular fossa and the direction and amount of movement is demonstrated. In cases of trauma, the position can illustrate dislocation or small fractures of the cortex of the condyle. Both sides are usually taken in both the open and closed mouth positions.

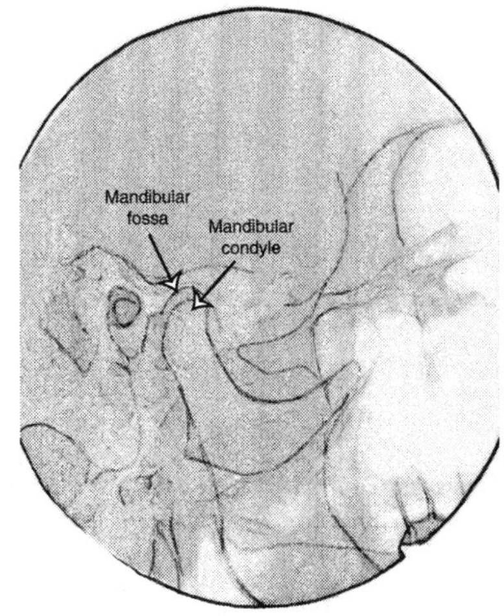

Technical Considerations
- Regular screen/film
- Grid
- kVp range: 70–80
- SID: 40 inch (100 cm)

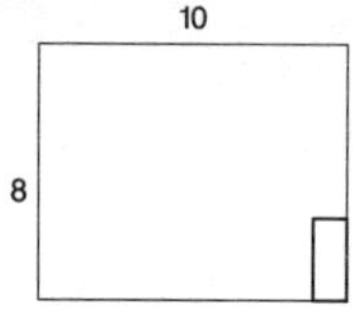

10

8

Radiation Protection

AEC (Phototiming)

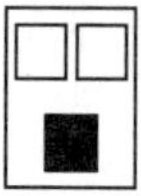

N DENSITY

Patient Position In a lateral position; all potential artifacts removed.

Part Position With the side to be demonstrated closest to the film, rest the cheek against the cassette holder; cassette is centered to the TMJ; rotate the head toward the film until MSP forms a 15° angle to the film; acanthiomeatal line is parallel to the transverse axis of the film.

Central Ray 15° caudal exiting through the TMJ.

Breathing Instructions
- Closed mouth: suspend respiration. Keep mouth closed.
- Open mouth: suspend respiration. Keep mouth open.

Example Exposure Techniques
Measure at CR and Use Chart (p.278)

Room	cm	kVp	mAs	mA	Sec	Beam	Film	Grid	1Ø3Ø
	11								
	12								
	13								
	14								
	15								
	16								
	17								
	18								
	19								
	20								

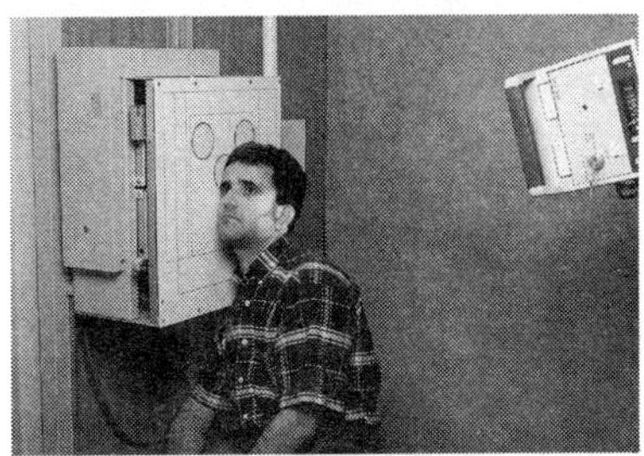

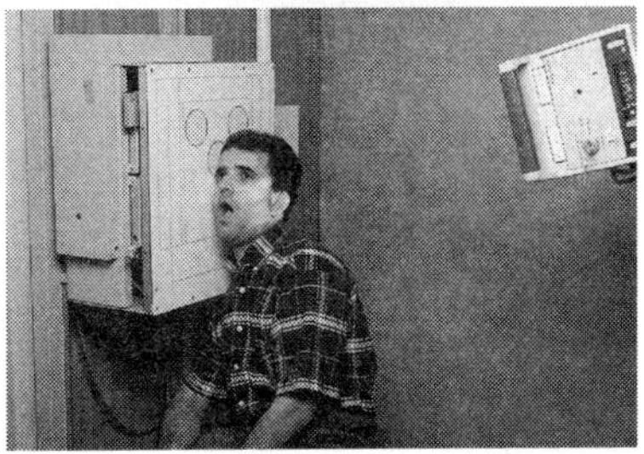

Evaluation Criteria

- Closed mouth position demonstrates the mandibular condyle in the mandibular fossa.
- In open mouth position condyle will move inferior and anterior.

Exam Rationale This position best demonstrates the TMJ closest to the film. The configuration of the condyle and mandibular fossa and the direction and amount of movement is demonstrated. The position also illustrates dislocation or small fractures of the cortex of the condyle. Both sides are usually taken in both the open and closed mouth positions.

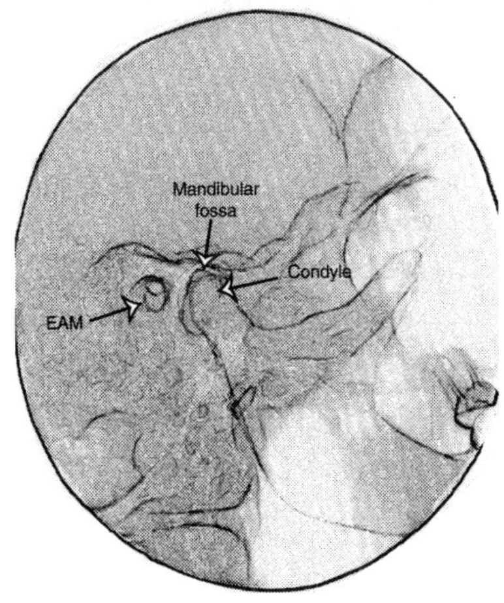

Technical Considerations

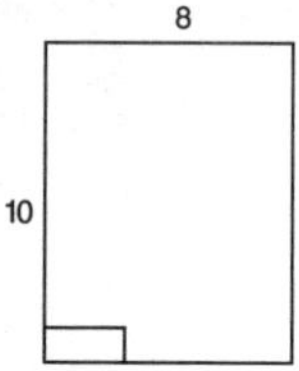

- Regular screen/film
- Grid
- kVp range: 70–80
- SID: 40 inch (100 cm)

8

10

Radiation Protection

AEC (Phototiming)

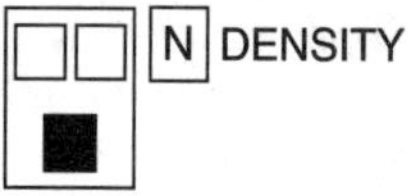

N DENSITY

Patient Position Facing the film; all potential artifacts removed.

Part Position Cassette is centered to the nasion; MSP is perpendicular to the midpoint of the grid; OML is perpendicular to the film.

Central Ray

15° caudal exiting at the nasion.

Breathing Instructions Suspend respiration.

Evaluation Criteria

- The petrous ridges are demonstrated in the lower third of the orbits.
- The frontal sinuses are situated above the frontonasal suture.

Example Exposure Techniques
Measure at CR and Use Chart (p.278)

Room	cm	kVp	mAs	mA	Sec	Beam	Film	Grid	1Ø3Ø
	16								
	17								
	18								
	19								
	20								
	21								
	22								
	23								
	24								
	25								

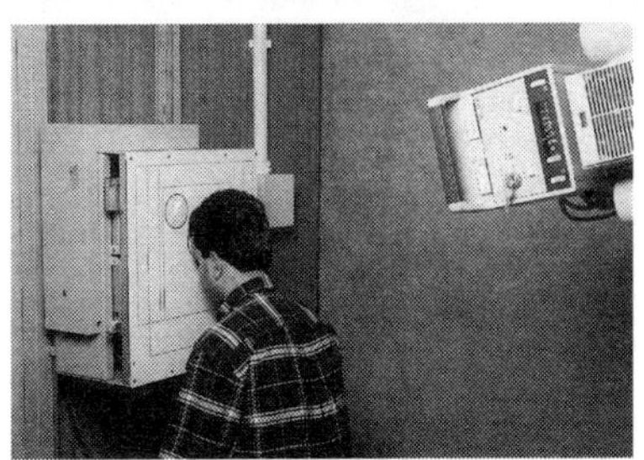

- The anterior ethmoid sinuses are demonstrated immediately lateral to the nasal bones and directly below the frontal sinuses.
- No rotation is evident.

Exam Rationale This projection best demonstrates inflammatory changes in the frontal sinuses and the ethmoid sinuses.

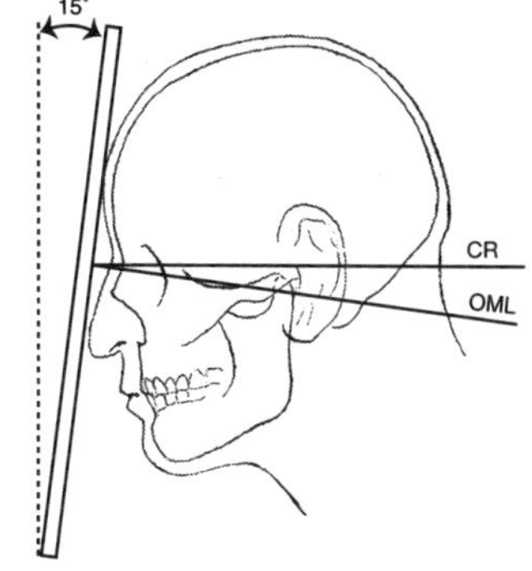

Tip To use a horizontal beam, tilt the film holder 15° with the superior edge toward the patient. Rest the nose and forehead on the holder and adjust the MSP perpendicular and OML perpendicular to the film.
This projection can be used to demonstrate the floor of the antra in those cases where it is difficult to demonstrate in other projections.

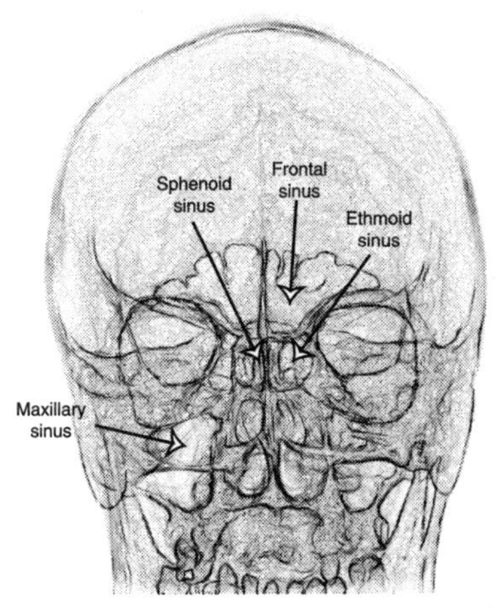

Technical Considerations

- Regular screen/film
- Grid
- kVp range: 70–80
- SID: 40 inch (100 cm)

8

10

Radiation Protection

AEC (Phototiming)

N DENSITY

Patient Position Facing the film; all potential artifacts removed.

Part Position Cassette is centered to the level of the acanthion; MSP is perpendicular to the midpoint of the grid; OML forms an angle of 37° to the plane of the film.

Central Ray Perpendicular to the film exiting at the acanthion.

Breathing Instructions Suspend respiration.

Evaluation Criteria

- The petrous ridges are projected immediately below the maxillary sinuses indicating proper extension.
- No rotation as evidenced by equal distance from the lateral border of the skull to the orbit on each side.

Example Exposure Techniques
Measure at CR and Use Chart (p.278)

Room	cm	kVp	mAs	mA	Sec	Beam	Film	Grid	1Ø3Ø
	16								
	17								
	18								
	19								
	20								
	21								
	22								
	23								
	24								
	25								

Exam Rationale This projection is used to demonstrate sinusitis of the maxillary sinuses, which are the most commonly infected. Retention cysts and nasal deviation can also be demonstrated.

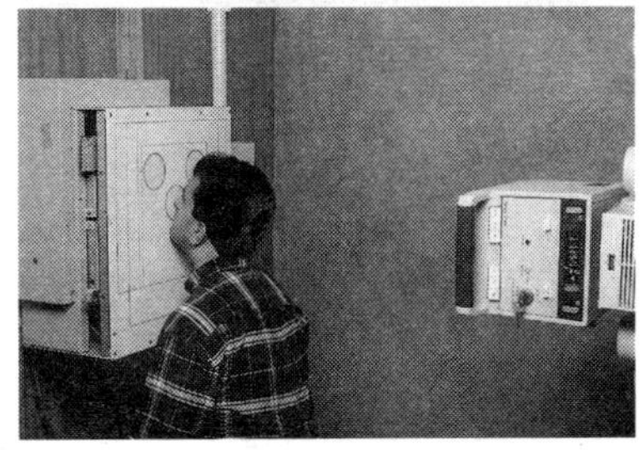

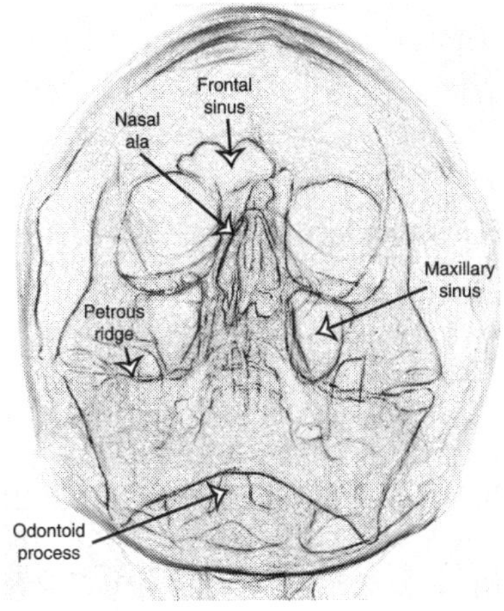

Technical Considerations

- Regular screen/film
- Grid
- kVp range: 70–80
- SID: 40 inch (100 cm)

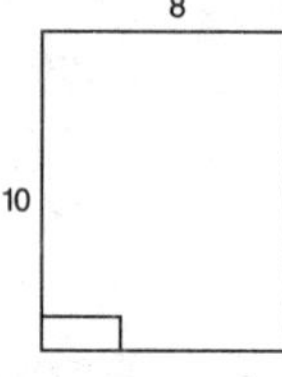

Radiation Protection

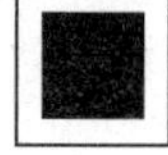

AEC (Phototiming)

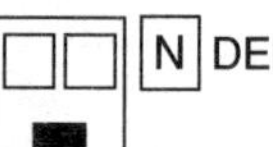

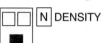

Patient Position In lateral position; all potential artifacts removed.

Part Position Side of interest closest to the film; cassette is centered to a point 1/2 to 1 inch (1–3 cm) posterior to the outer canthus; MSP is parallel to the film; interpupillary line is perpendicular to the film; IOML is parallel to the transverse axis of the film.

Central Ray Perpendicular to the film entering 1/2 to 1 inch (1–3 cm) posterior to the outer canthus.

Breathing Instructions Suspend respiration.

Evaluation Criteria

- All sinuses should be visualized.
- No rotation as evidenced by superimposition of the mandibular rami and orbital roofs and the sella turcica is seen without rotation.

Example Exposure Techniques **Measure at CR and Use Chart (p.278)**									
Room	**cm**	**kVp**	**mAs**	**mA**	**Sec**	**Beam**	**Film**	**Grid**	**1Ø3Ø**
	11								
	12								
	13								
	14								
	15								
	16								
	17								
	18								
	19								
	20								

Exam Rationale This is the best position to demonstrate the sphenoid sinuses; it also demonstrates the frontal, maxillary, and ethmoid sinuses.

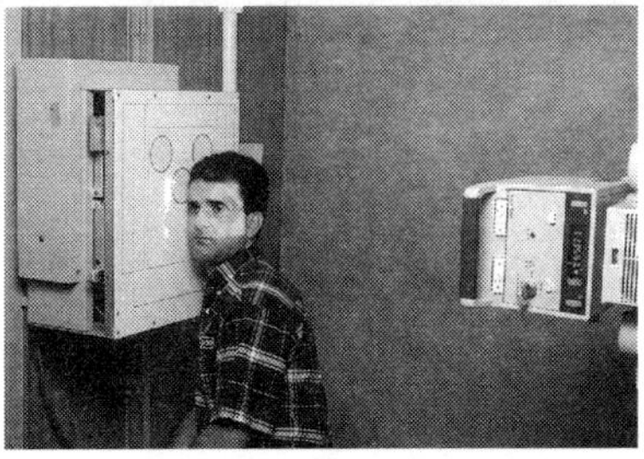

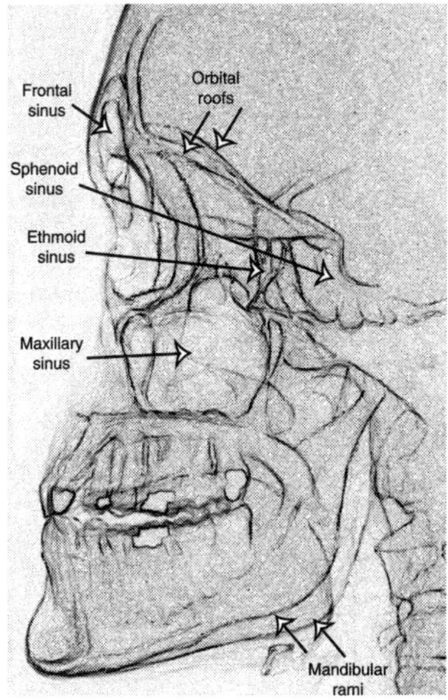

Technical Considerations
- Regular screen/film
- Grid
- kVp range: 70–80
- SID: 40 inch (100 cm)

8

10

Radiation Protection

AEC (Phototiming)

N DENSITY

Patient Position Facing the tube; all potential artifacts removed.

Part Position Vertex of the head is resting on the cassette holder; cassette is centered to the level of the sella turcica; MSP is perpendicular to the midpoint of the grid; IOML is parallel to the plane of the film.

Central Ray Perpendicular to the IOML entering midway between the angles of the mandible approximately 2 inches (5 cm) inferior to the mandibular symphysis.

Breathing Instructions Suspend respiration.

Evaluation Criteria
- The mandibular symphysis is superimposed on the anterior frontal bone indicating adequate extension or tube angle.

Example Exposure Techniques
Measure at CR and Use Chart (p.278)

Room	cm	kVp	mAs	mA	Sec	Beam	Film	Grid	1Ø3Ø
	16								
	17								
	18								
	19								
	20								
	21								
	22								
	23								
	24								
	25								

- There is no rotation as evidenced by symmetrical petrous ridges and equal distance between the mandible and the lateral border of the skull.

Exam Rationale This projection best demonstrates the sphenoid sinuses, the ethmoid sinuses, and the nasal passages.

Tip For the patient who is unable to assume this position, the verticosubmental is an option. With the patient seated at the end of the table, the cassette is placed on an angle sponge. The patient's chin rests on the cassette and the head is adjusted to place the MSP perpendicular to the film and the IOML parallel to the film. The central ray is perpendicular to the IOML.

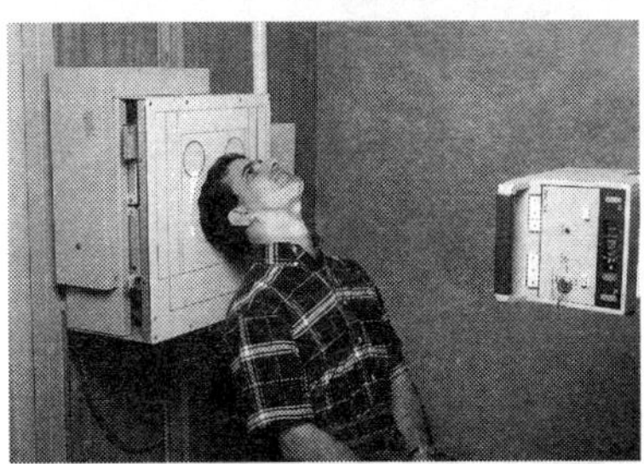

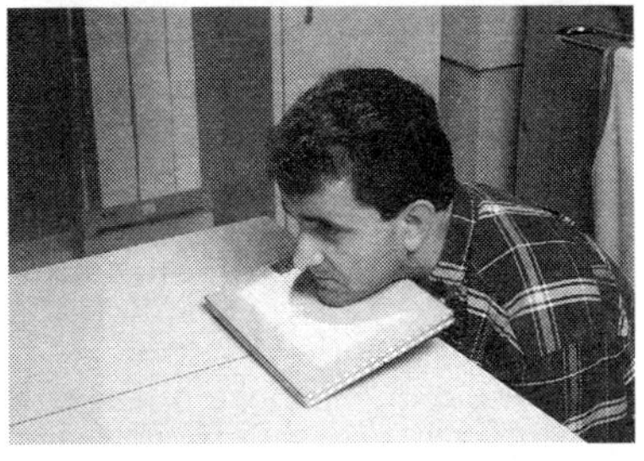

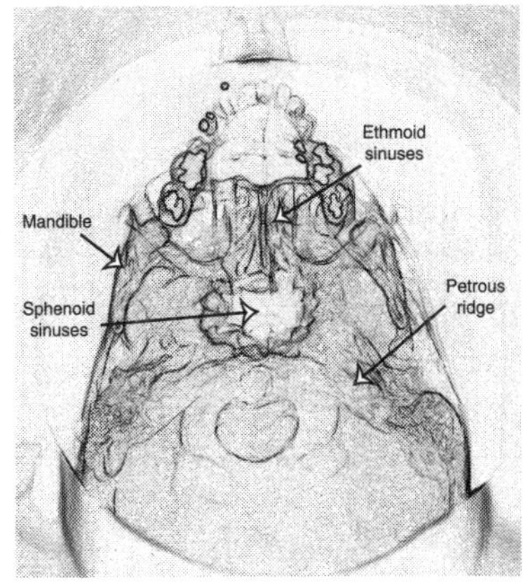

Technical Considerations

- Regular screen/film
- Grid
- kVp range: 70–80
- SID: 40 inch (100 cm)

8

10

Radiation Protection

AEC (Phototiming)

N DENSITY

Patient Position Facing the film; all potential artifacts removed.

Part Position Place the nose and chin on the cassette holder; the mouth is open and centered to the film; MSP is perpendicular to the film and centered to the grid.

Central Ray At a 30° caudal angle along a line extending from the sella turcica to the center of the open mouth.

Breathing Instructions Suspend respiration.

Evaluation Criteria

- Sphenoid sinuses demonstrated through the open mouth.

Exam Rationale This projection demonstrates the sphenoid sinuses projected through the open mouth. The maxillary sinuses and nasal fossae are also visualized.

Example Exposure Techniques **Measure at CR and Use Chart (p.278)**									
Room	**cm**	**kVp**	**mAs**	**mA**	**Sec**	**Beam**	**Film**	**Grid**	**1Ø3Ø**
	16								
	17								
	18								
	19								
	20								
	21								
	22								
	23								
	24								
	25								

Tips

1. The sella turcica is located at a level 3/4 inch (2 cm) anterior and 3/4 inch (2 cm) superior to the external auditory meatus.
2. It is especially important to clean the Bucky surface in the presence of the patient before positioning.

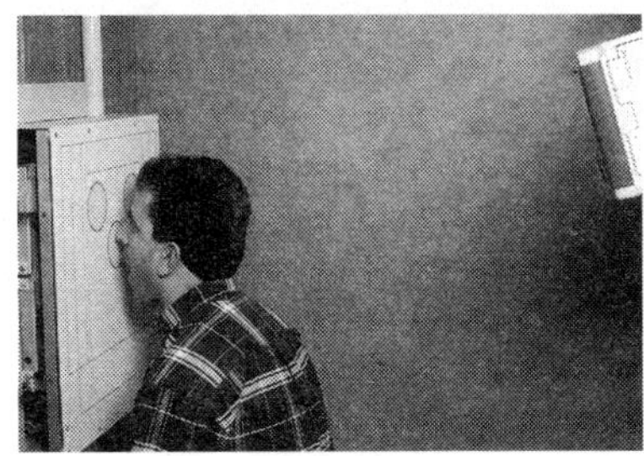

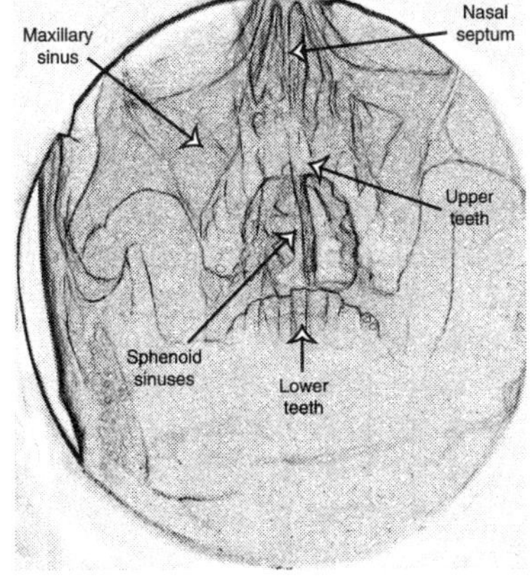

Technical Considerations
- Regular screen/film
- Grid
- kVp range: 70–80
- SID: 40 inch (100 cm)

8

10

Radiation Protection

AEC (Phototiming)

N DENSITY

Patient Position Facing the tube; all potential artifacts removed.

Part Position MSP is perpendicular to the midpoint of the film; OML is perpendicular to the film.

Central Ray At a 30° caudal angle exiting through the external auditory meatus.

Breathing Instructions Suspend respiration.

Evaluation Criteria
- The petrous ridges and mastoid air cells should be included.
- No rotation as evidenced by:
  —Symmetrical petrous ridges
  —Equal distance from lateral border of foramen magnum to lateral border of skull

Example Exposure Techniques
Measure at CR and Use Chart (p.278)

Room	cm	kVp	mAs	mA	Sec	Beam	Film	Grid	1Ø3Ø
	16								
	17								
	18								
	19								
	20								
	21								
	22								
	23								
	24								
	25								

- Dorsum sella and posterior clinoids should be visualized within the foramen magnum.

Exam Rationale This projection demonstrates a symmetrical image of the petrous portion of the temporal bone, the internal auditory canals, the arcuate eminences, labyrinths, mastoid antrum, and middle ear.

Tip If it is not possible to place the OML perpendicular to the film, the IOML can be placed perpendicular to the film, and the central ray angle is increased to 37°.

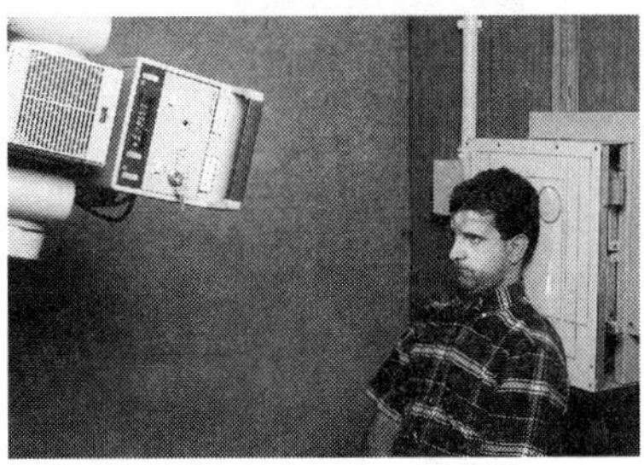

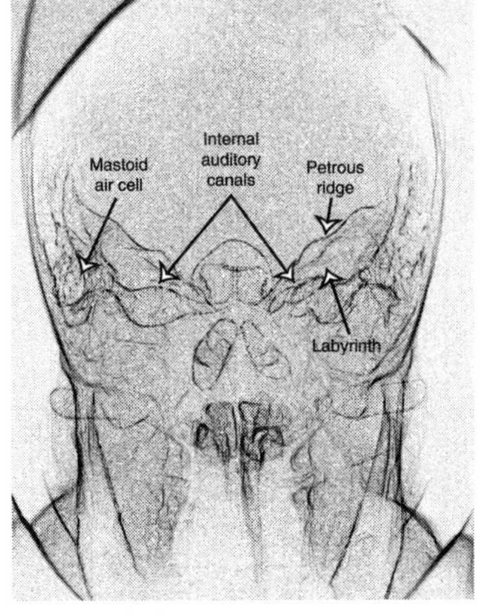

Technical Considerations
- Regular screen/film
- Grid
- kVp range: 70–80
- SID: 40 inch (100 cm)

10

8

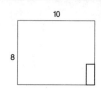

Radiation Protection

AEC (Phototiming)

N DENSITY

Patient Position In a lateral position; all potential artifacts removed. The auricle of the ear should be taped forward to prevent superimposition of it over the mastoid air cells.

Part Position Place head in lateral position and then rotate the face toward the film so the MSP is 15° to the plane of the film; center the film approximately 1 inch (3 cm) posterior to the EAM closest to the film.

Central Ray 15° caudal entering approximately 2 inches (5 cm) posterior and 2 inches (5 cm) superior to the uppermost EAM.

Breathing Instructions Suspend respiration.

Example Exposure Techniques **Measure at CR and Use Chart (p.278)**									
Room	**cm**	**kVp**	**mAs**	**mA**	**Sec**	**Beam**	**Film**	**Grid**	**1Ø3Ø**
	11								
	12								
	13								
	14								
	15								
	16								
	17								
	18								
	19								
	20								

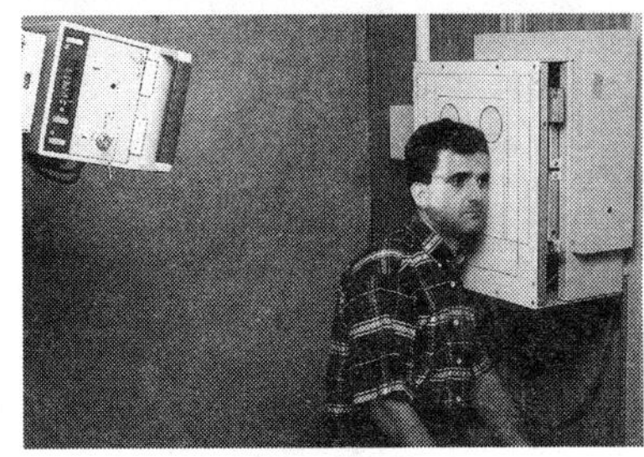

Evaluation Criteria

- The mastoid air cells of interest are located in the center of the film without superimposition of the opposite side.
- The internal and external meatuses are superimposed.
- The TMJ is located anterior to the mastoid air cells.
- The auricle of the ear should not superimpose the mastoid air cells.

Exam Rationale This position demonstrates the mastoid air cells and the internal auditory canal of the side closest to the film. Both sides should be done for comparison.

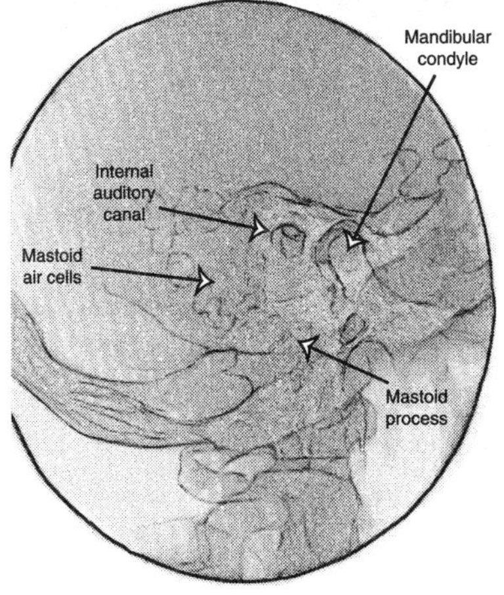

Technical Considerations

- Regular screen/film
- Grid
- kVp range: 70–80
- SID: 40 inch (100 cm)

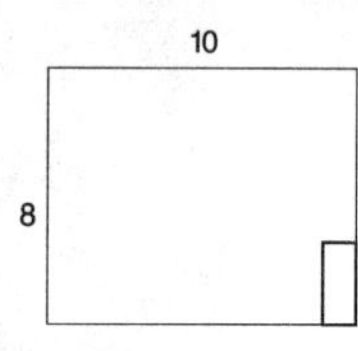

Radiation Protection

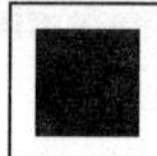

AEC (Phototiming)

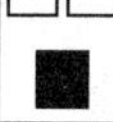

Patient Position Facing the film; all potential artifacts removed.

Part Position Rest the patient's head on the forehead, nose, and zygoma; center the film 1 inch (3 cm) anterior to the external auditory canal closest to the film; IOML is parallel to the transverse axis of the film; MSP forms an angle of 45° to the film.

Central Ray 12° cephalad entering approximately 2 inches (5 cm) posterior to the uppermost EAM.

Breathing Instructions Suspend respiration.

Evaluation Criteria

- The petrous ridge and mastoid process of the side of interest is included.

Example Exposure Techniques **Measure at CR and Use Chart (p.278)**									
Room	**cm**	**kVp**	**mAs**	**mA**	**Sec**	**Beam**	**Film**	**Grid**	**1Ø3Ø**
	16								
	17								
	18								
	19								
	20								
	21								
	22								
	23								
	24								
	25								

- The internal auditory canal and bony labyrinths are demonstrated below the petrous ridge.
- The mandibular ramus and condyle are superimposed on the cervical spine.

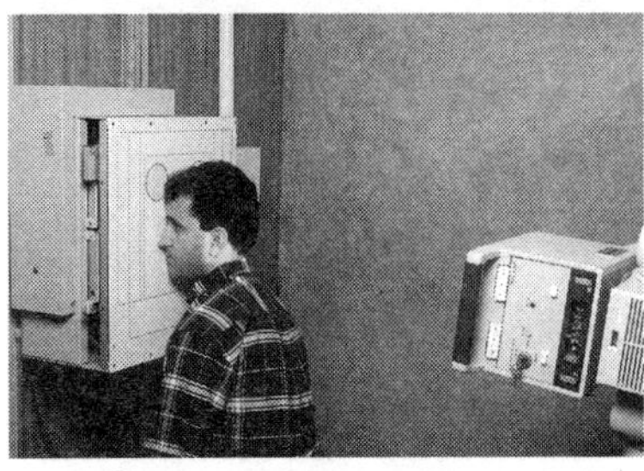

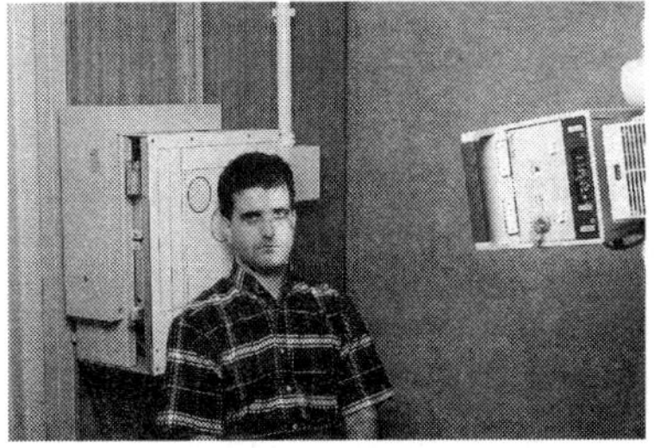

Exam Rationale This position demonstrates the dependent petrous portion parallel to the film. The petrous ridge, the mastoid air cells, the tip of the mastoid, the mastoid antrum, the labyrinth, and the internal auditory canal are visualized. Both sides should be done for comparison.

Tip For patients who cannot be placed in a prone position, the anterior profile (Arcelin method) can be used. Center the MSP to the midpoint of the film; rotate the head 45° away from the side of interest; place IOML perpendicular to the film; angle the central ray 10° caudal, entering approximately 1 inch (3 cm) anterior and slightly above the uppermost EAM.

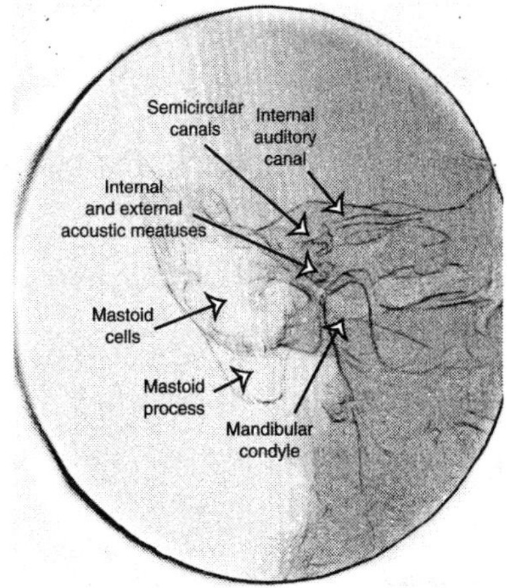

Technical Considerations
- Regular screen/film
- Grid
- kVp range: 70–80
- SID: 40 inch (100 cm)

8

10

Radiation Protection

AEC (Phototiming)

N DENSITY

Patient Position Facing the tube; all potential artifacts removed.

Part Position With the back of the patient's head against the cassette holder, rotate the head 45° toward the side of interest; the chin is depressed to place the IOML parallel to the transverse axis of the film.

Central Ray 45° caudal exiting through the EAM of interest.

Breathing Instructions Suspend respiration.

Evaluation Criteria
- The mastoid air cells of the side of interest are located in the center of the film.
- The external auditory meatus is demonstrated anterior to the petrosa.
- The TMJ is anterior to the EAM.

Example Exposure Techniques
Measure at CR and Use Chart (p.278)

Room	cm	kVp	mAs	mA	Sec	Beam	Film	Grid	1Ø3Ø
	16								
	17								
	18								
	19								
	20								
	21								
	22								
	23								
	24								
	25								

Exam Rationale An axial oblique position of the mastoid air cells is demonstrated. The external auditory meatus, the mastoid antrum, and bony labyrinth are visualized. Both sides should be done for comparison.

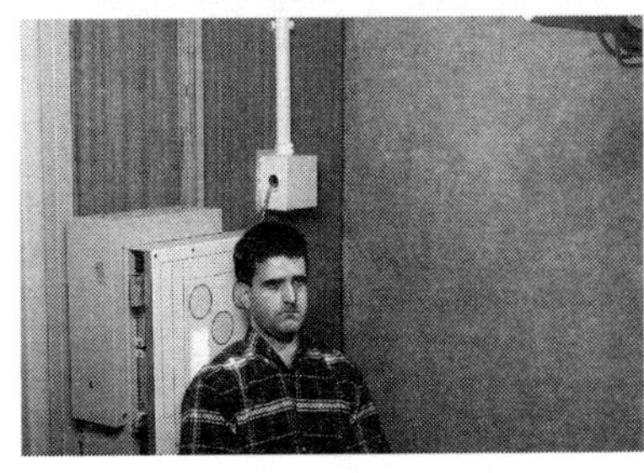

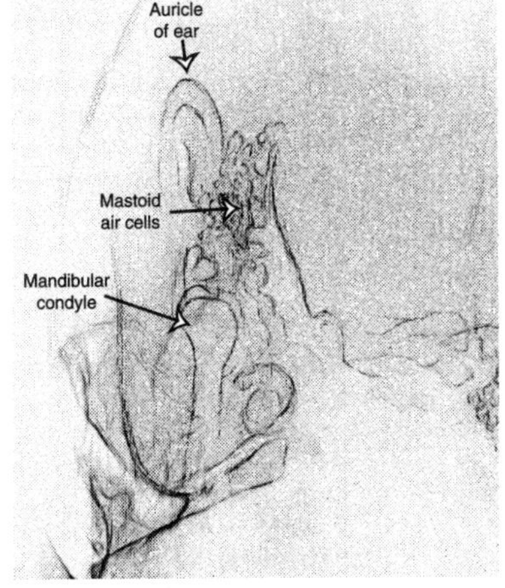

Technical Considerations
- Regular screen/film
- Grid
- kVp range: 70–80
- SID: 40 inch (100 cm)

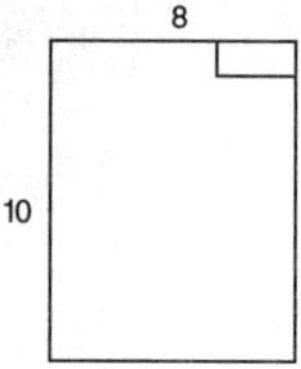

8

10

Radiation Protection

AEC (Phototiming)

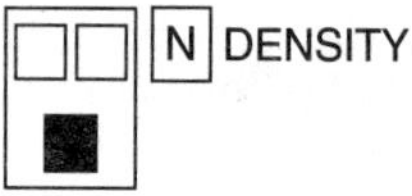

N DENSITY

Patient Position Facing the tube; all potential artifacts removed.

Part Position Patient's neck is extended until the head is resting on the vertex; cassette is centered to the level of the mandibular angles; IOML is parallel to the film.

Central Ray Perpendicular to IOML entering midway between the mandibular angles.

Breathing Instructions Suspend respiration.

Evaluation Criteria
- The mandibular condyles should be demonstrated anterior to the petrous ridges and the external auditory canals.

Example Exposure Techniques **Measure at CR and Use Chart (p.278)**									
Room	**cm**	**kVp**	**mAs**	**mA**	**Sec**	**Beam**	**Film**	**Grid**	**1Ø3Ø**
	16								
	17								
	18								
	19								
	20								
	21								
	22								
	23								
	24								
	25								

- The distance from the lateral border of the mandibular condyle to the lateral border of the cranium should be equal on both sides demonstrating no rotation.
- The petrosa should be symmetrical.

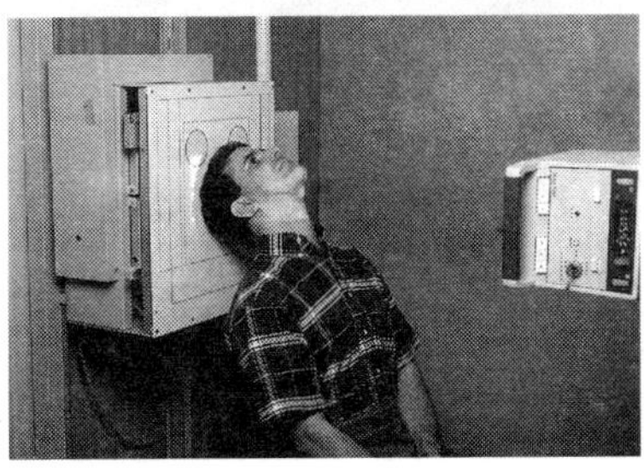

Exam Rationale This projection demonstrates symmetrical petrosa, the auditory canals, the mastoid processes, the labyrinths, and the tympanic cavities.

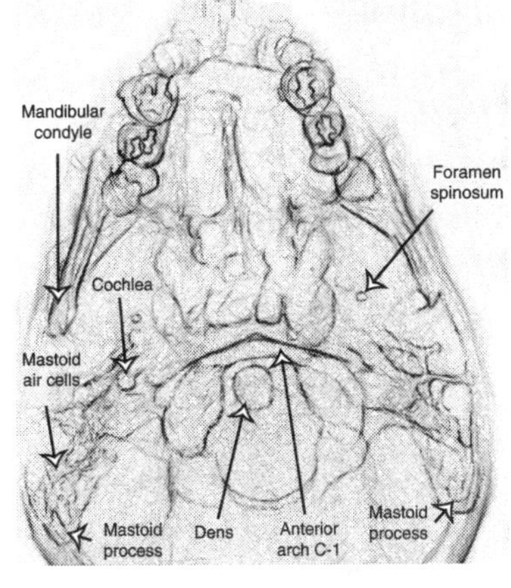

Technical Considerations
- Regular screen/film
- Grid
- kVp range: 70–80
- SID: 40 inch (100 cm)

8

10

Radiation Protection

AEC (Phototiming)

N DENSITY

Patient Position Facing the tube; all potential artifacts removed.

Part Position MSP is perpendicular to the midpoint of the film; IOML is perpendicular to the film; center the cassette to coincide with the central ray.

Central Ray 30° caudal if the anterior clinoids are of interest or 37° caudal if the dorsum sella and posterior clinoids are of interest. The central ray should exit through the foramen magnum.

Breathing Instructions Suspend respiration.

Example Exposure Techniques **Measure at CR and Use Chart (p.278)**									
Room	cm	kVp	mAs	mA	Sec	Beam	Film	Grid	1Ø3Ø
	16								
	17								
	18								
	19								
	20								
	21								
	22								
	23								
	24								
	25								

Evaluation Criteria

- No rotation as evidenced by symmetrical petrous ridges.
- 30° caudal angle:
  —The dorsum sella and anterior clinoids are projected through the occipital bone and are visualized above the foramen magnum.
- 37° caudal angle:
  —The dorsum sella and posterior clinoids are projected through the foramen magnum.

Exam Rationale This projection demonstrates the dorsum sella, anterior and posterior clinoids, the petrous pyramids, and the foramen magnum.

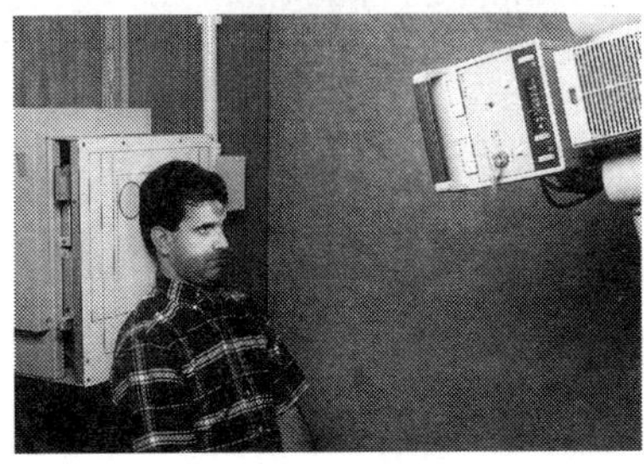

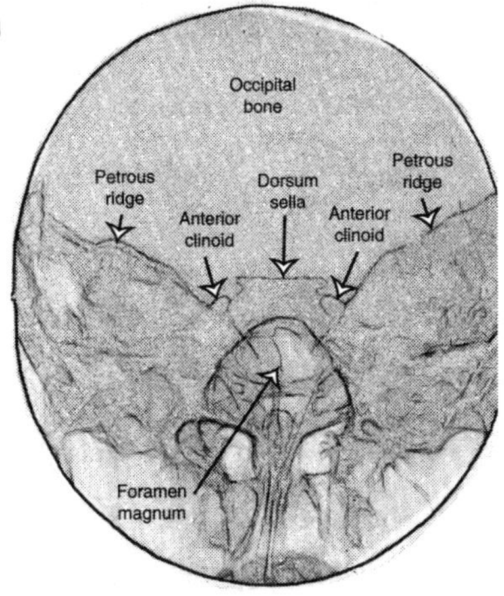

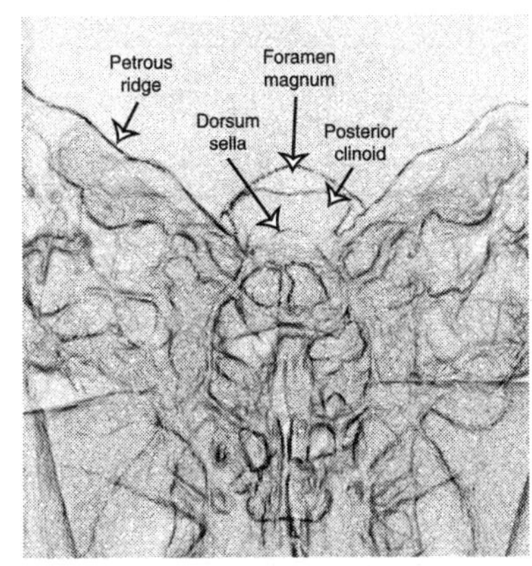

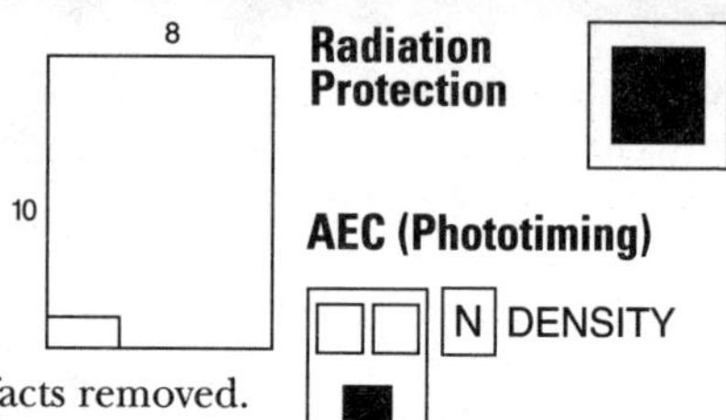

Technical Considerations

- Regular screen/film
- Grid
- kVp range: 70–80
- SID: 40 inch (100 cm)

Patient Position In lateral position; all potential artifacts removed.

Part Position Cassette is centered to a point 3/4 inch (2 cm) anterior and 3/4 inch (2 cm) superior to the EAM; MSP is parallel to the film; interpupillary line is perpendicular to the film; IOML is parallel to the transverse axis of the film.

Central Ray Perpendicular to the film entering 3/4 inch (2 cm) anterior to and 3/4 inch (2 cm) superior to the EAM.

Breathing Instructions Suspend respiration.

Evaluation Criteria

- The sella turcica is centered to the film.
- No rotation is visualized as evidenced by superimposition of the anterior clinoids and of the posterior clinoids.
- Sella turcica is seen in profile.

Example Exposure Techniques
Measure at CR and Use Chart (p.278)

Room	cm	kVp	mAs	mA	Sec	Beam	Film	Grid	1Ø3Ø
	11								
	12								
	13								
	14								
	15								
	16								
	17								
	18								
	19								
	20								

Exam Rationale This position demonstrates a lateral view of the sella turcica, the anterior and posterior clinoids, the dorsum sella, and the clivus.

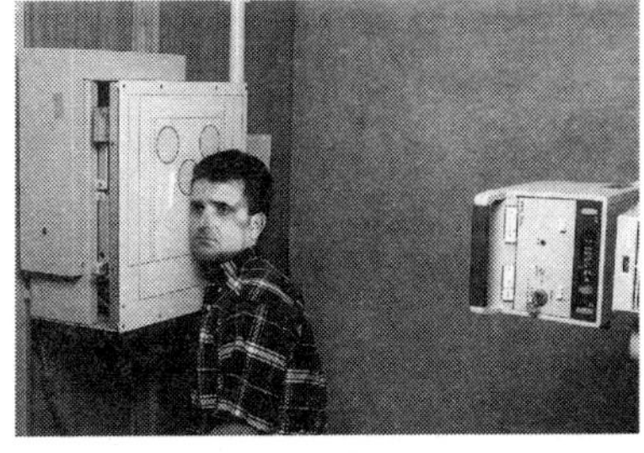

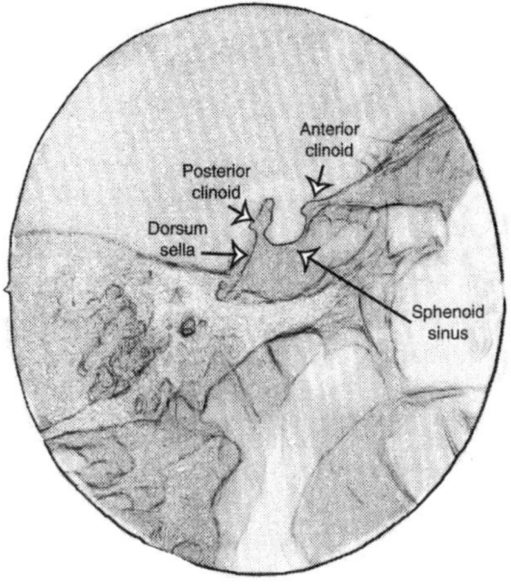

Technical Considerations

- Regular screen/film
- Grid
- kVp range: 70–80
- SID: 40 inch (100 cm)

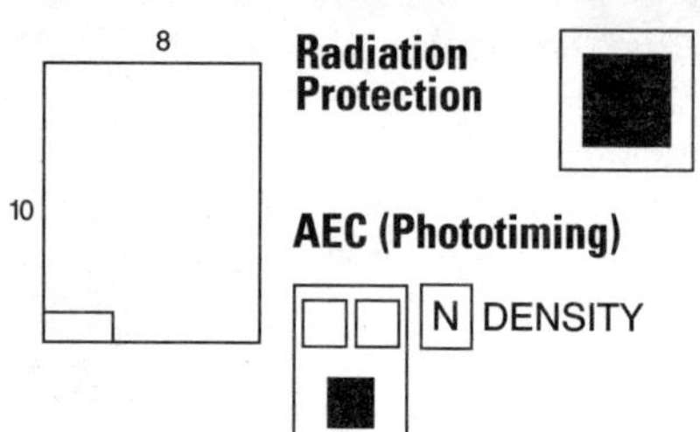

Patient Position Facing the film; all potential artifacts removed.

Part Position Patient's forehead and nose rest against the cassette holder; cassette is centered 1 inch (3 cm) superior to the superciliary arch; MSP is perpendicular to the midline of the film; OML is perpendicular to the film.

Central Ray 25° cephalic entering 1 1/2 inch (4 cm) inferior to the inion.

Breathing Instructions Suspend respiration.

Evaluation Criteria

- The dorsum sellae and the posterior clinoids should be demonstrated within the shadow of the foramen magnum.
- No rotation should be demonstrated.
- Symmetrical petrous pyramids are visualized.

Example Exposure Techniques **Measure at CR and Use Chart (p.278)**									
Room	cm	kVp	mAs	mA	Sec	Beam	Film	Grid	1Ø3Ø
	16								
	17								
	18								
	19								
	20								
	21								
	22								
	23								
	24								
	25								

Exam Rationale This is an alternate projection for demonstrating the dorsum sella, posterior clinoids, foramen magnum, and petrous ridges.

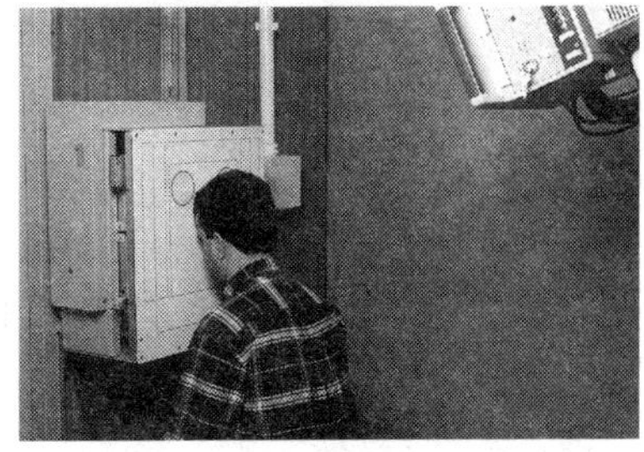

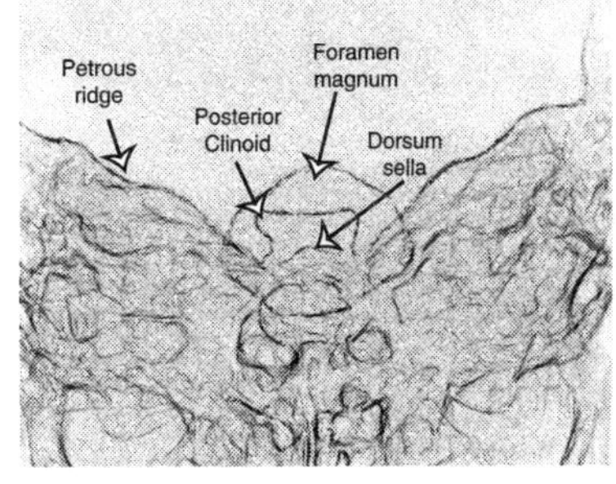

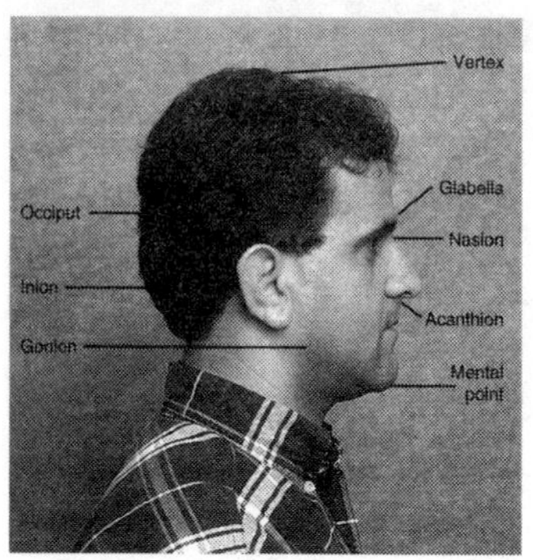

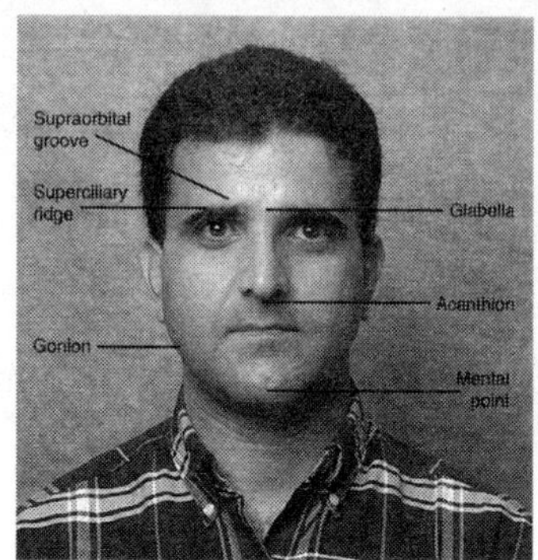

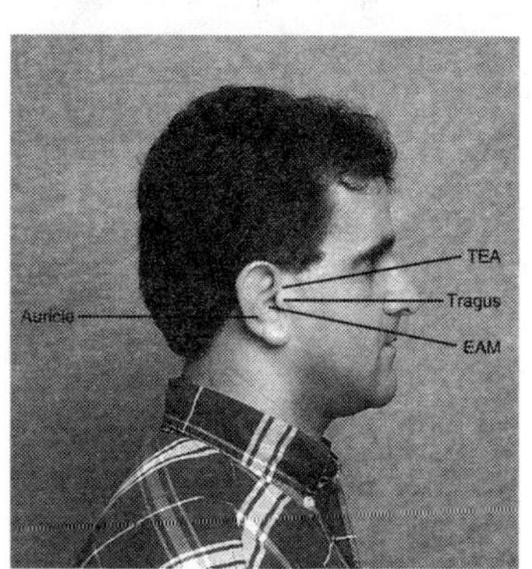

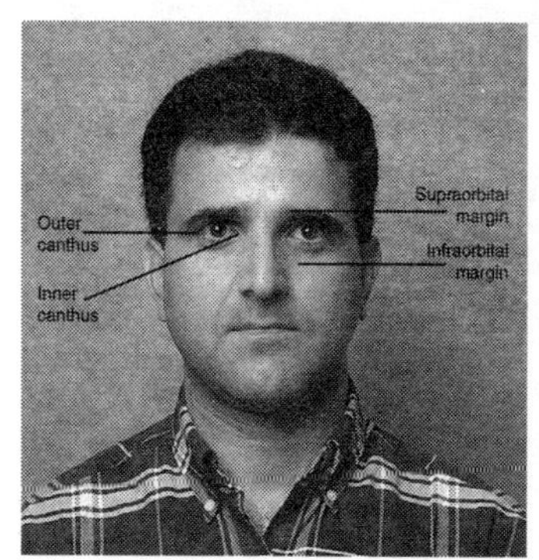

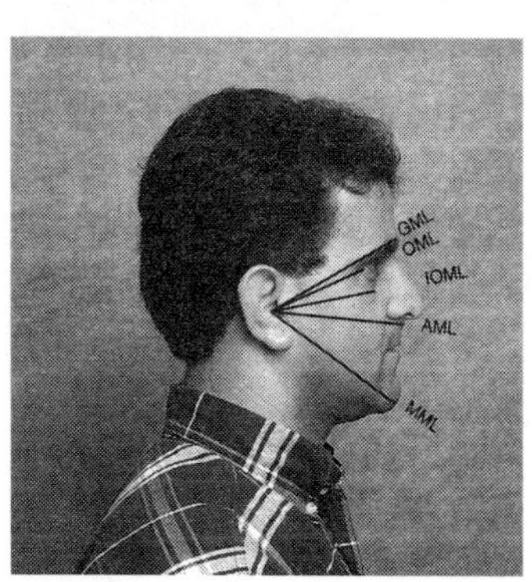

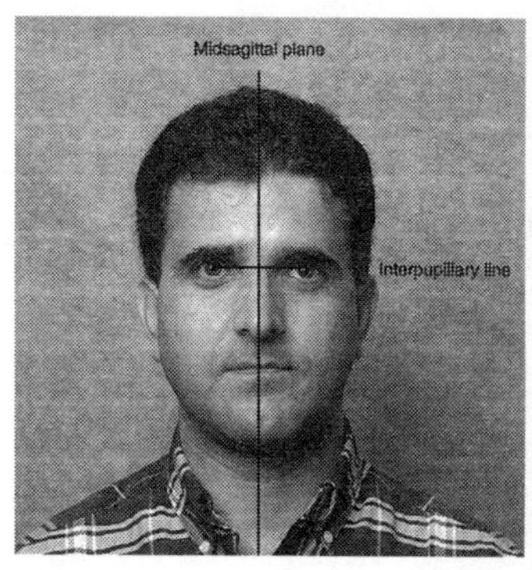

For further information refer to Appendix D.

ALTERNATIVE POSITIONS/PROJECTIONS

Part	Alternative	Page
Skull (trauma)	AP	352
	Axial AP (Grashey/Townes)	354
	Lateral	356

Fundamental Principles Always, if there is any concern about cervical spine injury, trauma skull films should not be attempted until a lateral cervical spine radiograph has been completed and interpreted by a physician.

When performing trauma radiography, two basic principles should be kept in mind. First, it is important to obtain two views 90° apart. For most situations this will include an AP and lateral. If true AP and lateral projections cannot be obtained, then two projections as close to 90° apart should be attempted.

The second principle concerns the alignment between the central ray, the part being radiographed, and the film. As with routine skull radiography, the relationship between these three variables must be maintained. The radiographer must be creative in adjusting the standard routines to maintain these relationships.

Technical Considerations

- Regular screen/film
- Grid
- kVp range: 70–80
- SID: 40 inch (100 cm)

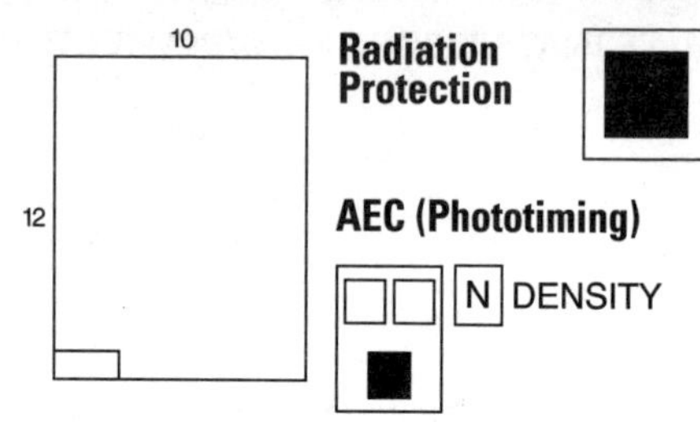

Patient Position

Supine on stretcher or table.

Part Position With minimal movement of the patient, place the cassette under the patient's head or in the table Bucky to position the top of the cassette slightly above the top of the patient's head and perpendicular to the MSP; adjust the patient's head to place the OML perpendicular to the cassette.

Central Ray Perpendicular to the film, entering at the nasion.

Breathing Instructions Suspend respiration.

Example Exposure Techniques
Measure at CR and Use Chart (p.278)

Room	cm	kVp	mAs	mA	Sec	Beam	Film	Grid	1Ø3Ø
	16								
	17								
	18								
	19								
	20								
	21								
	22								
	23								
	24								
	25								

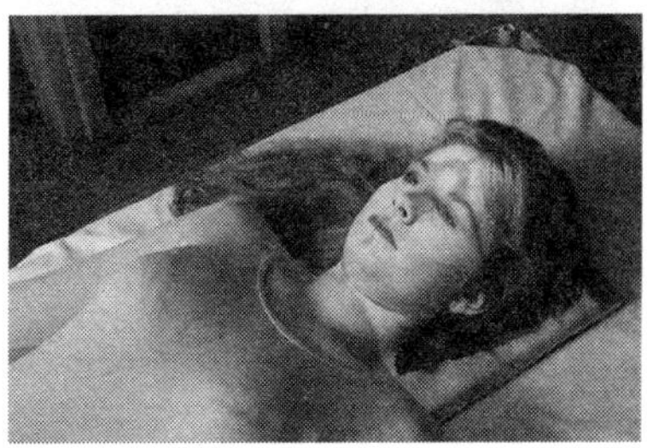

Evaluation Criteria

- Entire cranium is demonstrated.
- No rotation or tilt as evidenced by equal distance between lateral border of orbit and edge of skull on each side and equal distance between midpoint of cranium and edge of film on each side.
- Petrous ridges fill the orbits.
- Sufficient density to visualize the frontal bone.
- No motion.

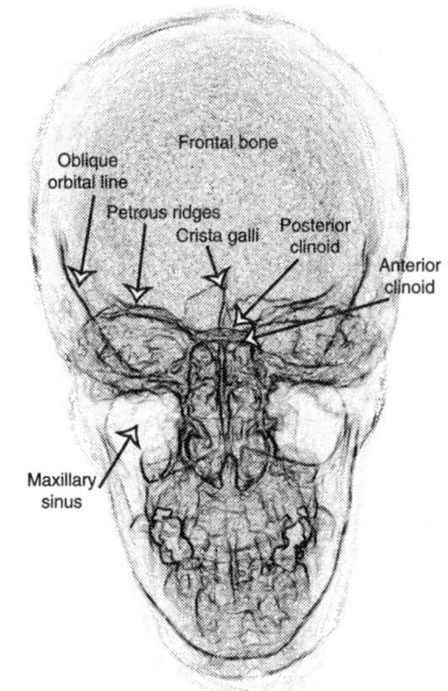

Exam Rationale This projection is used to evaluate the condition or status of the cranial bones in patients who have experienced trauma or are in unstable condition. Structures demonstrated are the frontal and parietal bones. It is comparable to a routine PA projection.

Tips

1. When the patient's condition will not allow movement of the head, angle the central ray until it is parallel to the OML.
2. Pediatric patients may require extension of the neck to place OML perpendicular to the cassette.

Technical Considerations

- Regular screen/film
- Grid
- kVp range: 70–80
- SID: 40 inch (100 cm)

Patient Position
Supine on stretcher or table.

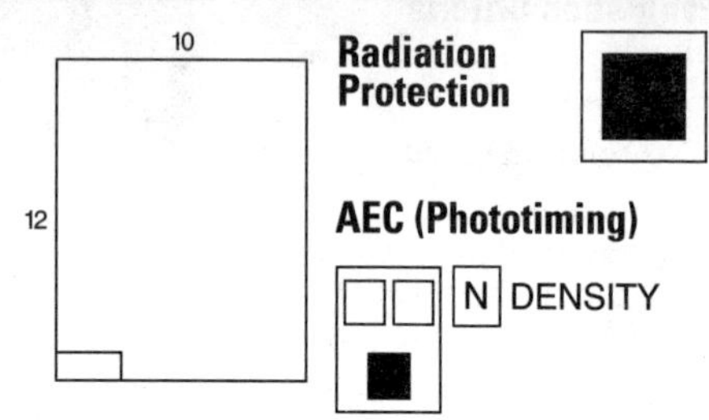

Part Position With minimal movement of the patient, place the cassette under the patient's head or in the table Bucky to place the top of the cassette at the top of the patient's head and perpendicular to the MSP; adjust the patient's head to place the OML perpendicular to the cassette.

Central Ray 30° caudad to enter the upper forehead and exit the foramen magnum.

Breathing Instructions Suspend respiration.

Example Exposure Techniques **Measure at CR and Use Chart (p.278)**									
Room	**cm**	**kVp**	**mAs**	**mA**	**Sec**	**Beam**	**Film**	**Grid**	**1Ø3Ø**
	16								
	17								
	18								
	19								
	20								
	21								
	22								
	23								
	24								
	25								

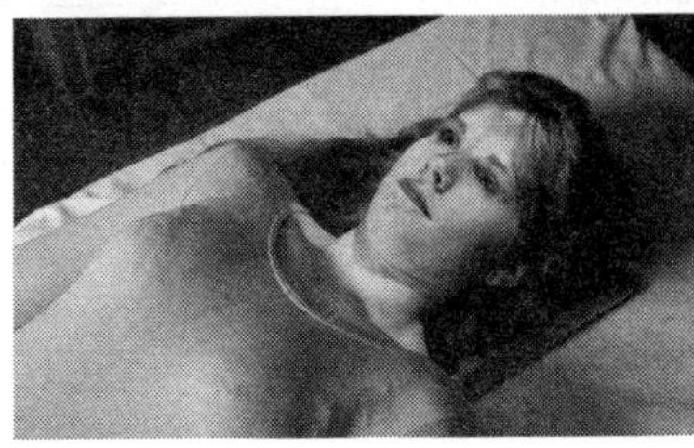

Evaluation Criteria

- Entire skull, including occipital and parietal bones, is demonstrated.
- No rotation or tilt as evidenced by equal distance between foramen magnum and edge of skull on each side, and equal distance between midpoint of cranium and edge of film on each side.
- Petrous ridges superior to mastoids.
- Dorsum sellae and posterior clinoid processes projected through shadow of foramen magnum.
- Sufficient density to visualize the occipital bone.
- No motion.

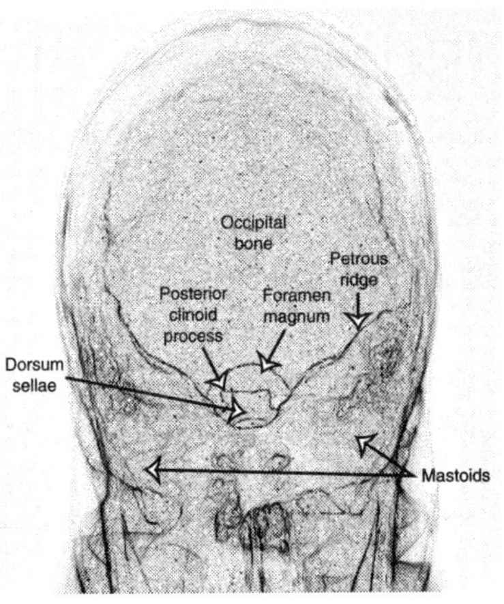

Exam Rationale This projection is used to evaluate the condition or status of the cranial bones in patients of unstable condition or who have experienced trauma. Structures demonstrated are the occipital bone, petrous ridges, and dorsum sellae and posterior clinoid processes projected within the shadow of the foramen magnum.

Tips

1. When the patient's condition will not allow movement of the head, increase the central ray angle (not to exceed 45°), to compensate for the angle between the OML and the vertical. For example, if the OML is angled 7° from the vertical (IOML perpendicular), increase the central ray angle to 37°, the angle between the OML and CR should always be 30°.
2. Pediatric patients may require extension of the neck to place OML perpendicular to the cassette.

Technical Considerations
- Regular screen/film
- Grid
- kVp range: 60–70
- SID: 40 inch (100 cm)

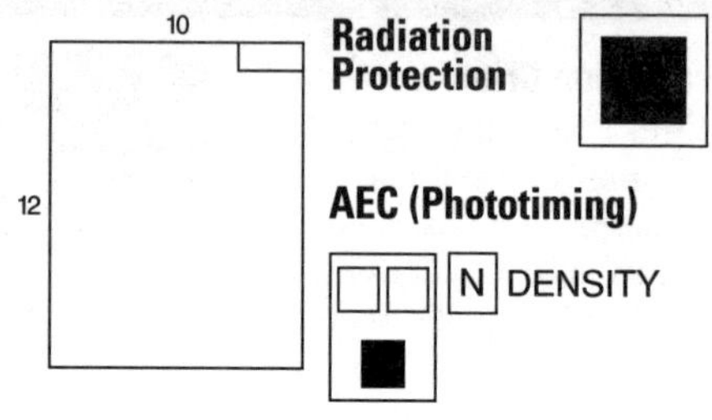

Patient Position Supine on stretcher or table.

Part Position With minimal movement of the patient, elevate the head on a radiolucent support; place the cassette vertical and in contact with the side of interest and parallel to the MSP; adjust the patient's head to place the interpupillary line perpendicular and IOML parallel to the cassette.

Central Ray Horizontal; perpendicular to cassette to enter 2 inches (5 cm) superior to the EAM.

Breathing Instructions Suspend respiration.

Evaluation Criteria
- Entire cranium is demonstrated.
- No rotation as evidenced by mandibular rami, orbital roofs, sphe-

Example Exposure Techniques **Measure at CR and Use Chart (p.278)**									
Room	**cm**	**kVp**	**mAs**	**mA**	**Sec**	**Beam**	**Film**	**Grid**	**1Ø3Ø**
	11								
	12								
	13								
	14								
	15								
	16								
	17								
	18								
	19								
	20								

noid wings, and external auditory canals superimposed.
- Sella turcica in profile without rotation.
- Sufficient density to visualize parietal bone.
- No motion.

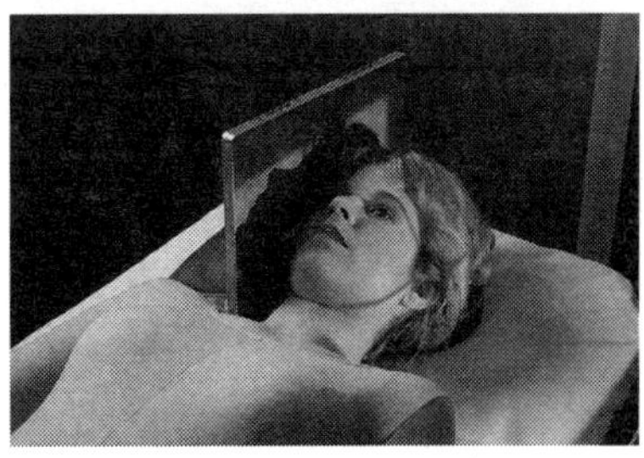

Exam Rationale This position is used to evaluate the condition or status of the cranial bones in patients who have experienced trauma or who are in unstable condition. The parietal bone closest to the cassette is best demonstrated.

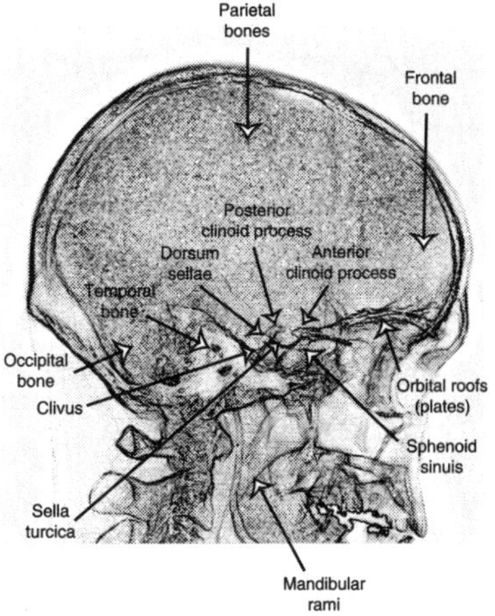

Tips

1. When the patient's condition will not allow the head to be elevated on a radiolucent sponge, place the bottom of the cassette slightly below the stretcher or table and occiput region. If this cannot be done, place the cassette vertical on stretcher or table and center the central ray 2 inches (5 cm) superior to and slightly posterior to EAM, open collimation to include the entire cranium. This off-centering will allow for the divergent beam to project the occipital region onto the film.
2. When doing only one lateral view, the side of the skull presenting the greatest injury should be radiographed.

UPPER GASTROINTESTINAL TRACT

ROUTINE AND ALTERNATIVE POSITIONS/PROJECTIONS

Part	Routine	Page	Alternative	Page
Esophagus	AP/PA	360		
	Lateral	362		
	Oblique	364		
			Lateral neck	366
Stomach	PA/AP	368		
	Oblique	370		
	Lateral	372		
Small bowel	Ileocecal valve spot filming	374		

Patient Preparation Before beginning the radiographic procedure, the radiographer should obtain a brief medical history and ensure that appropriate preparation procedures were followed. The patient should remove all clothing except shoes and socks, and dress in a patient gown. The radiographer should explain all aspects of the procedure, including the expected length. This is particularly important in small-bowel studies, which can take several hours.

Technical Considerations

- Regular film/screen
- Bucky/grid
- kVp range: 75–85
- SID: 40 inch (100 cm)

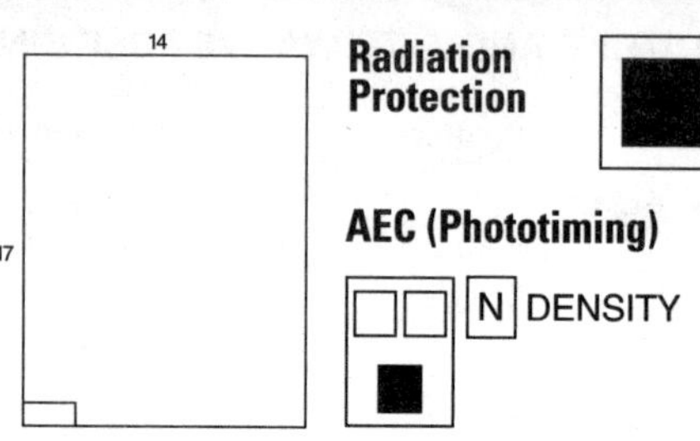

Patient Position

Back against the upright Bucky with the MSP parallel to the long axis of the film; no rotation of the shoulders or pelvis; head may be turned to the side to aid in swallowing of contrast during filming.

Central Ray Perpendicular to the film at the level of T-6.

Patient Instructions Have patient drink through the straw.

Evaluation Criteria

- Demonstrates the entire esophagus.
- No rotation of the body.
- Short scale of contrast to enhance visualization of the esophagus.

Example Exposure Techniques
Measure at CR and Use Chart (p.370)

Room	cm	kVp	mAs	mA	Sec	Beam	Film	Grid	1Ø3Ø
	14								
	16								
	18								
	20								
	22								
	24								
	26								
	28								
	30								
	32								

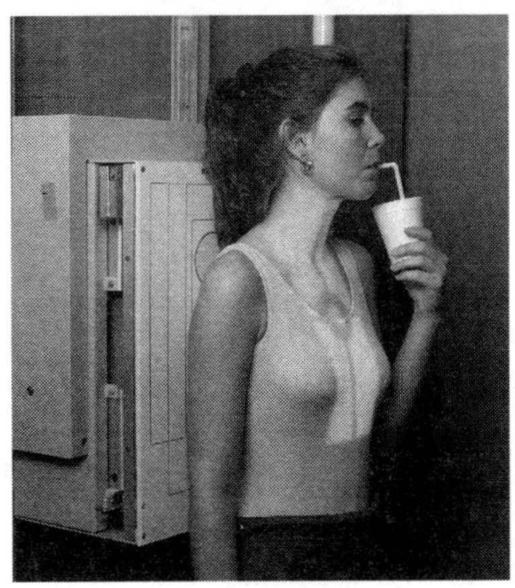

Exam Rationale The radiographic examination of the esophagus attempts to image the swallowing process and the route of transmission for ingested material to the stomach. Common clinical indications are dysphagia, mediastinal pain, esophageal reflux, dyspepsia, dysphonia, a feeling of stricture or not being able to clear one's throat, and obstruction of food.

Tips

1. To ensure a contrast-filled esophagus, instructions to the patient must be very clear. Take time for explanation and check the patient's comprehension.
2. The PA projection may be used and gives similar results.
3. This may also be done in the recumbent position.

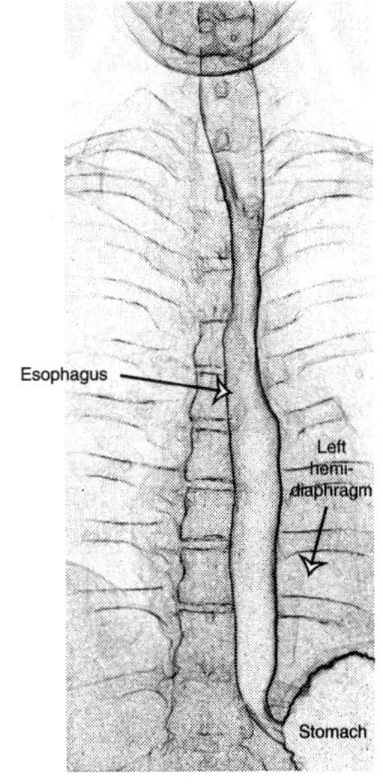

Technical Considerations

- Regular film/screen
- Bucky/grid
- kVp range: 80–90
- SID: 40 inch (100 cm)

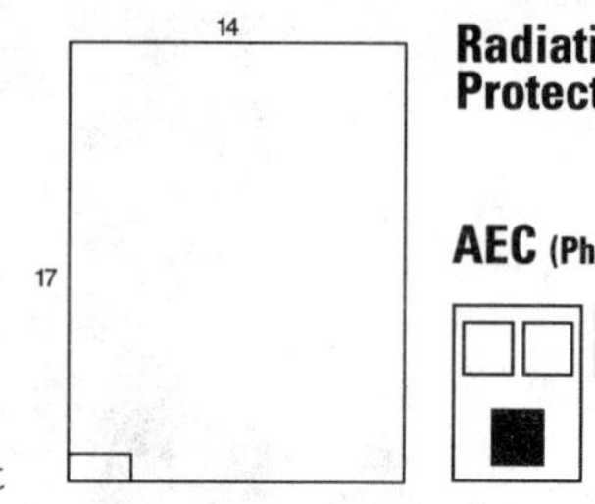

Radiation Protection

AEC (Phototiming)

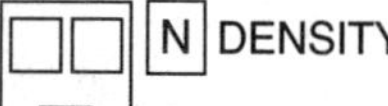

Patient Position Left lateral with the arms up and out of the way of the chest.

Central Ray Perpendicular to the film at the level of T6 and 1 inch (3 cm) anterior to the midcoronal plane.

Patient Instructions Have patient drink through the straw.

Evaluation Criteria

- Should demonstrate entire esophagus filled with contrast.
- Little or no rotation of the thoracic cavity.
- Arms should not superimpose the esophagus.
- Short scale of contrast to enhance visualization of esophagus.

Example Exposure Techniques **Measure at CR and Use Chart (p.370)**									
Room	**cm**	**kVp**	**mAs**	**mA**	**Sec**	**Beam**	**Film**	**Grid**	**1Ø3Ø**
	20								
	22								
	24								
	26								
	28								
	30								
	32								
	34								
	36								
	38								

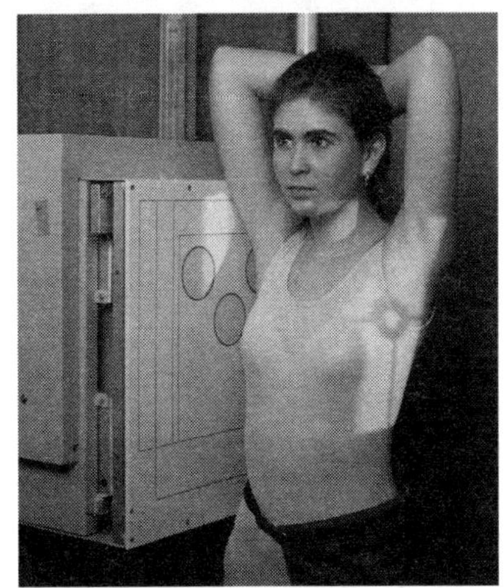

Exam Rationale This position demontrates the esophagus free from superimposition of the thoracic spine and heart. The left lateral is usually done.

Tips

1. To ensure a contrast-filled esophagus, instructions to the patient must be very clear. Take time for explanation and check the patient's comprehension.
2. This may also be done in the recumbent position.

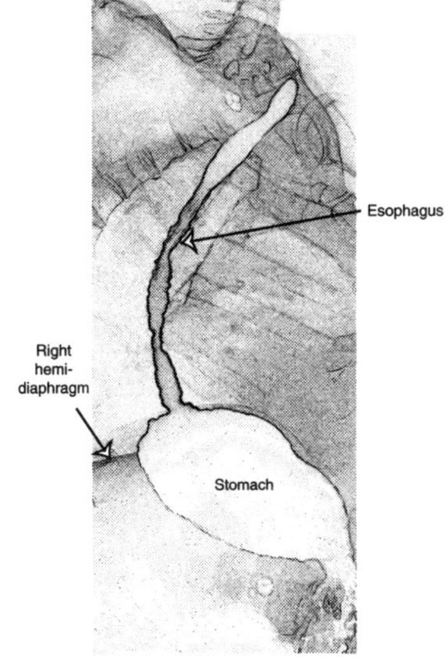

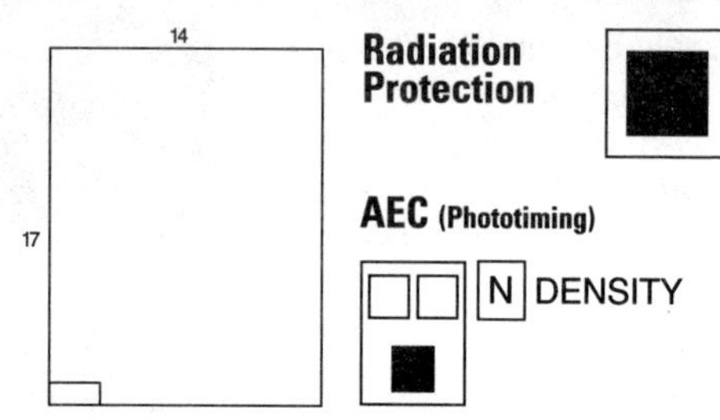

Technical Considerations

- Regular film/screen
- Bucky/grid
- kVp range: 80–90
- SID: 40 inch (100 cm)

Patient Position

RAO (approximately 40°) with the right arm down by the body and the left arm up by the elevated shoulder; MSP 2 inches (5 cm) to left of spinous processes is centered to the midline of the upright Bucky.

Central Ray Two to 3 inches (5–8 cm) lateral to the MSP at the level of T6.

Patient Instructions Have patient drink through the straw.

Evaluation Criteria

- Entire contrast-filled esophagus should be visible and demonstrated between the thoracic spine and the heart for the RAO.
- Hips and shoulders should be in the same plane.
- Short scale of contrast to enhance visualization of the esophagus.

Example Exposure Techniques **Measure at CR and Use Chart (p.370)**									
Room	**cm**	**kVp**	**mAs**	**mA**	**Sec**	**Beam**	**Film**	**Grid**	**1Ø3Ø**
	20								
	22								
	24								
	26								
	28								
	30								
	32								
	34								
	36								
	38								

Exam Rationale The oblique positions demonstrate the esophagus between the vertebrae and heart. One or both obliques may be done.

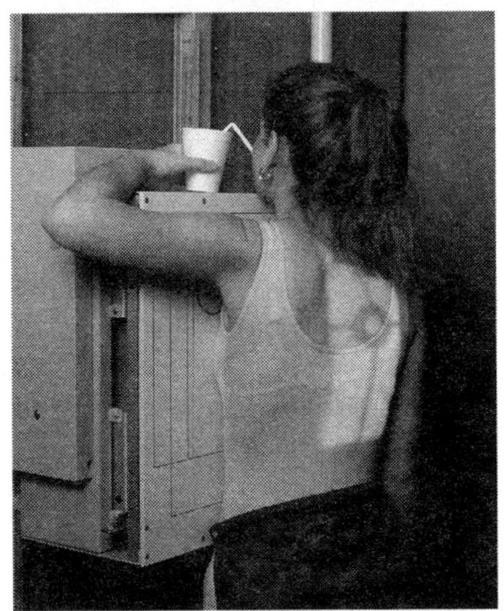

Tips

1. An LPO will produce a comparable image and may be indicated by department protocol or patient condition.
2. An angle sponge may be used to obtain proper obliquity and patient cooperation when this is done in the recumbent position.

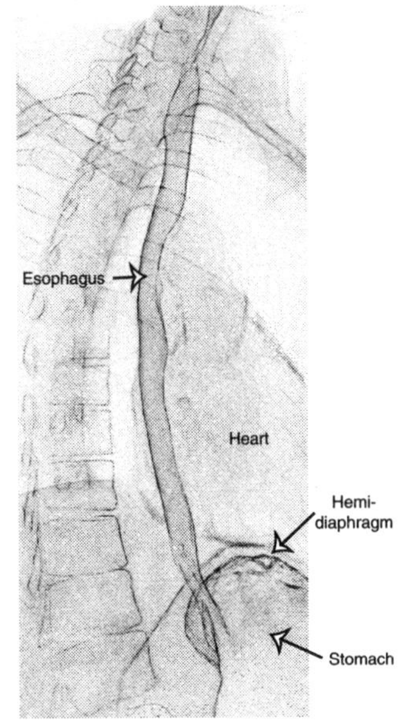

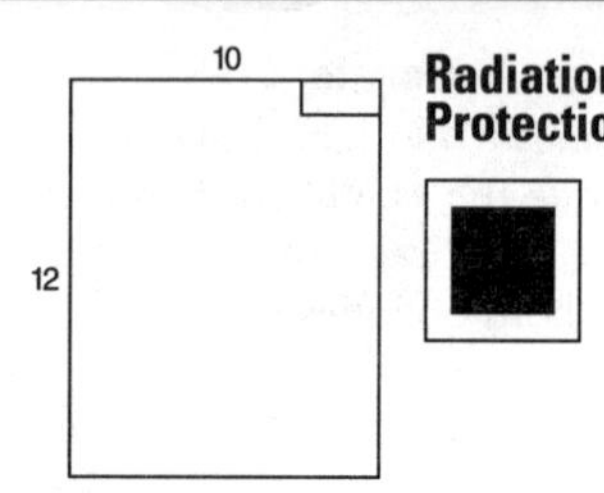

Technical Considerations

- Regular film/screen
- Bucky/grid
- kVp range: 60–65
- SID: 40 inch (100 cm)

Patient Position Erect in the left lateral position; chin is slightly extended; midsagittal and interpupillary lines are perpendicular to the film; midcoronal plane is centered to the midline of the film.

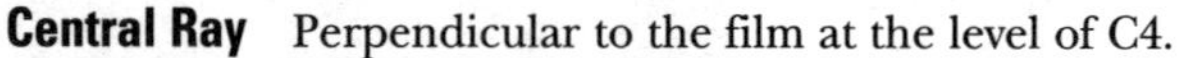

Central Ray Perpendicular to the film at the level of C4.

Patient Instructions Have patient close mouth and breathe through nose. Suspend on inspiration.

Evaluation Criteria

- Sides of the mandible superimposed.
- Limited or no rotation.
- Soft tissues demonstrated.

Example Exposure Techniques **Measure at CR and Use Chart (p.370)**									
Room	**cm**	**kVp**	**mAs**	**mA**	**Sec**	**Beam**	**Film**	**Grid**	**1Ø3Ø**
	9								
	10								
	11								
	12								
	13								
	14								
	15								
	16								
	17								
	18								

Exam Rationale This position demonstrates the pharynx and upper esophagus and may be done to visualize opaque foreign bodies, lesions, or calcifications.

Tip This may also be done with the patient in a left lateral recumbent position.

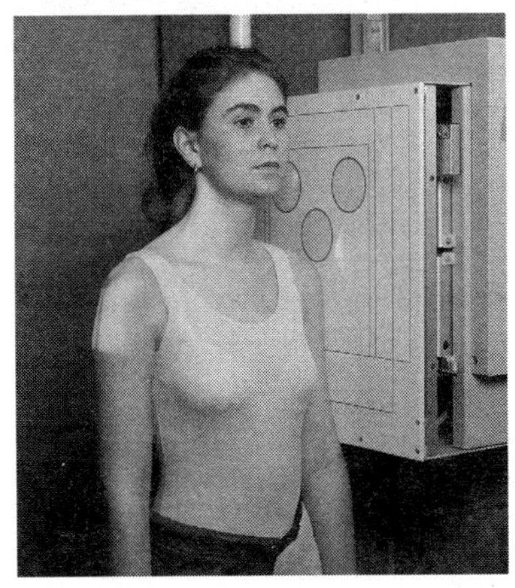

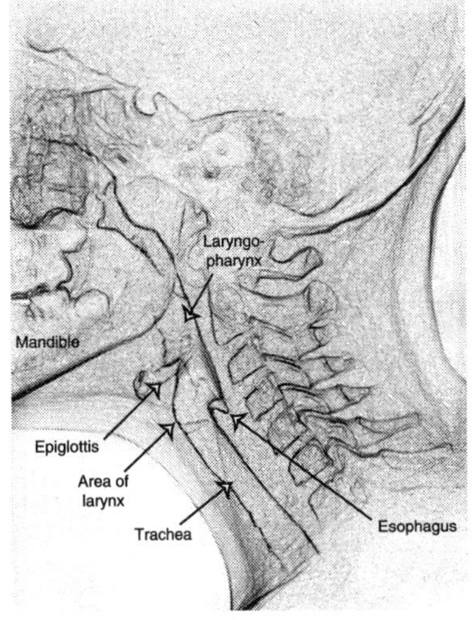

Technical Considerations

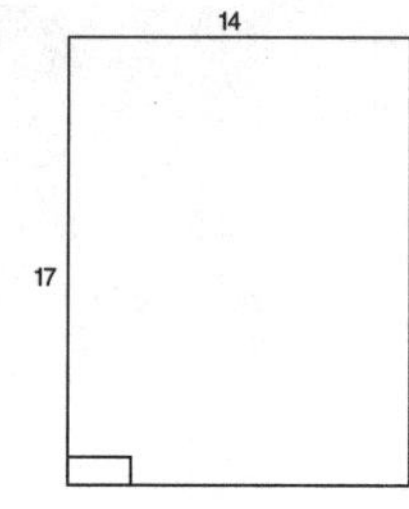

- Regular film/screen
- Bucky/grid
- kVp range: preliminary—70–75; opacified—90–95
- SID: 40 inch (100 cm)

Radiation Protection

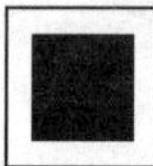

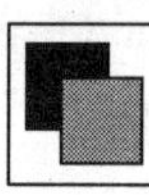

Yes if protocol allows; most protocols require visualization of the entire abdomen.

AEC (Phototiming)

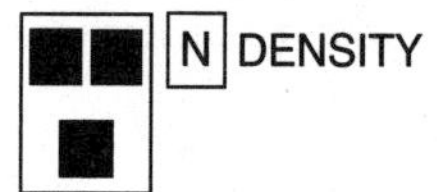

Patient Position Supine with the MSP parallel to the long axis of the table.

Central Ray Perpendicular to the film with the central ray entering the patient on the midline at the level of L1.

Breathing Instructions Suspend on expiration.

Evaluation Criteria

- Spine straight.
- No rotation of iliac crests or rib cage.
- Diaphragm elevated to demonstrate gastric area.
- Centered to body to demonstrate gastric area.

Example Exposure Techniques
Measure at CR and Use Chart (p.370)

Room	cm	kVp	mAs	mA	Sec	Beam	Film	Grid	1Ø3Ø
	10								
	14								
	18								
	22								
	26								
	30								
	34								
	38								
	42								
	46								

- No abdominal or respiratory motion.
- Barium will appear in the fundus and upper body, air in the lower body, pylorus, and duodenum.

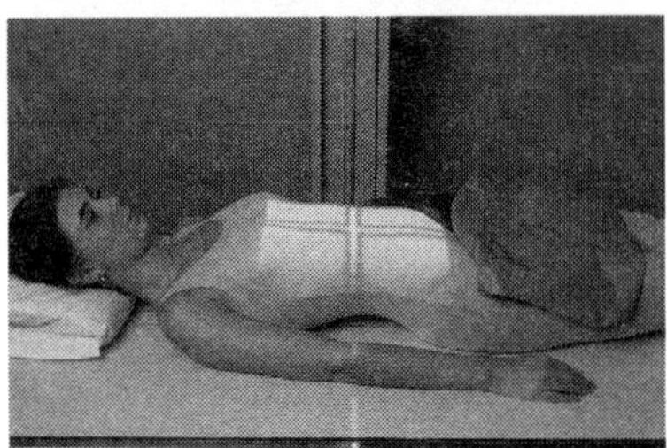

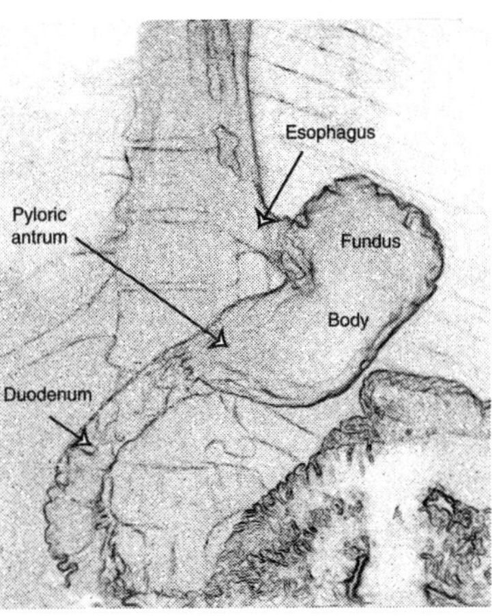

Exam Rationale This projection can be used as a preliminary film to overview the area and check for adequate preparation or, after administration of contrast, to demonstrate the entire stomach and the duodenal loop.

Tips

1. This may be done PA; this would show barium in the lower body, pylorus, and duodenum with air in the fundus and upper body of stomach.
2. For extremely large patients, two 14 × 17 (36 × 43 cm) crosswise films may be used and centered to include anatomy from the axilla to the symphysis pubis.
3. A sponge may be placed under the knees to lessen back strain and place the back in contact with the table.
4. This may be done erect.
5. By observing the location of anatomic structures during the fluoro procedure, the radiographer can gain insight into the location of the stomach relative to other landmarks.

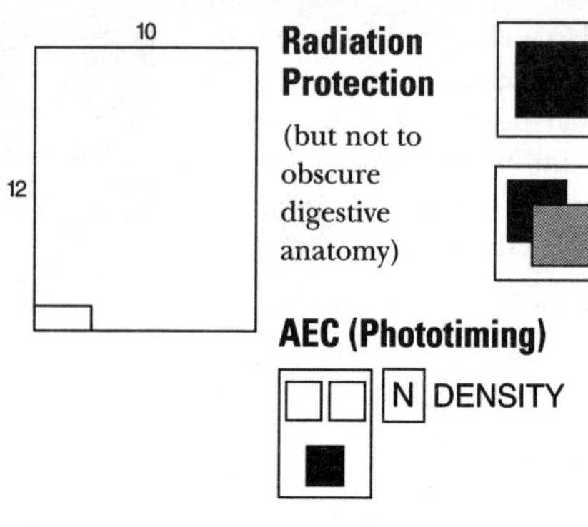

Technical Considerations
Note: Due to body habitus and the position of the stomach, filming may also use 10 × 12 crosswise (25 × 30 cm) or 11 × 14 (28 × 36 cm) lengthwise or crosswise film sizes.

- Regular film/screen
- Bucky/grid
- kVp range: 90–95
- SID: 40 inch (100 cm)

Patient Position RAO—rotated approximately 45°.

Central Ray RAO—perpendicular to the film at the level of ASIS on the left side (side up) of the patient at a point midway between the vertebral column and the lateral border of the body.

Breathing Instructions Suspend on expiration.

Example Exposure Techniques **Measure at CR and Use this Chart**									
Room	**cm**	**kVp**	**mAs**	**mA**	**Sec**	**Beam**	**Film**	**Grid**	**1Ø3Ø**
	12								
	16								
	20								
	24								
	28								
	32								
	36								
	40								
	44								
	48								

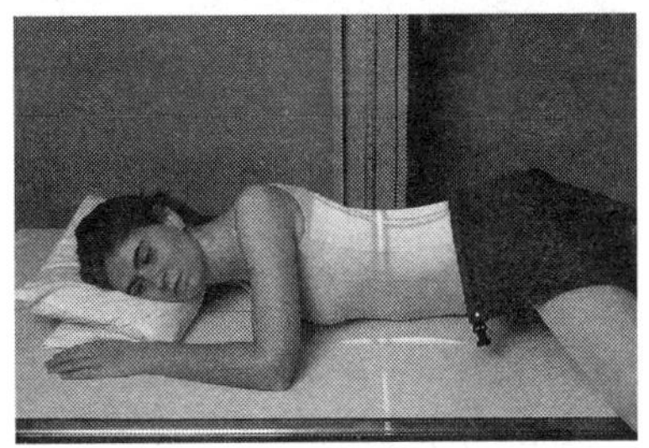

Evaluation Criteria

- Entire stomach is visualized; fundus is well seen.
- Duodenal bulb is shown without superimposition of the pylorus.
- Duodenal loop is shown in profile.
- Contrast is adequately penetrated.
- Air is in the fundus and barium is in the body, pylorus, and duodenum.

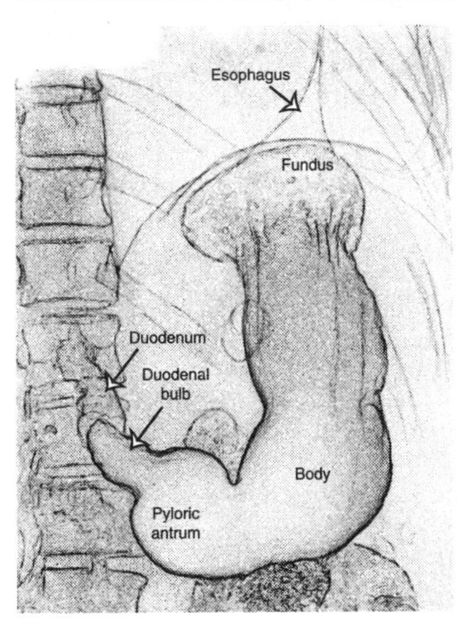

Exam Rationale The obliques are performed to demonstrate the stomach, especially the fundus and the duodenal loop. The duodenal bulb is also projected free of superimposition of the pylorus.

Tips

1. An LPO will demonstrate the same anatomy and may be indicated by patient condition.
2. Obliquity can vary from 30° to 60°, with thinner patients requiring less rotation.
3. Sponges may be used to achieve correct positioning angles.

Technical Considerations

Note: Due to body habitus and the position of the stomach, filming may also use 10 × 12 (25 × 30 cm) crosswise or 11 × 14 (28 × 36 cm) lengthwise or crosswise film sizes.

- Regular film/screen
- Bucky/grid
- kVp range: 90–95
- SID: 40 inch (100 cm)

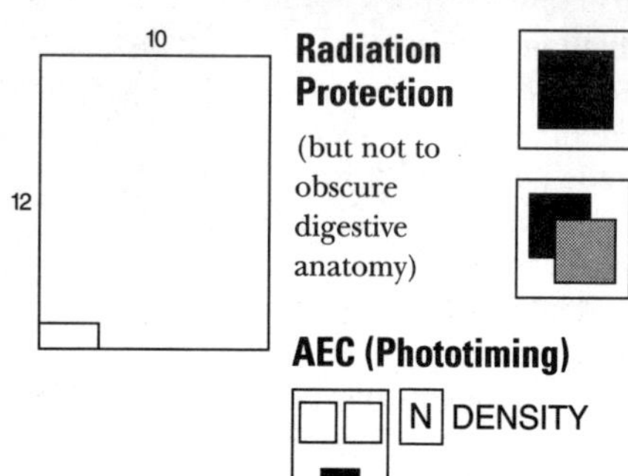

Radiation Protection

(but not to obscure digestive anatomy)

AEC (Phototiming)

Patient Position Right lateral recumbent; for average patients center at a point midway between the midcoronal plane and the anterior surface of the body to the midline of the table.

Central Ray Perpendicular at a point midway between the midcoronal plane and the anterior surface of the body to the center of the film.

Breathing Instructions Suspend on expiration.

Example Exposure Techniques **Measure at CR and Use Chart (p.370)**									
Room	**cm**	**kVp**	**mAs**	**mA**	**Sec**	**Beam**	**Film**	**Grid**	**1Ø3Ø**
	26								
	28								
	30								
	32								
	34								
	36								
	38								
	40								
	42								
	44								

Evaluation Criteria

- Patient is in a true lateral position, no rotation.
- Visualization of the entire stomach and the duodenal loop.
- Contrast is adequately penetrated.

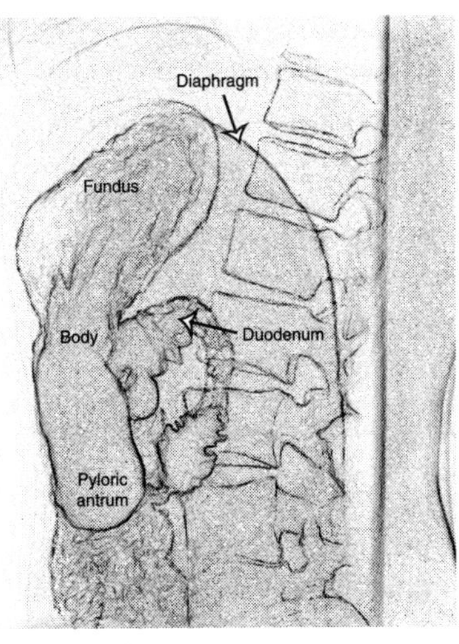

Exam Rationale The right lateral affords a look at the anterior and posterior aspects of the stomach as well as an unobstructed view of the pylorus, duodenal bulb, and loop. Visualization of the duodenal loop is essential due to the anatomic location of the head of the pancreas nestled in the C-shaped loop and the joining of the second segment of the small intestine, the jejunum.

Tips

1. Placing small sponges between the knees and elbows of the patient may create more stable positioning and less opportunity for movement. Some very thin patients may also benefit from a small sponge placed under the right iliac crest.
2. For larger patients, watching the fluoroscopy monitor to locate the stomach in relation to a landmark (vertebral level, ribs, etc.) will be helpful in positioning the patient for overhead films.

Technical Considerations
(for fluoroscopic spot filming)

- Regular film/screen
- Bucky/grid
- kVp range: 90–95
- Fluoroscopic kVp: 80
- SID: 40 inch (100 cm) unless fluoroscopic spot filming

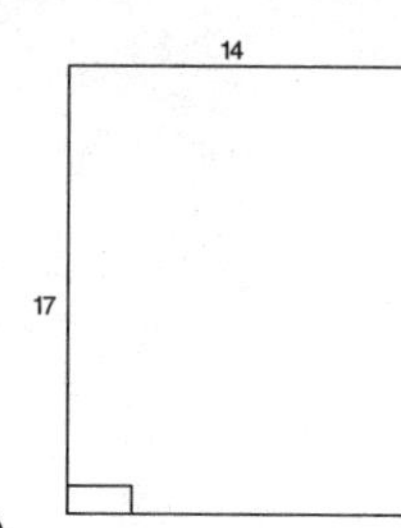

Radiation Protection
(if small bowel anatomy is not obscured)

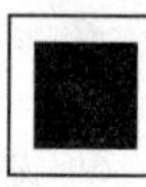

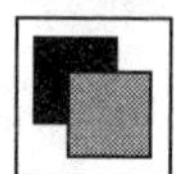

AEC (Phototiming)

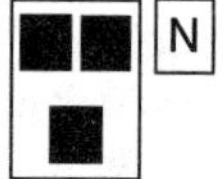

N DENSITY

Patient Position Prone with the MSP centered to the table. A small sponge or paddle device is placed under the patient, in the lower right quadrant, at approximately the lower level of the sacroiliac joint.

Central Ray Perpendicular to the film centered at the level of the iliac crests on the MSP.

Breathing Instructions Suspend on expiration.

Example Exposure Techniques **Measure at CR and Use Chart (p.370)**									
Room	**cm**	**kVp**	**mAs**	**mA**	**Sec**	**Beam**	**Film**	**Grid**	**1Ø3Ø**
	10								
	14								
	18								
	22								
	26								
	30								
	34								
	38								
	42								
	46								

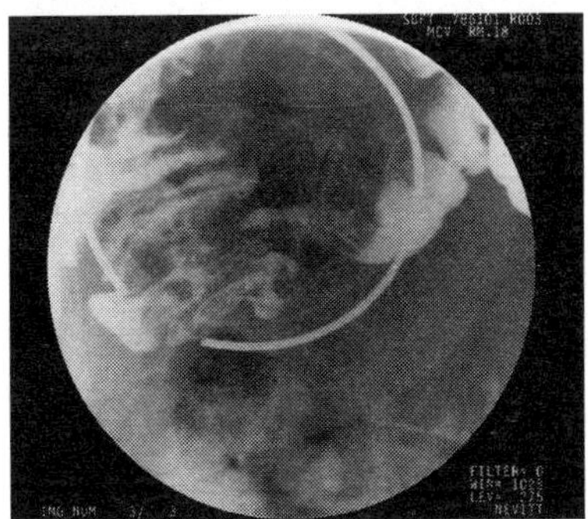

Evaluation Criteria

- Terminal ileum visible.
- Compression, if used, visible.
- Contrast is adequately penetrated.

Exam Rationale When the barium contrast reaches the cecum of the large intestine, the radiologist may choose to demonstrate the terminal area of the ileum by using one of two filming methods: a PA projection with compression or fluoroscopic spot filming.

ROUTINE AND ALTERNATIVE POSITIONS/PROJECTIONS

Part	Routine	Page	Alternative	Page
Large Intestine	PA/AP	378		
	Axial PA/AP	380		
	Obliques	382		
	Lateral decubitus	384		
	Lateral rectum	386		
			Axial oblique	388

Technical Considerations The use of high kVp technique (100–120 kVp) is recommended with the use of high-density contrast media. For air-contrast studies or studies using water-soluble contrast, a mid-range kVp (80–90) should be used.

Gonadal shielding is not possible for female patients undergoing examination of the lower digestive tract. Gonadal shielding is always recommended for male fluoroscopy patients. However, due to the placement of the enema tip, this type of shielding may hinder the examination. A shadow shield is ideal for radiographic imaging of the large intestine in male patients. It is also possible to reduce male gonadal dose by consistently keeping the primary beam above the level of the symphysis pubis.

Technical Considerations

- Regular screen/film
- Grid
- kVp range:
  —Opacified: 100–120 (single contrast); 80–90 (double contrast)
  —Preliminary or postevacuation: 80–90
- SID: 40 inch (100 cm)

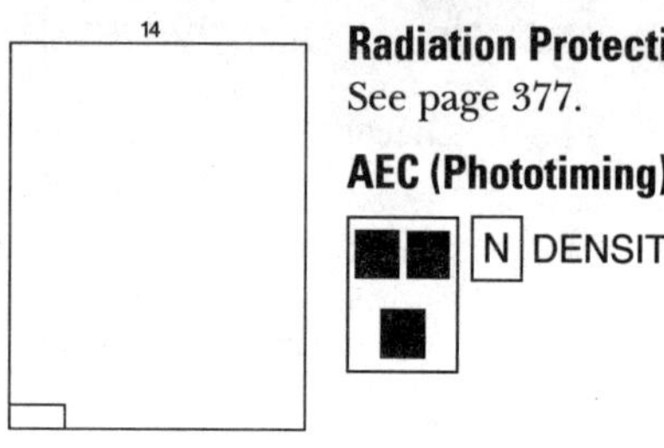

Radiation Protection

See page 377.

AEC (Phototiming)

Patient Position Supine or prone with the MSP centered to the midline of the table.

Part Position Adjust so there is no rotation of the body.

Central Ray Perpendicular to iliac crest.

Breathing Instructions Suspend on expiration.

Example Exposure Techniques
Measure at CR and Use Chart (p.370)

Room	cm	kVp	mAs	mA	Sec	Beam	Film	Grid	1Ø3Ø
	10								
	14								
	18								
	22								
	26								
	30								
	34								
	38								
	42								
	46								

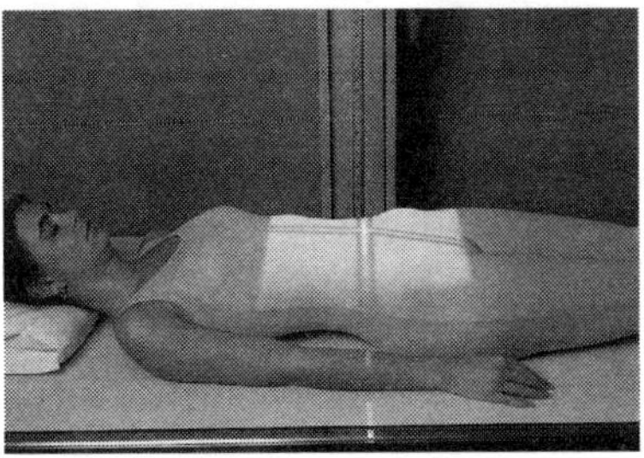

Evaluation Criteria

- Should demonstrate entire large intestine.
- There should be no rotation as evidenced by symmetry of hips and wings of ilium.

Exam Rationale This projection is used in one or more of the following ways: as a preliminary film to check for adequate bowel cleansing, as a pre-evacuation film to demonstrate all of the barium-filled large intestine, or as a postevacuation film to demonstrate the extent of bowel emptying.

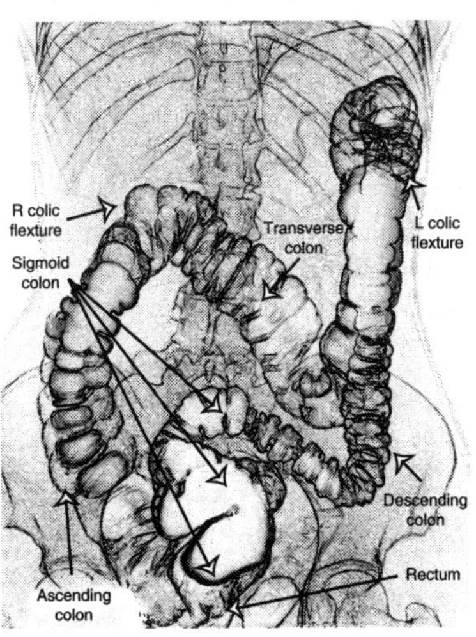

Tips

1. For a hypersthenic or asthenic patient, the central ray should be adjusted 1 inch (3 cm) higher or lower respectively.
2. For a patient with a large, wide colon, it may be necessary to use two 14 × 17 (36 × 43 cm) films crosswise to include all of the colon.
3. Do not ask the patient to take in a deep breath and let it out. This may relax the abdominal muscles and result in poor retention of the barium.

Technical Considerations

- Regular screen/film
- Grid
- kVp range: 100–200 (single contrast); 90–100 (double contrast)
- SID: 40 inch (100 cm)

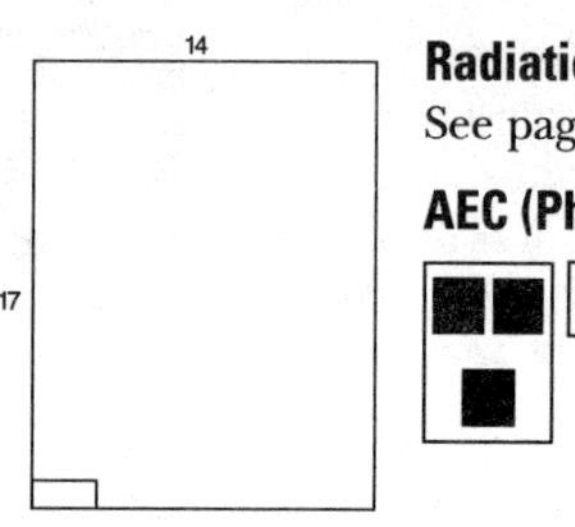

Radiation Protection

See page 377.

AEC (Phototiming)

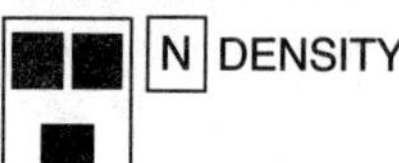

Patient Position Supine or prone with the MSP centered to the midline of the table.

Part Position Adjust so there is no rotation of the body.

Central Ray

- Supine: 2 inches (5 cm) inferior to the ASIS at a 30° to 40° cephalic angle.
- Prone: To exit at the level of the ASIS with a 30° to 40° caudal angle.

Breathing Instructions Suspend on expiration.

Example Exposure Techniques **Measure at CR and Use Chart (p.370)**									
Room	**cm**	**kVp**	**mAs**	**mA**	**Sec**	**Beam**	**Film**	**Grid**	**1Ø3Ø**
	10								
	14								
	18								
	22								
	26								
	30								
	34								
	38								
	42								
	46								

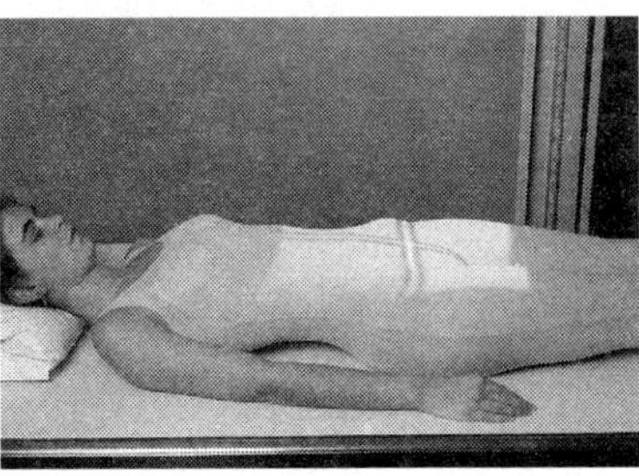

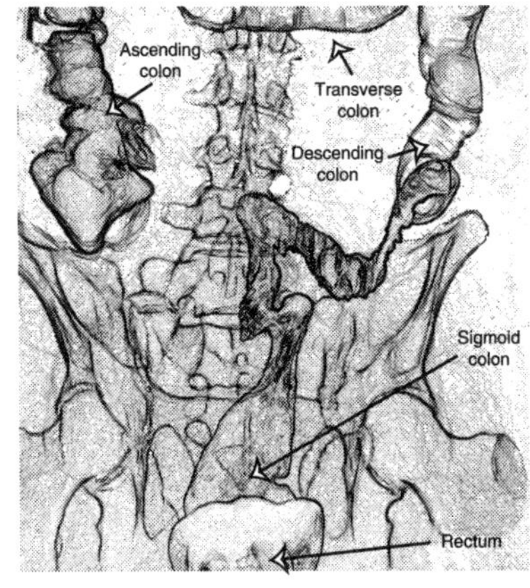

Evaluation Criteria

- Should be no rotation as evidenced by symmetrical appearance of hips.
- Rectal and sigmoid portions of colon should be elongated and less superimposed than on PA or AP.
- Not necessary to include transverse colon and flexures.

Exam Rationale This projection gives an elongated view of the rectosigmoid area of the colon.

Technical Considerations

- Regular screen/film
- Grid
- kVp range: 100–200 (single contrast); 80–90 (double contrast)
- SID: 40 inch (100 cm)

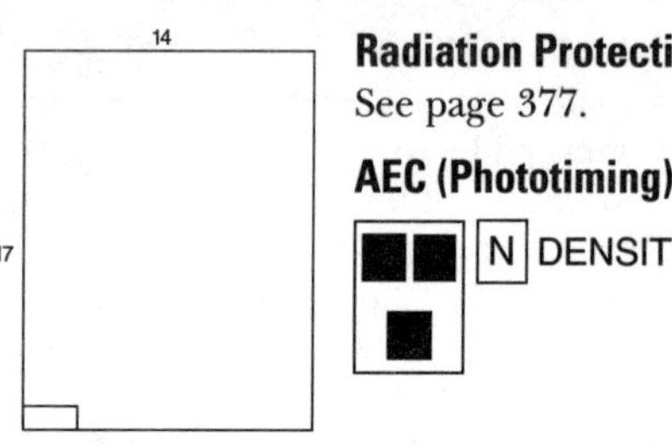

Radiation Protection

See page 377.

AEC (Phototiming)

Patient Position Supine or prone with the MSP centered to the midline of the table.

Part Position Rotate the body 35° to 45° from the supine or prone position.

Central Ray Perpendicular at the level of the iliac crest about 1 inch (3 cm) anterior to the MSP.

Breathing Instructions Suspend on expiration.

Evaluation Criteria

- Entire colon should be included.
- RAO (LPO) should demonstrate ascending colon and right colic flexure.

Example Exposure Techniques **Measure at CR and Use Chart (p.370)**									
Room	**cm**	**kVp**	**mAs**	**mA**	**Sec**	**Beam**	**Film**	**Grid**	**1Ø3Ø**
	12								
	16								
	20								
	24								
	28								
	32								
	36								
	40								
	44								
	48								

- LAO (RPO) should include descending colon and left colic flexure.

Exam Rationale The RAO (or LPO) demonstrates the right colic (hepatic) flexure and the ascending colon. The LAO (or RAO) demonstrates the left colic (splenic) flexure and the descending colon.

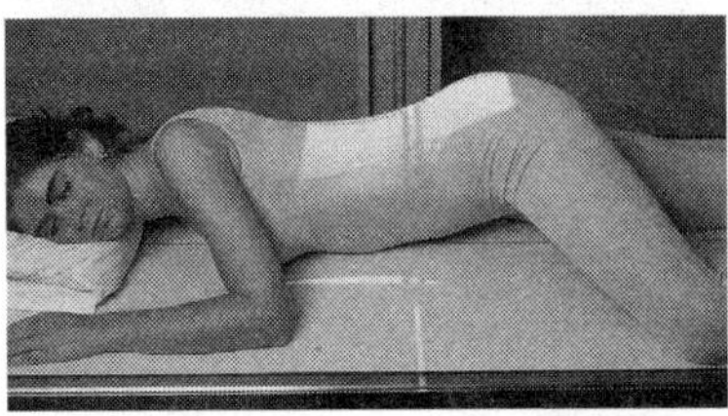

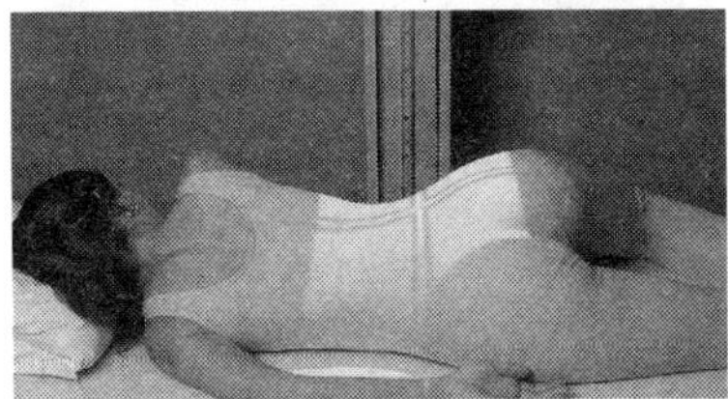

Tips

1. For a hypersthenic or asthenic patient, the central ray should be adjusted 1 inch (3 cm) higher or lower, respectively.
2. For a patient with a large, wide colon, it may be necessary to use two 14 × 17 (36 × 43 cm) films crosswise to include all of the colon.

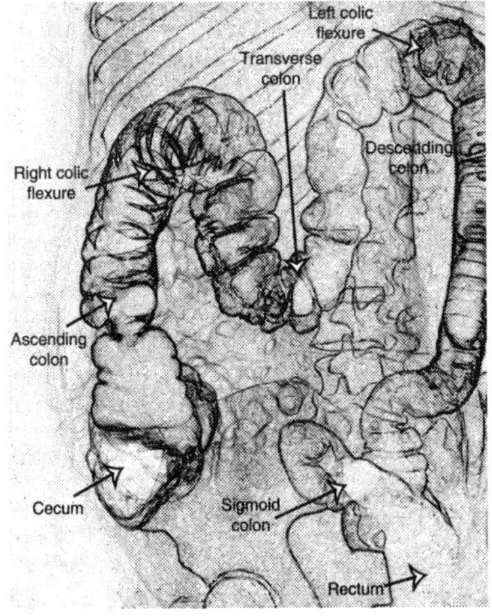

Technical Considerations

- Regular screen/film
- Grid
- kVp range: 80–90 (double contrast)
- SID: 40 inch (100 cm)

Radiation Protection

See page 377.

AEC (Phototiming)

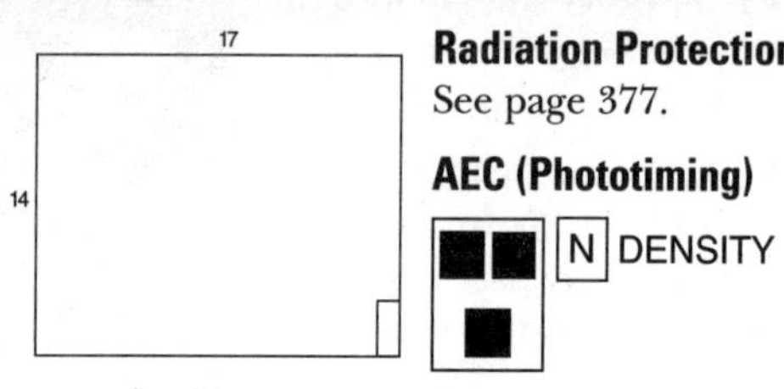

Patient Position Left lateral and right lateral recumbent positions with iliac crest centered to the midline of the table or film holder; patient's knees should be flexed to aid in maintaining the position.

Part Position Adjust so there is no rotation of the body.

Central Ray Horizontal; perpendicular to the iliac crest.

Breathing Instructions Suspend on expiration.

Evaluation Criteria

- Should demonstrate entire large intestine.
- There should be no rotation as evidenced by symmetry of wings of ilium.

Example Exposure Techniques **Measure at CR and Use Chart (p.370)**									
Room	**cm**	**kVp**	**mAs**	**mA**	**Sec**	**Beam**	**Film**	**Grid**	**1Ø3Ø**
	10								
	14								
	18								
	22								
	26								
	30								
	34								
	38								
	42								
	46								

Exam Rationale The right and left lateral decubiti are done in conjunction with a double-contrast barium enema to demonstrate the entire contrast-filled colon. These projections are particularly useful in the evaluation of polyps. Both sides are typically done, with the "up" side (air-filled) portion best demonstrated.

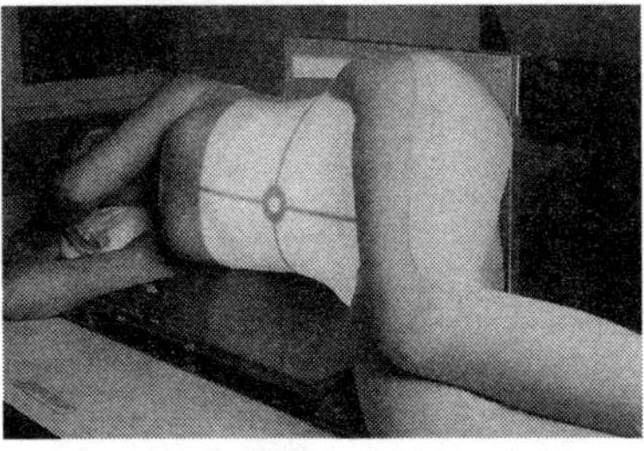

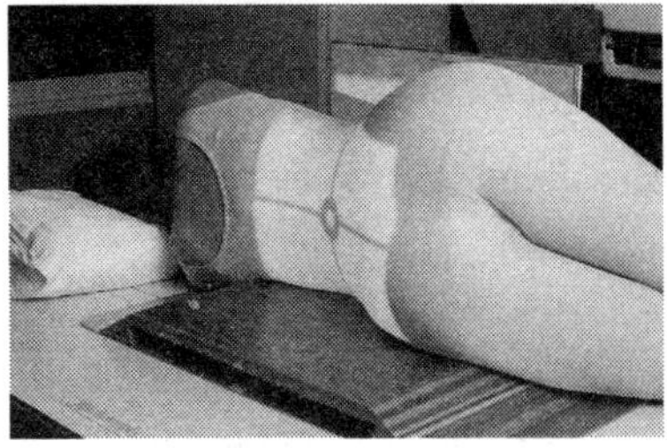

Tips

1. To ensure visualization of "down" side, patient should be slightly elevated with some type of radiolucent support.
2. Projections may be done with patient facing either toward or away from the film holder; facing away from the film is generally more comfortable for the patient.
3. Use AEC only with upright Bucky device.

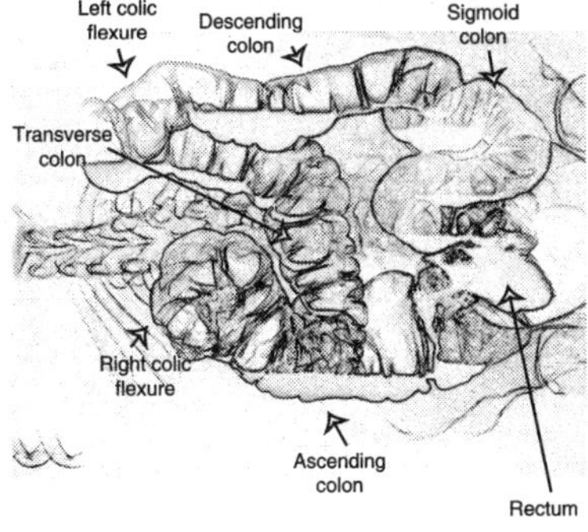

Technical Considerations
- Regular screen/film
- Grid
- kVp range: 100–125
- SID: 40 inch (100 cm)

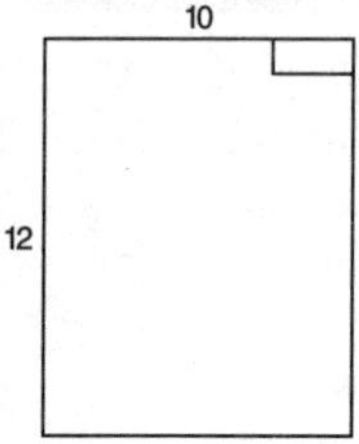

10

12

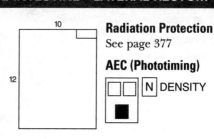

Radiation Protection
See page 377

AEC (Phototiming)

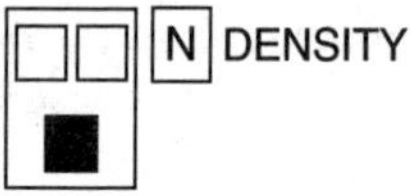

N DENSITY

Patient Position Lateral recumbent position with midaxillary plane centered to the midline of the table.

Part Position Adjust so there is no rotation of the body.

Central Ray Perpendicular to iliac crest.

Breathing Instructions Suspend on expiration.

Evaluation Criteria
- Rectosigmoid area should be in center of film.
- There should be no rotation as evidenced by superimposition of the hips and femurs.

Exam Rationale The lateral position demonstrates the rectum and rectosigmoid areas.

Example Exposure Techniques **Measure at CR and Use Chart (p.370)**									
Room	**cm**	**kVp**	**mAs**	**mA**	**Sec**	**Beam**	**Film**	**Grid**	**1Ø3Ø**
	14								
	18								
	22								
	26								
	30								
	34								
	38								
	42								
	46								
	50								

Tips

1. Although the left lateral is more commonly used, either a right or left lateral may be done.
2. Tight collimation is essential to minimize scatter radiation. The placement of a lead strip behind the patient's buttocks will also help reduce scatter.

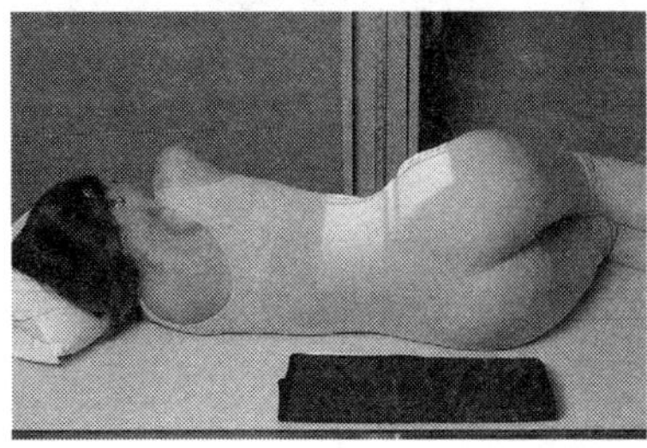

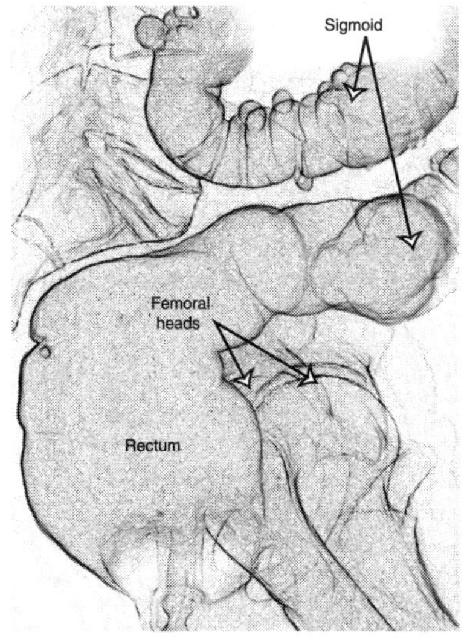

Technical Considerations

- Regular screen/film
- Grid
- kVp range: 100–200 (single contrast); 80–90 (double contrast)
- SID: 40 inch (100 cm)

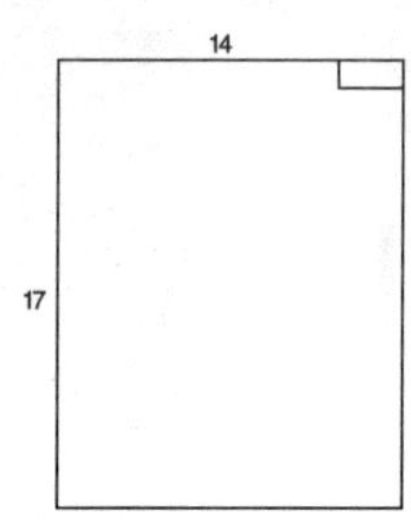

Radiation Protection
See page 377.

AEC (Phototiming)

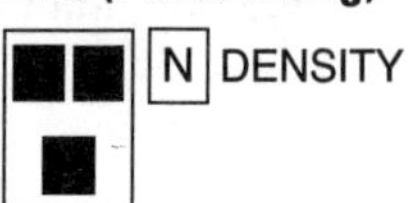

Patient Position Supine or prone with the MSP centered to the midline of the table.

Part Position Rotate the body 30° to 40° from the supine or prone position.

Central Ray

- Supine: 2 inches (5 cm) inferior to the ASIS and 2 inches (5 cm) anterior to the MSP at a 30° to 40° cephalic angle.
- Prone: At the level of the ASIS and 2 inches (5 cm) anterior to the MSP at a 30° to 40° caudal angle.

Breathing Instructions Suspend on expiration.

Example Exposure Techniques **Measure at CR and Use Chart (p.370)**									
Room	**cm**	**kVp**	**mAs**	**mA**	**Sec**	**Beam**	**Film**	**Grid**	**1Ø3Ø**
	12								
	16								
	20								
	24								
	28								
	32								
	36								
	41								
	44								
	48								

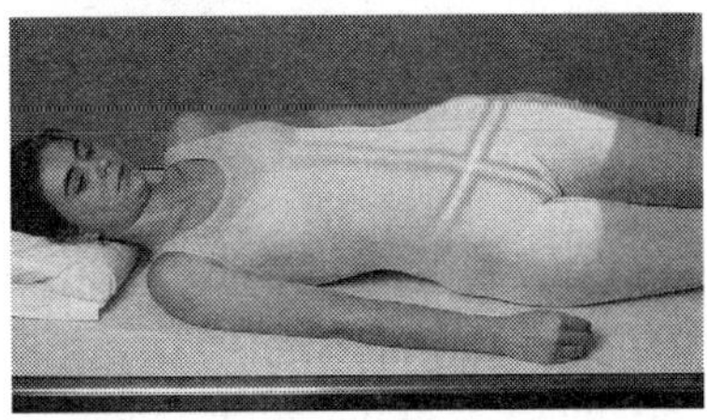

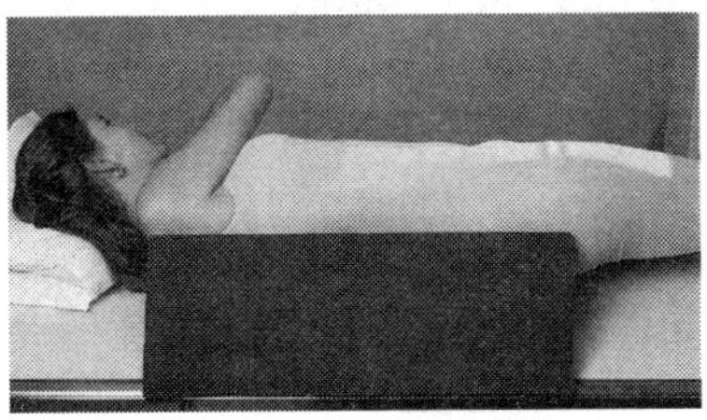

Evaluation Criteria

- Should have sufficient obliquity of patient and angulation of the central ray to elongate the rectosigmoid area and to minimize superimposition.

Exam Rationale These projections provide an elongated view of the rectosigmoid portion of the colon with less superimposition than on other views.

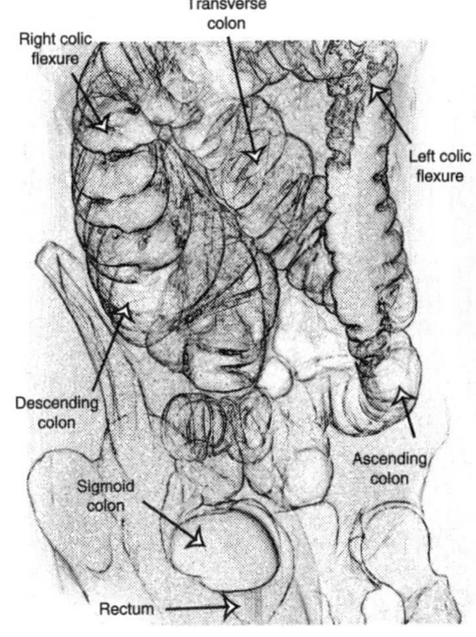

Pediatric Considerations Less stringent bowel preparation is needed for pediatric patients. A circumcision board or Octastop restraint board can be invaluable during a barium enema procedure on younger children. The octagonal restraint device has the advantage of allowing easy rotation of the child into various degrees of obliquity.

Geriatric Considerations As patients age, muscle control decreases. Thus, it is important for older patients to clearly understand the barium enema procedure and the need for their cooperation in retaining the enema. If the patient is concerned about the ability to retain the enema, a retention tip should be used.

Due to reduced mobility and flexibility, geriatric patients may have difficulty in moving quickly from one position to another. Assistance in slow, gentle movements is required, even given the urgency to complete filming.

Appendix A Abbreviations

AP	anteroposterior
BaE	barium enema
b.i.d.	twice daily
BP	blood pressure
C	centigrade or Celsius
c̄	with
cc	cubic centimeter (equal to milliliter)
CHF	congestive heart failure
cm	centimeter
CT	computed tomography
D.C.	discontinue
DNR	do not resuscitate
ECG	electrocardiogram
ER	emergency room
FFD	focus-film distance
FOD	focus-object distance
G.B.	gallbladder
g	gram
gr	grain
gtt.	drop/s
GU	genitourinary
Gy	gray
Gyn	gynecology
hr/s	hour/s
H_2O	water
HVL	half value layer
Hz	Hertz (cycles per second)
ICU	intensive care unit
IM	intramuscular
IV	intravenous
keV	kilo electron volts
kg	kilogram
KUB	kidneys, ureters, bladder
kV	kilovolts, kilovoltage

kVp	kilovoltage peak
kW	kilowatts, kilowattage
L	left
LAO	left anterior oblique
LAT	lateral
LET	linear energy transfer
LLQ	left lower quadrant of the abdomen
LPO	left posterior oblique
LUQ	left upper quadrant of the abdomen
mA	milliampere/s
mAs	milliampere-seconds
meV	million electron volts
mg	milligram
MI	myocardial infarction
ml	milliliter (equal to cubic centimeter)
mm	millimeter
MPD	maximum permissible dose
mR	milliroentgen
mrad	millirad
mrem	millirem
mSv	millisievert
m	microgram
nm	nanometer
NPO	nothing by mouth
OFD	object-film distance
OR	operating room
PA	posteroanterior
pH	hydrogen ion concentration
prn	as necessary
q.d.	every day
q.h.	every hour
q.i.d.	4 times daily
q.2 h.	every 2 hours
q.4 h.	every 4 hours
R	right
R	roentgen
rad	radiation absorbed dose
RAO	right anterior oblique
rem	radiation equivalency in man

RLQ	right lower quadrant of the abdomen
RPO	right posterior oblique
RUQ	right upper quadrant of the abdomen
Rx	therapy
s	second
$\bar{s}$	without
stat	at once
Sv	sievert
t.i.d.	3 times daily
URI	upper respiratory infection
WBC	white blood cell
WC	wheelchair
x	times

Appendix B
Exposure Conversion Tables

Effects of Radiographic Exposure Variable on the Primary Factors

This table summarizes the effects of the major variables.

Variable	Density	Contrast	Recorded Detail	Distortion
EQUIPMENT				
Generator Phase	D	I	0	0
Kilovoltage	D	I	0	0
Milliamperage-seconds	D	0	0	0
SID	I	0	D	I
OID	I	D	I	D
TUBE				
Focal Spot Size	0	0	I	0
Filtration	I	I	0	0
Beam Restriction	I	D	0	0
SUBJECT				
Part Thickness	I	I	I	D
Tissue Type	I	I	0	0
Additive Pathology	I	I	0	0
Destructive Pathology	D	D	0	0
IMAGE RECEPTOR				
Grid Ratio	I	D	0	0
Film/Screen				
Relative Speed	D	0	I	0
Film Processing				
Developer Time	D	I	0	0
Developer Temperature	D	I	0	0
Developer Replenishment	D	I	0	0

D = direct relationship (when the variable changes, the effect changes in the same direction).

I = inverse relationship (when the variable changes, the effect changes in the opposite direction).

NOTE: Many effects are not linearly proportional.

0 = no effect.

Major Exposure Conversion Rules

Exposure conversions are primarily concerned with maintaining acceptable image density. These conversion tables are all designed to convert to a new condition from exposure factors known to produce an acceptable image. Conversions are affected by a wide range of complex variables interacting with one another. The following conversions may vary considerably from one clinical situation to another but are generally accepted as valid under many conditions. **Under no circumstances should a conversion be first attempted with a patient.** Always test conversions in the clinical setting with anatomical phantoms.

These conversions work from an acceptance limit of -50% to +100% because it is expected that actual results will be fine-tuned from the initial exposure to assure a high level of image quality.

All the guidelines given in this section have been both laboratory- and field-tested. Full explanations and discussion are included in Carlton and Adler's *Principles of Radiographic Imaging.*

This following standard encourages the radiographer to choose one of the following three basic choices when converting technical factors:

- **Double mAs**
- **Halve mAs**
- **No Change**

The following rules are also valid:

- **2 kVp/cm Rule**
  Maintains density by changing kVp for different part sizes.
  Change by 2 kVp for every cm of part size.
  EXAMPLE: 60 kVp for 10 cm = 64 kVp for 12 cm

- **4-5 cm Rule**
  Maintains density by changing mAs for different part sizes.
  Double or halve mAs for every 4-5 cm of part size.
  EXAMPLE: 10 mAs for 20 cm = 20 mAs for 24 cm

- **15% Rule**
  Maintains density when kVp is changed.
  Increase kVp 15% and (decrease mAs to half) halve mAs.
  EXAMPLE: 60 kVp and 10 mAs = 69 kVp and 5 mAs

Decrease kVp 15% and (increase mAs double) double mAs.
EXAMPLE: 60 kVp and 10 mAs = 51 kVp and 20 mAs

- **Distance**
  40" to 56" to 72"
  Double mAs for each distance increase above
  Halve mAs for each distance decrease above
  EXAMPLE: 40" at 2 mAs = 72" at 8 mAs
  Note: 10% error in distance produces an image within normal acceptance limits (Example: 40" permits SID from 38" to 42") This does not consider the affect of magnification on image detail.

- **Generator Phase**
  Single phase to multi-phase (3 phase, high frequency, etc.)
  Halve mAs
  EXAMPLE: Single phase at 10 mAs = Three phase at 5 mAs
  Multi-phase to single phase
  Double mAs
  EXAMPLE: Multi-phase at 10 mAs = Single phase at 20 mAs

- **Grid Conversion**
  Grid conversion charts are notoriously inaccurate because they are especially dependent on part size and kVp range (of which both dramatically affect the amount of scatter radiation). The following chart is only a starting point for most clinical settings. It does not take into consideration the grid frequency or weight, interspace material, etc. Its single advantage is that it is easy to remember.

Grid Ratio	Change mAs By
No Grid	1×
6:1	2×
8:1	3×
10:1	4×
12:1	5×
16:1	6×

It is not recommended that grid conversions be attempted with kVp changes.

EXAMPLE: No grid at 5 mAs = 8:1 grid at 15 mAs

NOTE: When converting from one grid ratio to another, it is recommended that the mAs be converted from the 1st grid technique to No Grid and then to the 2nd grid.

EXAMPLE: 8:1 grid at 15 mAs to 12:1 grid
8:1 grid at 15 mAs = No grid at 5 mAs
No grid at 5 mAs = 12:1 grid at 25 mAs

- **Film-Screen Speed**

  Double Film-Screen Relative Speed (RS)
  Halve mAs

  EXAMPLE: 200 RS at 10 mAs = 400 RS at 5 mAs

  Halve Film-Screen Relative Speed (RS)
  Double mAs

  EXAMPLE: 200 RS at 10 mAs = 100 RS at 20 mAs

- **Casts**

  Plaster (Wet or Dry) - equivalent to same size part
  (Measure part including cast and set mAs as if tissue was the same total thickness.)

  Fiberglass or Air Splint - equivalent to part size only
  (Estimate actual part size and set mAs accordingly.)

- **Tube Angle**

  Measure part at thickest side of primary beam (not central ray).

- **Collimation Field Size**

  No compensation is required for field sizes from 8 × 10" to 14 × 17".

  Collimation from any standard film size to spot film sizes of 4 × 4" and smaller requires a 50% to 200% increase in mAs The exact amount depends not so much on collimation as on grid ratio, kVp level, and part size.

Time In seconds	mA 50	75	100	150	200	250	300	400	500	600	800
1/500 .002	.1	.15	.2	.3	.4	.5	.6	.8	1	1.2	1.6
1/200 .005	.25	.38	.5	.75	1.0	1.25	1.5	2	2.5	3	4
1/120 .008	.4	.6	.8	1.2	1.6	2	2.4	3.2	4	4.8	6.4
1/100 .01	.5	.75	1	1.5	2	2.5	3	4	5	6	8
1/80 .012	.65	.98	1.3	1.95	2.6	3.25	3.9	5.2	6.5	7.8	10.4
1/60 .016	.8	1.2	1.6	2.4	3.2	4	4.8	6.4	8	9.6	12.8
1/50 .020	.95	1.43	1.9	2.85	3.8	4.75	5.7	7.6	9.5	11.4	15.2
1/40 .025	1.25	1.88	2.5	3.75	5	6.25	7.5	10	12.5	15	20
1/30 .033	1.65	2.48	3.3	4.95	6.6	8.25	9.9	13.2	16.5	19.8	26.4
1/24 .04	2.05	3.08	4.1	6.15	8.2	10.25	12.3	16.4	20.5	24.6	32.8
1/20 .05	2.5	3.75	5	7.5	10	12.5	15	20	25	30	40
1/15 .06	3.2	4.8	6.4	9.6	12.8	16	19.2	25.6	32	38.4	51.2
1/12 .08	4	6	8	12	16	20	24	32	40	48	64
1/10 .1	5	7.5	10	15	20	25	30	40	50	60	80
1/8 .125	6.25	9.38	12.5	18.8	25	31.25	37.5	50	62.5	75	100
1/6 .16	8	12	16	24	32	40	48	64	80	96	128
1/5 .2	10	15	20	30	40	50	60	70	100	120	160
3/10 .3	15	22.5	30	45	60	75	90	120	150	180	240
2/5 .4	20	30	40	60	80	100	120	160	200	240	320
1/2 .5	25	37.5	50	75	100	125	150	200	250	300	400
3/5 .6	30	45	60	90	120	150	180	240	300	360	480
4/5 .8	40	60	80	120	160	200	240	320	400	480	640

Appendix C References and Recommended Reading

Primary References

Carlton R., & Adler, A. (1996). *Principles of radiographic imaging: An art and a science.* (2nd ed.). Albany, NY: Delmar Publishers.

Greathouse, J. (1998). *Delmar's radiographic positioning and procedures Volume I: Basic positioning and procedures.* Albany, NY: Delmar Publishers.

Principles of Exposure Additional Suggested Readings

Carroll, Q. B. (1997). *Fuchs's radiographic exposure, processing and quality control.* (6th ed.). Springfield, IL: Charles C. Thomas Publishers.

Carroll, Q. B. (1993). *Evaluating radiographs.* Springfield, IL: Charles C. Thomas Publishers.

Cullinan, A. & Cullinan, J. (1994). *Producing quality radiographs.* (2nd ed.). Philadelphia: J. B. Lippincott.

Eastman, T. R. (1979). *Radiographic fundamentals and technique guide.* St. Louis: C. V. Mosby.

Hiss, S. S. (1993). *Understanding radiography.* (3rd ed.). Springfield, IL: Charles C. Thomas Publishers.

Positioning Procedures Additional Suggested Readings

Ballinger, P. W. (1995). *Merrill's atlas of radiographic positions and radiologic procedures.* (8th ed.). St. Louis: C. V. Mosby.

Bontrager, K. L. (1997). *Textbook of radiographic positioning and related anatomy.* (4th ed.). St. Louis: C. V. Mosby.

McInnes, J. (1973). *Clark's Positioning in radiography.* (9th ed.). Chicago: Yearbook/C. V. Mosby.

Appendix D Surface Landmarks and Lines of the Skull

CRANIAL TOPOGRAPHY, LINES, AND PLANES

The following cranial topography, lines, and planes provide localization points important for positioning and centering of the cranium. Accurate adjustment or centering of these visual, palpable, and imaginary localization points will assist in producing optimal radiographs of the cranium.

Surface Landmarks Used in Skull Positioning (Figures D1 and D2)

- **Glabella**—smooth flat surface just *above* the midpoint of the eyebrows
- **Acanthion**—point where the upper lip joins the base of the nose
- **Mental point**—tip of the chin
- **Superciliary ridge/arch**—ridge of bone at the eyebrow
- **Supraorbital groove**—depression in bone *above* the eyebrow
- **Nasion**—point where the right and left nasal bones meet
- **Angle of mandible/gonion**—junction of the mandibular body and ramus

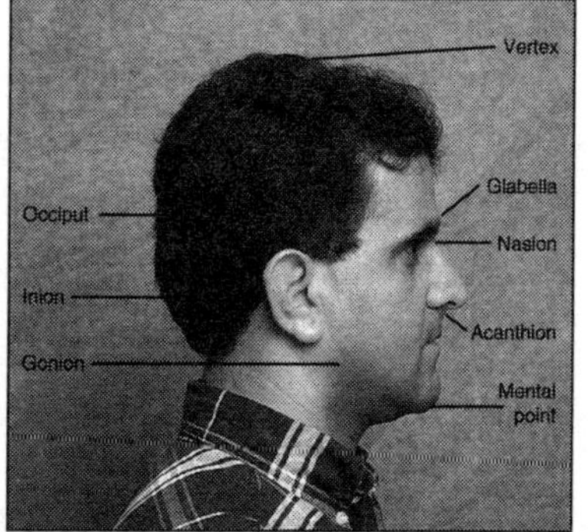

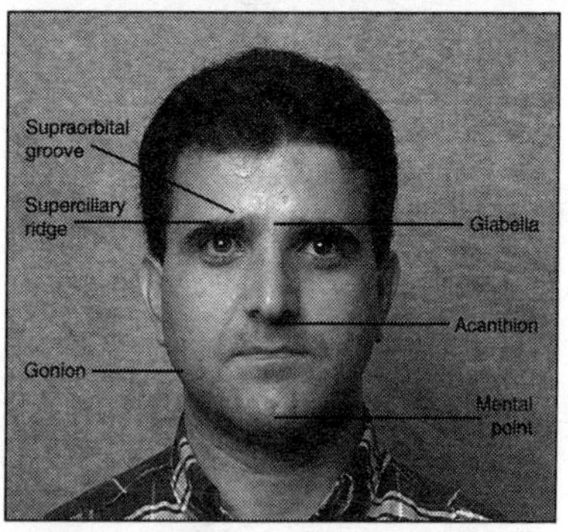

Figures D1 and D2 Cranial Topography

- **Vertex**—most superior surface of cranium
- **Inion**—external protuberance on occipital bone
- **Occiput**—most posterior surface of cranium

Base of Orbit (Figure D3)

- Inner and outer **canthi**—points where the upper and lower eyelids meet (singular-**canthus**)
- Supraorbital margin (SOM)—ridge of bone *above* orbit
- Infraorbital margin (IOM)—ridge of bone *below* orbit

Ear (Figure D4)

- **External auditory meatus** (EAM)—opening of the external ear canal
- **Auricle/pinna**—cartilage protecting the ear canal
- **Tragus**—cartilage flap at the opening of the EAM
- Top of ear attachment (TEA)—point where the auricle attaches to the cranium

Planes/Lines

These are imaginary surfaces or set of points used to adjust the position of the cranium (Figures D5 and D6).

- Midsagittal (median) plane (MSP)—divides the body

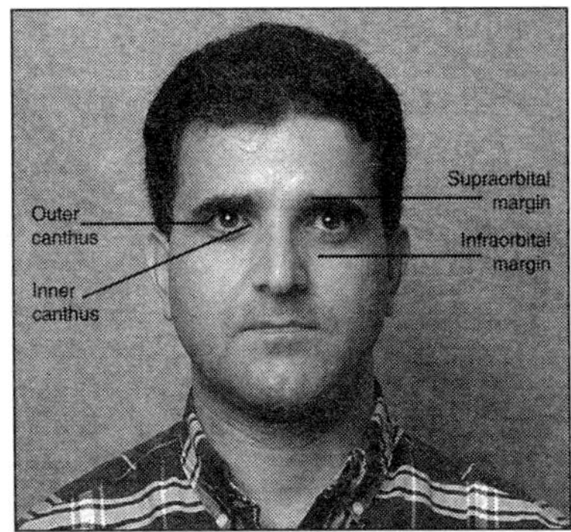

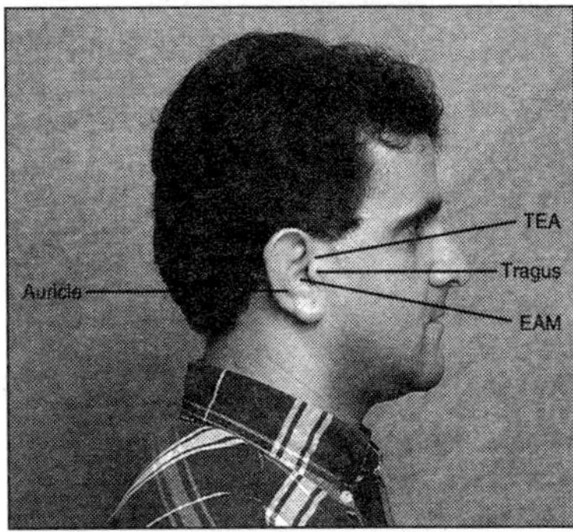

Figures D3 and D4 Cranial Topography

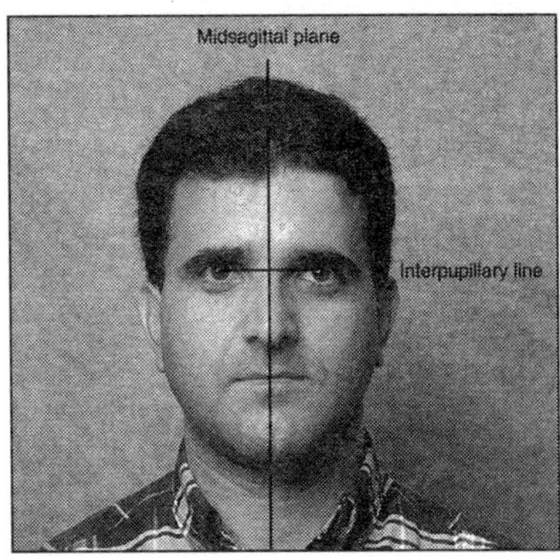

Figure D5 Positioning Lines

into equal right and left halves
- **Interpupillary (interorbital) line**—drawn between the pupils
- **Acanthiomeatal line**—drawn between the junction of upper lip/nose and the EAM
- **Mentomeatal line** (MML)—drawn between the tip of chin and the EAM
- **Infraorbitomeatal line** (IOML)—drawn between the infraorbital margin and the EAM

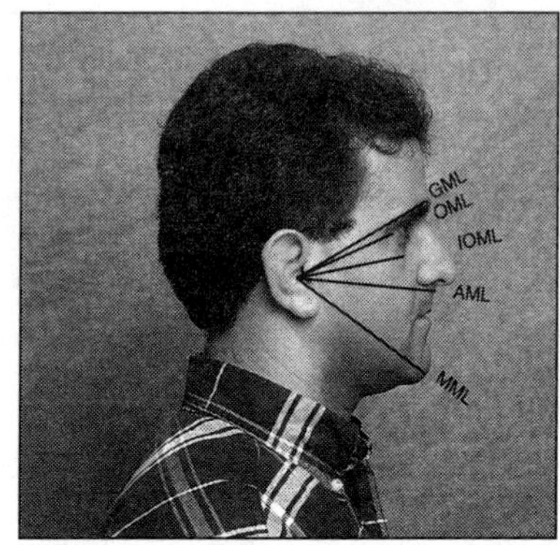

Figure D6 Positioning Lines

- **Glabellomeatal line**—drawn between the glabella and the EAM
- **Orbitomeatal line** (OML)—drawn between the outer orbital margin and the EAM

PATIENT AND POSITIONING CONSIDERATIONS

Erect versus Recumbent

Comparable skull radiographs can be obtained in either the upright or recumbent position as long as the tube-part-film relationship is maintained. The equipment available will in part determine whether skull radiography is performed erect or recumbent. A head unit or upright Bucky device offers two advantages. The erect position is easier for the patient and, secondly, it allows for visualization of air/fluid levels with a horizontal beam.

The age and condition of the patient must be assessed and considered before attempting upright skull radiography. Pediatric patients may not be able to remain still in the upright position. Unstable or injured patients may not be able to tolerate an upright position for skull radiography.

When performing skull radiography with the patient recumbent, it is important to maintain patient comfort with the use of positioning sponges. For example, hyposthenic or asthenic patients require a sponge under their chest for comfort during skull radiography. The sponge elevates the chest to assist in positioning and provides a cushion between the patient's chest and table. Hypersthenic patients may need to rest their head on a sponge to aid in positioning. Elevating the head will provide more flexibility to properly align the head to the film.

Every effort should be made to perform radiography of the sinuses in the upright position. This allows for the visualization of air/fluid levels within the sinuses (Figure D7).

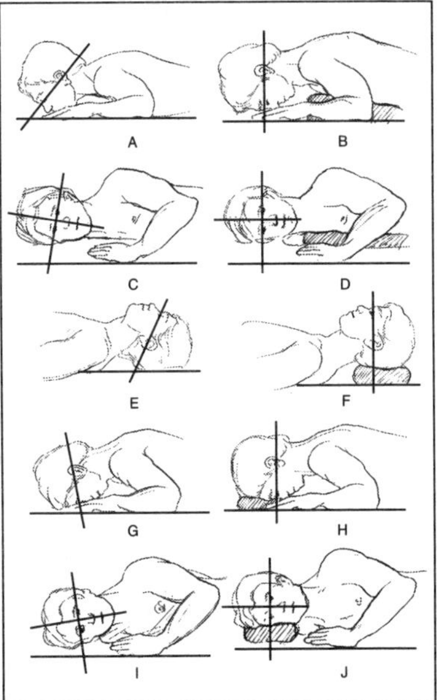

Figure D7 (A) Hyposthenic/asthenic patient prone; (B) Hyposthenic/asthenic prone positioning adjustment; (C) Hyposthenic/asthenic patient lateral; (D) Hyposthenic/asthenic lateral positioning adjustment; (E) Hypersthenic patient supine; (F) Hypersthenic supine positioning adjustment; (G) Hypersthenic patient prone; (H) Hypersthenic prone positioning adjustment; (I) Hypersthenic patient lateral; (J) Hypersthenic lateral positioning adjustment.

Pediatric versus Adults

Pediatric patients typically have an adult size skull attached to a small body. Alternate use of flexion or extension may be needed to achieve the proper alignment of positioning lines and planes. For example, the neck of a pediatric patient may need to be extended to place the orbitomeatal line perpendicular when positioning an AP skull. Immobilization devices are often helpful in reducing motion when radiographing a pediatric skull.

Positioning Errors

When alignment of the patient's head and body is not properly maintained, positioning errors result. To prevent misalignment, the long axis of the patient's head and body must coincide with or be parallel to the midline of the table and the cervical spine must remain at the level of the foramen magnum. Asymmetry of cranial and facial features may hinder efforts to align structures during positioning. It is best to palpate landmarks such as the mastoid tips and orbital margins instead of visualizing alignment of variable facial features. Additionally, the use of an angligner or skull protractor will aid in positioning the cranium and its alignment with the cervical spine.

Common Positioning Errors

Rotation and **tilt** are the most common positioning errors during skull radiography. Motion of the head around the longitudinal axis results in rotation. On the resulting frontal image, this can be demonstrated by unequal distances between the lateral border of the orbit and edge of the cranium on the right or left sides. When the longitudinal axis of the head is no longer aligned with the longitudinal axis of the body the cranium is tilted. On a frontal projection, this is seen as unequal distance between the midline of the anatomic part and the edge of the film. Both rotation and tilt positioning errors will separate structures that should be superimposed in a lateral position. It is important to distinguish between rotation and tilt of the cranium, so when presented, the radiographer can make the appropriate adjustment.

Appendix E Clinical Competency Requirement Forms

There are core clinical competencies that all individuals must demonstrate to establish eligibility for ARRT certification. These requirements are in addition to graduation from an educational program accredited by a mechanism acceptable to ARRT. The requirements listed are the *minimum* core clinical competencies necessary to establish eligibility for participation in the ARRT Radiography Examination. ARRT encourages individuals to obtain education and experience beyond these core requirements. This document will be periodically updated to reflect changes in the requirements of professional practice.

Students must demonstrate competency in all 39 of the **mandatory** *Radiological Procedures.* At least 30 of the 39 **mandatory** *Radiological Procedure* competencies must be demonstrated on patients (not phantoms or simulated). Students must demonstrate competency in at least 10 of the 23 **elective** *Radiological Procedures.* **Electives** may be demonstrated on patients or phantoms or as simulations.

In addition to the *Radiological Procedure* competencies, the four *General Patient Care* competencies are mandatory. These competencies may be simulated.

ARRT recommends that educational programs include a mechanism of continuing and terminal competency evaluation to assure students maintain proficiency during the course of the program. Competency demonstration should incorporate patient-specific variations such as age and pathology.

The checklist should be used to record completion of competencies. The checklist should NOT be sent to ARRT. Only the Program Director's signature in the Verification Section of the *Application for Examination* attesting to completion of these requirements is needed.

Competency Requirement: Perform the *Radiological Procedures* listed demonstrating appropriate:

- evaluation of requisition and patient assessment
- physical facilities readiness
- patient care and management
- equipment operation and technique selection
- positioning skills
- radiation protection for patient, self and others
- image processing

and evaluate whether the resulting images demonstrate proper:

- anatomical part(s)
- alignment
- radiographic techniques
- image identification
- radiation protection

Note: For an example of further delineation of these steps, see the *ASRT Clinical Education Competency Evaluation Model,* Appendix C "Sample Clinical Competency Competency Evaluation Form."

RADIOLOGICAL PROCEDURES

THORAX	Mandatory	Elective	Date Completed	Patient or Simulated	Verified By
Chest, routine					
Chest, age 6 or younger					
Chest, wheelchair or stretcher					
Ribs					
Chest, decubitus					
Sternum					
EXTREMITIES					
Finger or Thumb					
Hand					
Wrist					
Forearm					
Elbow					
Humerus					
Shoulder					
Foot					
Ankle					
Tibia and Fibula					
Knee					
Patella					
Femur					
Trauma Extremity					
Extremity, age 6 years or younger					
Scapula					
Clavicle					
Acromioclavicular Joints					
Trauma Shoulder (for example, Y view or transthoracic)					
Toes					
Os Calcis					

Continued

HEAD AND NECK	Mandatory	Elective	Date Completed	Patient or Simulated	Verified By
Facial Bones					
Nasal Bones					
Paranasal Sinuses					
Skull					
Orbits					
Zygomatic Arches					
Mandible					
Larynx (Soft Tissue Neck)					
SPINE AND PELVIS					
Cervical Spine					
Trauma Cervical Spine (cross-table lateral)					
Thoracic Spine					
Lumbosacral Spine					
Pelvis					
Hip					
Trauma Hip (cross-table lateral)					
Scoliosis Series					
Sacrum and/or Coccyx					
Sacroiliac Joints					
ABDOMEN AND GI TRACT					
Esophagus Study					
Abdomen, supine and upright					
Abdomen, decubitus					
Upper G.I. Series					
Small Bowel Series					
Barium Enema (single or double contrast)					
OTHER					
Intravenous Urography					
Myelography					
Cystography or Cystourethrography					
Digital Fluoroscopy					
Digital Radiography					

MOBILE AND SURGICAL	Mandatory	Elective	Date Completed	Patient or Simulated	Verified By
Portable Chest					
Portable Abdomen					
Portable Orthopedics					
C-Arm Procedure (surgical)					
Operative Cholangiography					
Retrograde Urography					

GENERAL PATIENT CARE

In addition to the Radiological Procedures, students must complete the following mandatory General Patient Care simulations.

	Date Completed	Verified By
CPR		
Vital Signs (blood pressure, pulse, respiration, temperature)		
Venipuncture		
O_2 Administration		

VERIFICATION SECTION
(Note: The Verification Section will appear on the examination application)

The applicant has demonstrated the competency requirements as identified in the *Radiography Clinical Competency Requirements* document.

______________________________ ______________

Program Director Signature Date

RADIOLOGICAL PROCEDURES

	Mandatory	Elective	Date Completed	Patient or Simulated	Verified By

RADIOLOGICAL PROCEDURES

	Mandatory	Elective	Date Completed	Patient or Simulated	Verified By

RADIOLOGICAL PROCEDURES					
	Mandatory	Elective	Date Completed	Patient or Simulated	Verified By

RADIOLOGICAL PROCEDURES					
	Mandatory	Elective	Date Completed	Patient or Simulated	Verified By
69 1/2					
61					
20 1/2					
20					
I Q	AND RANGE				
221 W	Crogan		St	963-6586	
Lville	GA	30045			
AR15	A1	$599			
[illegible] Plus					
		14	209		

RADIOLOGICAL PROCEDURES					
	Mandatory	Elective	Date Completed	Patient or Simulated	Verified By

RADIOLOGICAL PROCEDURES

	Mandatory	Elective	Date Completed	Patient or Simulated	Verified By

Index